Abnormal
Laboratory Results

Edited by Geoffrey Kellerman

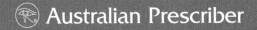 Australian Prescriber

Third Edition

The McGraw-Hill Companies

Sydney New York San Francisco Auckland
Bangkok Bogotá Caracas Hong Kong
Kuala Lumpur Lisbon London Madrid
Mexico City Milan New Delhi San Juan
Seoul Singapore Taipei Toronto

Notice

Medicine is an ever-changing science. As new research and clinical experience broaden our knowledge, changes in treatment and drug therapy are required. The editors and the publisher of this work have checked with sources believed to be reliable in their efforts to provide information that is complete and generally in accord with the standards accepted at the time of publication. However, in view of the possibility of human error or changes in medical sciences, neither the editors, nor the publisher, nor any other party who has been involved in the preparation or publication of this work warrants that the information contained herein is in every respect accurate or complete. Readers are encouraged to confirm the information contained herein with other sources. For example, and in particular, readers are advised to check the product information sheet included in the package of each drug they plan to administer to be certain that the information contained in this book is accurate and that changes have not been made in the recommended dose or in the contraindications for administration. This recommendation is of particular importance in connection with new or infrequently used drugs.

Reprinted 2011, 2013
This third edition published 2011
First edition published 2001
Second edition published 2006

Text © 2011 Commonwealth Government of Australia and National Prescribing Service
Illustrations and design © 2011 McGraw-Hill Australia Pty Limited
Additional owners of copyright are acknowledged on the Acknowledgments page

Every effort has been made to trace and acknowledge copyrighted material. The authors and publishers tender their apologies should any infringement have occurred.

National Library of Australia Cataloguing-in-Publication Data
Title: Abnormal laboratory results / edited by Geoffrey Kellerman.
Edition: 3rd ed.
ISBN: 9780070998421 (pbk.)
Notes: Includes index.
Subjects: Diagnostic errors.
            Diagnosis, Laboratory—Evaluation.
            Clinical chemistry.
Other Authors/Contributors: Kellerman, Geoffrey.
Dewey Number: 616.0756

Published in Australia by
McGraw-Hill Australia Pty Ltd
Level 33 World Square, 680 George Street Sydney, NSW 2000, Australia
Associate editor: Fiona Richardson
Art director: Astred Hicks
Internal design: Peta Nugent
Production editor: Claire Linsdell
Copyeditor: Kathy Kramer
Illustrator: Alan Laver, Shelly Communications
Proofreader: Vicki Deakin
Indexer: Barbara Bessant
Typeset in Zapf Humanist 8/10.5pt by Midland Typesetters, Australia
Printed in Australia by Pegasus Media & Logistics

Foreword

A bewildering array of laboratory tests is available to today's health professionals, and there is more to these tests than ticking a box on a request form and looking at the normal range of results. To provide more detail about commonly ordered tests, *Australian Prescriber* runs a series called 'Abnormal Laboratory Results'. Although this may seem an odd topic for a journal mainly concerned with drugs, laboratory tests have an important role in therapeutics.

Australian Prescriber first published a booklet on laboratory tests in 1987. Over the ensuing years more articles appeared in the series, so there was a need to update the booklet. Compiling and revising all the material was beyond the resources of *Australian Prescriber* but McGraw-Hill was able to help and gave Dr Robert Dunstan the responsibility of updating all of the articles published since 1978. The result was the first edition of *Abnormal Laboratory Results*, which appeared in 2001.

By 2006, *Australian Prescriber* had published enough articles on new topics to warrant a second edition of the book. This was edited by Professor Geoffrey Kellerman, who not only added the new chapters but also ensured that the earlier chapters were brought up to date.

Australian Prescriber has published more articles in the *Abnormal Laboratory Results* series over the past four years. I am pleased that Professor Kellerman has again agreed to prepare these articles for the third edition of the book.

This 2011 edition is timely because NPS, the publisher of *Australian Prescriber*, has recently established a Quality Diagnostic Referrals program. This has the aim of improving the use of laboratory tests. *Abnormal Laboratory Results* will be a perfect complement to these educational activities. The third edition has already proven to be very popular, going into reprint within six months of publication.

Dr John S. Dowden
Editor, *Australian Prescriber*
Canberra
www.australianprescriber.com

Australian Prescriber is published by NPS, an independent, not-for-profit organisation funded by the Australian Government Department of Health and Ageing.

Contents

Contents

Preface to the third edition

Since the publication of the second edition of this work in 2006 there have been 13 further articles in *Australian Prescriber* in the 'Abnormal Laboratory Results' series. These articles, and the 39 from the second edition of McGraw-Hill's *Abnormal Laboratory Results*, have been collected in this new edition, and almost every one has been updated. These updates have been made by the original author, or authors, with the exception of the few, identified at the beginning of the chapter, where the original author was unable to perform the task and another expert did so.

In most articles the changes are still relatively minor, so that the book can maintain its role as a reissue of articles originally published in *Australian Prescriber*. However, research gradually adds to or changes accepted knowledge and practice and this is especially noticeable in the areas of hyperlipidaemia, calcium and bone metabolism, cardiac troponins, vitamin B_{12} metabolism, rheumatoid arthritis and viral diseases such as Hepatitis B and C and HIV, where extensive rewriting has occurred. Chapters from new authors have replaced two of the original articles, and a single chapter combines the original two on serum creatinine and creatinine clearance. Most articles include some key references so that interested readers can extend their study and understanding of areas of special interest.

I am grateful to the authors for their cooperation and to the publishers for their help and advice during the writing and production periods. It is our hope that this volume will prove to be of ongoing value to all readers who are involved, or preparing to become involved, in patient care in any aspect of the health care system.

While it includes nearly 50 chapters, this book is not yet a complete cover of all laboratory testing procedures; however, further articles are planned for *Australian Prescriber* to cover important aspects that have not yet been addressed. There is a real lack of a suitable entry-level textbook for students and new graduates in the area of test ordering and interpretation. This gap could be filled by a fourth edition of this publication if the requisite articles can be identified and selected over the next four to five years.

We welcome suggestions from readers for priority areas for future topics.

Geoffrey M. Kellerman

Contributors

T. I. Robertson   Chapter 1
Late Visiting Physician
Westmead Hospital, Sydney, Australia

J. Fowler   Chapter 1
Retired Consulting Physician, Newcastle, Australia

C. G. Fraser   Chapter 2
Retired Clinical Leader
Department of Biochemical Medicine
NHS Tayside, Ninewells Hospital and Medical School,
Dundee, Scotland

G. M. Kellerman   Chapter 3
Emeritus Professor of Medical Biochemistry
University of Newcastle
VMO in Clinical Chemistry
Hunter Area Pathology Service, Newcastle, Australia

P. Phillips   Chapter 4
Senior Director
Endocrinology Unit
Queen Elizabeth Hospital, Adelaide, Australia

J. Attia   Chapter 5
Academic Director, General Medicine
John Hunter Hospital, Newcastle, Australia

M. Shephard   Chapter 6
Associate Professor
Director and Senior Research Fellow
Community Point of Care Services
Flinders University Rural Clinical School
Bedford Park, SA, Australia

J. F. Mahony   Chapter 7
Former Renal Physician
Department of Renal Medicine
Royal North Shore Hospital, Sydney, Australia

T. H. Mathew   Chapter 8
Medical Director
Kidney Health Australia, Adelaide, Australia

G. S. Stokes   Chapter 9
Emeritus Professor
Hypertension Unit, Department of Cardiology
Royal North Shore Hospital, Sydney, Australia

E. P. MacCarthy   Chapter 9
Former Head
Hypertension Unit
University of Cincinnati Medical Centre, Cincinnati,
Ohio, United States of America

T. H. Mathew   Chapter 10
Medical Director
Kidney Health Australia, Adelaide, Australia

B. J. Nankivell   Chapter 11
Department of Renal Medicine
Westmead Hospital and University of Sydney, Sydney, Australia

A. K. Verma   Chapter 12
Resident, General Medicine
Gosford Hospital, Gosford, Australia

P. Roach   Chapter 12
Consultant Physician
Respiratory and Sleep Medicine
Gosford Hospital, Gosford, Australia

J. D. Wark   Chapter 13
Professor of Medicine
University of Melbourne
Head, Bone and Mineral Service
Royal Melbourne Hospital, Melbourne, Australia

C. J. Yates   Chapter 13
Research Fellow
Department of Diabetes and Endocrinology
Royal Melbourne Hospital, Melbourne, Australia

Contributors

J. Wu
Registrar, Chemical Pathology
Queensland Health Pathology Service
Brisbane, Australia

Chapter 14

A. Carter
Director Chemical Pathology
Queensland Health Pathology Service
Brisbane, Australia

Chapter 14

B. T. Emmerson
Emeritus Professor
Department of Medicine, University of Queensland
and Honorary Research Consultant
Princess Alexandra Hospital, Woolloongabba, Australia

Chapter 15

L. W. Powell
Director of Clinical Research
Royal Brisbane and Women's Hospital, Brisbane, Australia

Chapter 16

M. L. Bassett
Australian National University Medical School
Gastroenterology and Hepatology Unit
Canberra Hospital, Canberra, Australia

Chapter 16

W. G. E. Cooksley
Professorial Research Fellow
Discipline of Medicine
University of Queensland, Royal Brisbane and Women's Hospital
Brisbane, Australia

Chapter 16

A. M. Dart
Professor, Clinical Program Director
Cardiorespiratory/Intensive Care
Alfred Hospital, Melbourne, Australia

Chapter 17

C. M. Reid
Principal Research Fellow and Head
Clinical Informatics and Data Management Unit
School of Public Health and Medicine
Monash University, Melbourne, Australia

Chapter 17

G. L. Jennings Chapter 17
Professor and Director
Baker IDI Heart and Diabetes Institute
Head, WHO Collaborating Centre for Research and
Training in Cardiovascular Disease
Professor (Honorary)
Faculty of Medicine Nursing & Health Sciences
Monash University, Melbourne, Australia

R. A. J. Conyers Chapter 17
Professor, Department of Immunology
Monash University, Melbourne, Australia

E. M. Nicholls Chapter 17
The Alfred Hospital and Baker Medical Research Institute
Melbourne, Australia

H-G. Schneider Chapter 17
Director of Pathology
Alfred Hospital, Melbourne, Australia

P. Nestel Chapter 18
Professor, Senior Faculty, Baker IDI Heart and Diabetes Institute
Melbourne, Australia

P. E. Hickman Chapter 19
Director of Chemical Pathology
ACT Pathology
Associate Professor
Australian National University Medical School
Canberra, Australia

J. M. Potter Chapter 19
Professor of Pathology
Australian National University Medical School
Executive Director
ACT Pathology
Canberra, Australia

Contributors

B. Ewald   Chapter 20
General Practitioner and
Senior Lecturer
Centre for Clinical Epidemiology and Biostatistics
University of Newcastle, Australia

R. H. Mortimer   Chapter 21
Department of Endocrinology
Royal Brisbane and Women's Hospital
Professor, University of Queensland, Brisbane, Australia

J. T. Ho   Chapter 22
Consultant Endocrinologist
Royal Adelaide Hospital, Adelaide, Australia

D. J. Torpy   Chapter 22
Associate Professor
Senior Consultant Endocrinologist
Royal Adelaide Hospital, Adelaide, Australia

S. K. Gan   Chapter 23
Associate Professor in Medicine
Royal Perth Hospital and University of Western Australia,
Perth, Australia

D. J. Chisholm   Chapter 23
Emeritus Professor and Head Clinical Diabetes Research
Diabetes and Obesity Research Program, Garvan Institute of
Medical Research and St Vincent's Hospital, Sydney, Australia

G. Jones   Chapter 24
Head, Department of Chemical Pathology
St Vincent's Hospital, Sydney, Australia

D. J. Chisholm   Chapter 24
Emeritus Professor and Head Clinical Diabetes Research
Diabetes and Obesity Research Program, Garvan Institute of
Medical Research and St Vincent's Hospital, Sydney, Australia

H-G. Schneider   Chapter 24
Director of Pathology
Alfred Hospital, Melbourne, Australia

R. J. Norman   Chapter 25
Director, Research Centre for Reproductive Health,
Academic Head, Repromed Pty Ltd
Professor, Department of Obstetrics and Gynaecology
University of Adelaide, Adelaide, Australia

H. A. Tran   Chapter 26
Head and Associate Professor
Division of Clinical Chemistry, Hunter Area Pathology Service
John Hunter Hospital and University of Newcastle, Newcastle, Australia

H. A. Tran   Chapter 27
Head and Associate Professor
Division of Clinical Chemistry, Hunter Area Pathology Service
John Hunter Hospital and University of Newcastle, Newcastle, Australia

P. Verras   Chapter 28
Complex Biochemistry Department
Division of Laboratory Services
Royal Children's Hospital, Melbourne, Australia

R. Greaves   Chapter 28
Senior Lecturer, Clinical Biochemistry
School of Medical Sciences
Royal Melbourne Institute of Technology
Melbourne, Australia

N. A. Buckley   Chapter 29
Professor of Medicine
University of NSW
Prince of Wales Hospital, Sydney, Australia

R. A. Ghiculescu   Chapter 30
Former Registrar
Department of Clinical Pharmacology
Princess Alexandra Hospital, Brisbane, Australia

Contributors

P. Pillans

Chapter 30

Professor and Director, Clinical Pharmacology
Princess Alexandra Hospital, Brisbane, Australia

W. R. Pitney

Chapter 31

Late Emeritus Professor
Department of Medicine
University of NSW, Sydney, Australia

M. Seldon

Chapter 31

Senior Haematologist
Hunter Haematology Unit, Mater Hospital and
Hunter New England Area Health Service, Newcastle, Australia

F. Firkin

Chapter 32

Associate Professor of Medicine
Senior Haematologist
St Vincents Hospital
Melbourne, Australia

B. Rush

Chapter 32

Former Director of Laboratory Haematology
St Vincent's Hospital, Melbourne, Australia

J. Metz

Chapter 33

Haematologist
Dorevitch Pathology, Fairfield, Australia

D. K. Bowden

Chapter 34

Associate Professor
Thalassaemia Service, Monash Medical Centre,
Melbourne, Australia

R. Baker

Chapter 35

Professor, Centre for Thrombosis and Haemophilia
Royal Perth Hospital
Murdoch University, Perth, Australia

J. McPherson   Chapter 36
Consultant and Honorary Professor of Medical Education
University of Papua New Guinea
Formerly Consultant Haematologist, Newcastle Mater Hospital,
Newcastle, Australia

A. Street   Chapter 36
Head, Haemostasis and Thrombosis Units
The Alfred Hospital, Melbourne, Australia

A. L. Greenway   Chapter 37
Paediatric Haematologist
Royal Children's Hospital, Melbourne, Australia

P. Monagle   Chapter 37
Stevenson Professor of Paediatrics
Head Department of Haematology
Royal Children's Hospital, Melbourne, Australia

D. S. Bowden   Chapter 38
Head, Molecular Microbiology
Victorian Infectious Diseases Reference Laboratory
Melbourne, Australia

S. A. Locarnini   Chapter 38
Head, Research and Molecular Development
Victorian Infectious Diseases Reference Library and
Director, WHO Collaborating Centre for Virus Reference
and Research Melbourne, Australia

D. S. Bowden   Chapter 39
Head, Molecular Microbiology
Victorian Infectious Diseases Reference Laboratory
Melbourne, Australia

A. M. Breschkin   Chapter 40
Senior Scientist
Victorian Infectious Diseases Reference Laboratory
Melbourne, Australia

Contributors

M. G. Catton
Medical Director and Head
Victorian Infectious Diseases Reference Laboratory
Melbourne, Australia

Chapter 40

C. J. Birch
Senior Scientist
Victorian HIV Reference Laboratory, VIDRL
Melbourne, Australia

Chapter 40

C. Ooi
Director, Sexual Health Service
Conjoint Lecturer
Faculty of Health
University of Newcastle, Australia

Chapter 41

D. Badov
Head of Gastroenterology and Consultant Gastroenterologist
Department of Gastroenterology
Frankston Hospital, Melbourne, Australia

Chapter 42

F. Firkin
Associate Professor of Medicine
Senior Haematologist
St Vincents Hospital, Melbourne, Australia

Chapter 43

S. Limaye
Immunologist
Concord Hospital, Sydney, Australia

Chapter 44

K. Cartwright
Clinical Associate Professor
Senior Consultant Haematologist
Wollongong Hospital, Wollongong, Australia

Chapter 45

R. M. O'Brien
Associate Professor of Medicine, Immunology and Rheumatology
Austin Hospital, Melbourne, Australia

Chapter 46

S. M. Chatfield   Chapter 47
Rheumatologist
Royal Melbourne Hospital, Melbourne, Australia

S. M. Chatfield   Chapter 48
Rheumatologist
Royal Melbourne Hospital, Melbourne, Australia

C. Lau   Chapter 49
Registrar, Genetics and Molecular Pathology
Women's and Children's Hospital, Adelaide, Australia

G. Suthers   Chapter 49
Head, Familial Cancer Unit
Women's and Children's Hospital, Adelaide, Australia

Acknowledgments

The editor would like to thank the following people for their assistance in the work which led to the production of this book:

- Each chapter's contributors who, despite their busy schedules, met the deadlines.
- J. S. Dowden and staff from *Australian Prescriber*, for their advice and encouragement.
- Staff from McGraw-Hill Australia, for their cheerful guidance.
- Kathy Kramer, for her copyediting.

Part 1

General Issues

1 What to do about abnormal laboratory results

The context

A note from the Editor

In the mosaic that represents the totality of the patient's problem and its management, laboratory results often play a minor part, sometimes are moderately important and occasionally are major contributors. These proportions depend on whether, for example, the patient is in general practice or a teaching hospital environment. Laboratory test results represent information and information serves to provide material for thought by the doctor: it is not a substitute for thought. Only in science fiction do machine tests make a magic assessment without human intervention. Dr Robertson (deceased) wrote initially from the point of view of the physician receiving results of laboratory tests. Dr Fowler has written recently from the point of view of the physician who is considering which tests to order. I believe that these two versions of the same introductory message are both worth reading.

○ T. I. Robertson

A biochemical profile in a symptomless male patient of 50 years shows a modestly elevated serum uric acid. Anti-gout medication lowers the level but causes a generalised skin rash that lasts for 3 months. A patient, 55 years old, in hospital with a myocardial infarct, is found on a routine blood count to have a haemoglobin level of 110 g/L. The stained film suggests iron deficiency. Follow up investigation uncovers a symptomless carcinoma of the caecum, which is successfully removed. These two examples, each initiated by a routine test, show on the one hand an annoying disability resulting from treatment that was probably unnecessary and on the other, a successful conclusion to the pursuit of an apparently minor abnormality.

We live in a maze of biochemical profiles, screening tests and routine investigations, a lot of them uncalled for and some presented to us by our patients themselves. A new category has been created: the symptomless patient with an investigational abnormality. These people are at special risk. Some of them have incipient, developing or subclinical disease and some have no disease at all. But all will be affected by the medical advice they receive. Neglect of an apparent triviality may be lethal, yet a clearly abnormal result may, in the patient's total interest, be best set aside. The advent of routine screening procedures has produced fresh problems and responsibilities and has tended to complicate rather than simplify medical management.

When should an abnormal result be considered undebatably abnormal? When should it be acted upon? How vigorously should it be pursued? When should it be ignored? The magnitude of the problem can be reduced at the source by discrimination in the investigations requested in the first place. The fewer tests ordered in isolation—that is, without proper integration with history, physical examination and general consideration of the clinical problem—the less difficult will be their interpretation. If a patient requires investigation of any type, he or she deserves the courtesy of proper history and examination first.

It is unrealistic to deny the ease, advantages and extra information provided by the automated blood count and multiple biochemical analysis. An investigation should, however, be mounted by way of a working diagnosis to be proved or disproved and the results of all tests viewed in that light. It should not be an undisciplined fishing expedition. If it is practical for only selective tests to be requested, to advance the working hypothesis, only these should be ordered. Secondary tests may be needed after analysis of the primary ones but this is the preferred approach. The practitioner advances his or her capabilities by being careful, even parsimonious, with investigations and by understanding them and their limitations. This applies to all levels of clinical practice, not least in the teaching hospitals.

Nevertheless the problem of interpreting more or less isolated abnormal results will always remain. Some of the difficulties in relation to particular tests are addressed by experts in the chapters that follow.

◯ J. Fowler

The clinical assessment, done with diligence, directs the investigations to support or refute a provisional diagnosis. A poor clinical history and physical examination (a time consuming process to do properly) does not permit you to ask the correct questions and poorly directed laboratory tests will not compensate for the omission. The solution of more difficult diagnostic dilemmas is dependent on your clinical assessment (that is, the pretest probability) as modified by the sensitivity and specificity of test results. When these test results are abnormal but do not support the provisional diagnosis, they do not of themselves become the problem. The clinical scenario is reconsidered by a further meticulous history and physical examination, which will often widen the differential diagnosis, encompassing the tests already done and perhaps suggesting further tests to enhance the probability of a diagnosis. The isolated discordant laboratory test(s) will then be incorporated into the final diagnosis or will need to be considered as a special pathological problem.

Patients and physicians want immediate answers but many diseases are subtle and at initial presentation are often incompletely developed. While there are clinical circumstances which demand immediate action on incomplete evidence (e.g. suspected bacterial meningitis), it is better where possible to allow time and observation to assist in solving the problem. The quick, dogmatic incorrect diagnosis closes off the thinking process. Honesty requires that we admit difficulty and doubt so that over time careful observation, with judicious laboratory tests, can give a more accurate final conclusion than the apparently brilliant guess.

Advances in the accuracy and range of laboratory investigations have enabled earlier and more exact definition of many clinical problems. Indeed modern medicine is dominated by X-ray reports, pathological profiles and tests, followed by more tests. The tests are interpreted by highly trained specialists, often unfortunately with no available clinical information, so the clinician should never believe these interpretations unless they can be integrated into the clinical assessment. Screening tests not linked to symptoms or a specific hypothesis pose a special problem. How can the clinician interpret and integrate such abnormal results? A good history, exploring such things as genetic predisposition and lifestyle risk factors, will often permit this integration.

Laboratory test results purely as numbers are prone to error. For example, a 'fasting glucose' taken after a fruit juice (not considered as food by many patients and therefore not reported by them) can give an incorrect diagnosis of diabetes mellitus. A urine sample to assess an albumin leak will give a spuriously high result if collected after heavy exercise or during menstruation. A normal glycated haemoglobin (HbA1c) does not mean good diabetic control if the red cell life span is shortened by, for example, haemolytic anaemia or slow blood loss. The clinician must know the limitations of tests ordered and the common causes of inaccurate results and must gather supporting evidence before acting on the result. When there is discordance a discussion with the laboratory expert can often be beneficial.

Patients commonly present with non-specific tiredness, exhaustion and lethargy, and the differential diagnosis is wide. A series of tests is ordered and the thyroid stimulating hormone (TSH) is found to be slightly elevated at, say, 6 (range 0.4–4). A possible answer is apparent—but no, the test result must answer the question and a TSH of 6 does not equate with major symptoms—so the clinician must think again.

The experts in the following chapters will discuss the range, specificity and sensitivity of their laboratory tests, which is the other half of the equation. Read on and enjoy the challenges.

2 Abnormal laboratory results

C.G. Fraser

The finding of an unexpected 'abnormal' laboratory result is not uncommon, particularly with current approaches in diagnosis, case finding and monitoring in which many different tests are often requested simultaneously, often in organ- or disease-related profiles. However, before clinical action is taken there are a number of logical reasons for the unexpected abnormal test result that should be considered.

Due to much international discussion and the wide dissemination of guidelines from the International Federation of Clinical Chemistry and Laboratory Medicine, the terms 'reference interval' or 'reference range' are now widely used in preference to 'normal range'. This supposedly minimises the many semantic difficulties associated with the word 'normal' and should clearly suggest that a result that is outside the limits of the reference interval does not necessarily imply that the person is diseased. Moreover, most will know that the reference interval is a statistical concept that simply ensures that the limits encompass the central 95% of the reference population. Thus, simply by definition, 5% of the apparently healthy population will have values outside the reference limits—2.5% will have high values and 2.5% will have low values. These individuals are not necessarily unhealthy, merely different from the bulk of the population. The unexpected laboratory result may well have arisen because the test has been done on one of these healthy but simply rather different individuals. Laboratories themselves may not help understanding or clinical interpretation because they often highlight or 'flag' these expected results that are outside the reference limits and, in fact, are either encouraged or required to do so by their accreditation bodies.

Purely on statistical grounds, the more tests that are done the higher the chance of finding an unexpected abnormal result. If one test is done, 5% of the population lie outside the reference limits. If two unrelated tests are done, over 9% of the population lie outside the reference limits for at least one test. When 20 tests are performed on the one patient there will be as high as a 60% chance of observing at least one result outside the reference interval.

Reference values are affected by many factors. There are endogenous factors such as age and gender and many exogenous factors such as time of day, relationship of sampling to food intake, exercise, posture, stress and immobilisation. Laboratories often do examine the effects of some of these factors on their reference values and, provided that the test requestor gives correct information, particularly about age and sex, modern laboratory information systems will insert the appropriately stratified or partitioned reference values on the test report, irrespective of whether this is paper or electronic. It is vital to note that reference values may be highly dependent on the analytical method that the laboratory uses, particularly for enzymes, drugs and hormones. Moreover, some reference values, such as glucose, are dependent on the type of sample—capillary blood is not the same as venous plasma which is not the same as serum. Thus, an unexplained abnormal laboratory result may arise because an inappropriate reference interval is used for comparison. Because reference values are dependent on population, laboratory methodology and workflow approaches, it is good practice to use only the values provided by the laboratory that performed the test. In certain parts of the world, significant effort is being made to harmonise reference values across geography: this is a laudable aim but technically difficult to achieve except for the common, easy-to-do tests. It is certainly totally inappropriate to use reference values found in texts, books, diaries and the like: these usually have no objective foundation. Undoubtedly, dependence on such sources will give rise to unexpected abnormal laboratory results.

Sometimes the unexpected abnormal laboratory result is said to be a 'laboratory error'. These are actually now very rare. Modern analytical equipment generally samples from the primary specimen tube used to collect the blood, so mix-ups are uncommon. The use of information technology and barcoding of patient identification, request forms and specimen tubes has also minimised errors. Laboratories have comprehensive internal quality control programs, which monitor all facets of performance. They also participate in regional, national and international external quality assessment schemes, which allow inter-laboratory comparisons of performance. In many countries laboratories have extensive accreditation procedures, and compliance with all the standards is mandatory. However, it is admitted that unexpected laboratory results caused by error do still occur. Most often these are caused by mistakes made before the laboratory receives the specimen, for example, through patient misidentification at test request entry, contamination of the sample by anticoagulants or IV fluids, incorrect specimen-to-anticoagulant ratio, prolonged venous stasis, delay in the delivery of unstable specimen and inadequate preservation or storage prior to or during transportation of the specimen to the laboratory.

Although analytical methodology continues to improve with time, certain test procedures are still not totally specific for the test they purport to measure. A number of commonly prescribed drugs do cross-react in current methods and the unexpected abnormal laboratory result may be due to such drug interference. Moreover, laboratory methods may profess to measure the same test but do not in reality do so: this is particularly relevant in the fields of hormone and drug analyses where many different types of similar molecules or metabolites may exist, which are measured in some analytical systems but not in others. The unexpected abnormal result may be due to measurement of an unusual molecule or metabolite of no real clinical significance. In addition, many quantities are protein bound in plasma and, if the carrier protein is abnormal, the test result for the quantity bound to that protein may appear abnormal when in fact it is physiologically still at an appropriate level. In particular, competition for binding sites on albumin can seriously affect free drug levels.

Laboratories report test results as single numbers. However, this number represents a range of values, the dispersion of which is dependent on inherent within-subject biological variation and on random analytical variation. Every analytical method has some random variation and this may be quite large for difficult-to-measure components, particularly those which are present in only very small amounts in body fluids. Thus, when a single numerical value is reported as being outside the reference interval, the range of readings that the single value actually refers to may, at least in part, overlap the reference interval. This is particularly so in borderline situations.

The natural history of many diseases is not fully understood as yet and it may be difficult to decide on the clinical implications of an unexpected abnormal result when no disease is apparent. Some would suggest that an abnormal result is a sign of unsuspected disease. However, there is little objective evidence to support such conclusions. A number of studies have examined the frequency with which unexpected laboratory results are found, particularly when the idea of performing a very comprehensive profile of common tests was in vogue. These studies have shown that in general the reasons for the unexpected abnormal laboratory results are far from clear.

Since there are many reasons for the unexpected abnormal result, the recommended approach is to seek the advice of the laboratory. Laboratory staff can assess whether the appropriate reference values were used and give advice on the many factors that influence such values—these are fully documented in the easily accessible literature of laboratory medicine. Moreover, laboratory staff can quickly check on the possibility of error as most laboratories retain all specimens for some time. Modern laboratories usually have excellent audit trailing and, using the laboratory computer system, can track everything that has happened to an individual specimen.

In addition, the possibility of an in vivo or in vitro drug–test interaction can be assessed—again, these are very fully documented in the literature of laboratory medicine. Furthermore, the possibility of the test result's being abnormal because of the presence of unusual molecular species or metabolites can often be explored. Laboratory staff will have knowledge of biological and analytical sources of variation and will be able to advise on the probability that the unexpected abnormal laboratory result does lie within the reference interval. Laboratory staff may be able to advise on the likelihood that a pathological process or latent disease is present and may well be able to suggest the most appropriate further investigations to clarify the situation.

○ Summary

Unexpected abnormal laboratory results are common. If there are no logical clinical reasons for the result, a carefully collected repeat specimen should always be submitted for analysis before other laboratory tests are requested, further diagnostic investigations (such as imaging) are instituted or clinical action initiated.

3 What does the reference range of a biochemical screen test mean?

G.M. Kellerman

The concept of a normal individual is one of the most difficult to define in clinical medicine. A working definition such as 'an individual who has no detectable disease and no demonstrable excess tendency to develop diseases relevant to the situation under discussion' has the benefit of leaving the uncertainty of undiagnosed disease in the definition, as well as permitting risk factor analysis at an appropriate level. But does such a normal individual have a normal value for a particular biochemical test? Normal individuals vary in many respects—age, sex, genetic make-up, lifestyle, body habits, preferred diet, exercise—and their values for a given test also vary, especially with such things as time of day, age, meals, exercise and menstrual cycle, generating a range of normal values. A few of these apparently normal individuals have as yet undiagnosed disease and, more importantly, others may be in a group as yet unrecognised, due to lack of appropriate research, with an increased risk for a particular disease to develop in, say, 20 years time. These people will surely be excluded when research has documented the risk factor—consider how the concepts of borderline hypertension, prediabetes or atherosclerosis have developed over the years. This is particularly germane with the current 'epidemic' of obesity.

The normal range for a particular test can be analysed statistically as described in standard textbooks.[1,2] If we assume a Gaussian distribution, simple prediction is possible of the proportion who will fall within so many standard deviations of the mean. Other types of distribution can be manipulated by special statistical methods. For many (but not all) tests, a given individual has a far narrower variation during health than does the population as a whole and an accurate knowledge of their personal normal range could be of value in assessing their state of health. Without such information we can use only the broader population-based normal range in our assessment of the patient, and our decision depends on where the person's own normal value happened to be and how far the value has moved with the disease process. There is uncertainty in decision making even if we have a previous normal value for the particular person. Furthermore, no analytical technique is perfect: there is always some error, leading either to non-reproducibility of a result on the same specimen (lack of precision) or an incorrect but reproducible answer (lack of accuracy). Using extensive and expensive quality control systems, clinical laboratories strive to minimise these errors and thus increase the predictive value of their results.

Clinical biochemists have accepted for some years the position described above and now define not a *normal* but a reference range. Values within the reference range do not raise suspicion of disease; nevertheless, they do not exclude the possibilty that disease may be affecting the parameter in question. Values outside the reference range are a signal that thought is necessary—and the further they are from the reference range, the more likely is the presence of a disease process. If the reference range is set too narrowly, too high a proportion of normal people will have suspicion cast on them (false positive results or low specificity); if the reference range is set too broadly, too many abnormal individuals will be missed (false negative results or low sensitivity). A compromise is always necessary in such circumstances between specificity and sensitivity, the exact decision depending on the prevalence of the disease in the population being studied.[3,4] In most hospital laboratories it is customary to set the reference range to include the central 95% of values of people presumed to be normal. Such a procedure yields only an index of suspicion—it is wrong to treat one in 20 of the population for a hypothetical condition with a treatment appropriate to a real condition: doctors should treat patients with problems, not analytical results. Further developments have occurred with some analytes, such as glucose, cholesterol and glycated haemoglobin, where a target range has been set based on outcome studies, as a result of which a higher proportion of the population are outside the range. A very similar set of considerations is used in setting appropriate therapeutic ranges for results of drug analyses, which are becoming more and more frequent as the pharmaceutical industry provides an ever increasing range of products for therapy.

Experienced clinicians, therefore, develop an index of increasing suspicion, combining the degree of deviation of a particular value from its reference range with results of other tests, observations of the patient and so on. They are really combining a number of probabilities, gained from their experience, appropriate for the community in which they work. They realise that a value within the reference range also has a given probability of being compatible with disease—less than for those outside the range but still not zero—and skilful manipulation of probabilities often can help in deciding between two possible diagnoses.[5] They avoid the trap whereby the more unrelated tests done on the one patient, the greater the chance that one or more will fall outside the reference range. They use their clinical judgment to avoid overreaction with further tests and investigations galore—the

QUICK FLICK 3

familiar investigation and treatment of the asterisks and not of the patient. Such clinicians can often combine results of several tests to add to their predictive accuracy (e.g. reciprocal movements of calcium and phosphate and appropriate changes in alkaline phosphatase) and research suggests that combining test results (even within the reference range) with sophisticated techniques such as discriminant function analysis may help to identify the probability of a given hypothesis. However, such analysis has proven to be very population dependent, so that even in neighbouring parts of a city coefficients may prove to be non-transferable, thus limiting the value of this method.

One final warning: how does a laboratory establish its reference range? Where do the normal subjects come from? Are the results from young, healthy, fit male football players (or doctors, nurses, blood donors, school children, volunteers or army conscripts) applicable to inhabitants of aged care facilities, pregnant women or newborn babies? There are numerous examples where it has been essential to establish age-specific reference ranges, especially for infants and children. Where a risk factor for a given result has been proposed (e.g. cholesterol and ischaemic heart disease), where does one draw the line of normality to establish the reference range? Can we use a hospital population, recognise that most results are normal and just throw away those from the obviously diseased? Current practice tends to either accept this last alternative or to collect a suitable set of apparently normal persons (age-matched, sex-matched and so on if appropriate), with statistical manipulations. Longitudinal studies—for example, Framingham—of a population group over years may permit identification of risk levels of various analytes.

However, we must not forget that any approach contains an element of personal value judgment, which may change in the future as methodology and knowledge improve. Long may it remain so, for our current use of laboratory test results is neither precise nor accurate, even if the tests themselves are. There is no substitute for thought, experience and research.

References

1. Kringle R.O. and Bogovich M. Statistical procedures. In: *Tietz Textbook of Clinical Chemistry*. 3rd edn. Philadelphia: WB Saunders, 1999, pp. 265–309.
2. Feinstein A.R. *Clinical Biostatistics*. St Louis: Mosby, 1977.
3. Henry R.J. and Reed A.H. Normal values and the use of laboratory results for the detection of disease. In: Henry R.J. and Reed A.H., eds. *Clinical Chemistry, Principles and Techniques*. Hagerstown: Harper and Row, 1974, pp. 343–71.

4. Watson R.A. and Tang D.B. The predictive value of prostatic acid phosphatase as a screening test for prostatic cancer. *NEJM* 1980; 303: 497–9.
5. Gorry G.A., Pauker S.G. and Schwartz W.B. The diagnostic importance of the normal finding. *NEJM* 1978; 298: 486–9.

4 Pitfalls in interpreting laboratory results

P. Phillips

Synopsis

The results of laboratory tests are affected by the collection and handling of the specimen, the particular laboratory and the method of analysis. They are also affected by variability within the individual and within the laboratory. Interpretation at one point in time should consider the position of the measurement within the laboratory reference range appropriate for the sample and the person being tested. Interpreting results over time should consider the likely variability of the measurement and the level of certainty required to identify a true change or absence of change. The more variable the measurement and the higher the required level of certainty, the larger the change between measurements needs to be before it can be considered clinically significant.

Introduction

Health professionals may find it hard to get clinically useful information from the barrage of figures, ranges, asterisks and comments in laboratory results. Some knowledge about the accuracy of laboratory results can help to sort out important clinical signals from the background noise. The laboratory does not know all the patient's details. Clinicians should consider test results in the context of the clinical presentation and not rely completely on the laboratory's interpretation.

Reference ranges

Quoted reference ranges depend on the method used in the laboratory and the population from which the reference range was derived. The results from one method may be systematically different from those of another and therefore the reference ranges will be different.

Some laboratories give the range quoted by the manufacturer of the test or derived from an easily accessible population such as blood donors. Others give ranges in terms of age, sex or biological phase. For example, the ranges quoted for female sex hormones are related to pre- and post-menopausal status and the phase of the menstrual cycle. Some important biological influences, such as seasonal effects on 25-hydroxyvitamin D, are often not included in the reference ranges. Perhaps this is because users would find it harder to interpret results if the reference ranges were changing all the time and because of the logistics and laboratory workload needed to derive such specific reference ranges.

The ideal reference range would relate to the individual being tested while healthy, at the same age and in the same biological phase and season. Clearly this is not possible but sometimes one gets insights from looking back through previous results (ideally reported by the same laboratory using the same method).

By tradition, laboratories quote a reference range that includes 95% of the reference population. If the results are normally distributed, this includes results within approximately two standard deviations above and two standard deviations below the mean value. The reference range therefore covers four standard deviations. Some results vary so much within the population that the laboratory may quote a reference range that includes a smaller proportion of the population. For example, the reference range commonly quoted for serum insulin may include only results within one standard deviation above and one standard deviation below the mean value. This covers 68% of the reference population. In this case, 16% of normal people will have 'abnormal' high insulin and 16% will have 'abnormal' low insulin according to the quoted reference range. Serum insulin is therefore not a useful test for assessing 'insulin resistance'.

Results have to be interpreted in terms of the particular laboratory's reference range. When monitoring results over time, clinicians also need to be aware that different laboratories will have different reference ranges.

As reference ranges are population based, a patient might have a result near the top or bottom of the normal range. Clinically significant changes could then occur without the results moving out of the population reference range. For example, if an elderly patient's plasma creatinine concentration is usually near the bottom of the reference range but then rises to the upper end of that range, the patient may have had a significant deterioration in renal function. Similar considerations apply to a haemoglobin concentration falling from a high normal to a low normal value.

QUICK FLICK

4

◐ **Specimen collection and handling**

Laboratory results can be affected by the procedures for specimen collection and handling (Table 4.1).[1] If a result is a surprise, check the patient's name and date of birth on the result report. You can also contact the laboratory and ask if the specimen looked normal and consider repeating the test.

Table 4.1 Abnormal laboratory results caused by incorrect collection and handling[†]

Step	Mechanism	Result	Measurement affected
Sample	Incorrect sample	Incorrect results	For example, random spot urine calcium:creatinine ratio instead of first voided
Venepuncture	Prolonged venostasis	Plasma filtration and concentration	Protein concentrations— globulins, albumins and lipoproteins and measurements affected by them (e.g. calcium)
	Difficult venepuncture	Haemolysis	Red cell leakage with high potassium, phosphate and lactate dehydrogenase
Specimen tube	Incorrect collection tube	Assay affected	• If potassium EDTA used for chemistry— potassium; calcium and enzymes (calcium binding and enzyme inhibition) • Lithium heparin anticoagulant— lithium assay

Step	Mechanism	Result	Measurement affected
Specimen handling	Delay in transport	Red cell use of glucose and leakage of contents	Blood glucose (if fluoride tube not used) Potassium, bicarbonate, phosphate, lactate dehydrogenase
	Specimen mislabelling	Incorrect results	Virtually everything
Laboratory	Machine malfunction Transcription error	Incorrect results	Virtually everything

†Derived from reference 1

◗ Why normal people often have abnormal results

A multiple biochemical analysis can be performed by one machine and produce 20 results. Assuming these results were all independent of each other (which they are not) and that results from the reference population are normally distributed (which they may not be), only 36% of normal people will have all 20 results in the reference range and 64% will have at least one abnormal result (Table 4.2). However, the more abnormal the result and the more related tests are abnormal, the more likely the abnormality is clinically significant.

Table 4.2 Normal results in normal people

If the reference range covers 95% of results for a normal population, the chance of a healthy individual having a certain number of normal tests is:
- Two out of two tests: $0.95 \times 0.95 = 90\%$
- All 20 of 20 tests: $0.95^{20} = 36\%$

If you consider the 99% reference range (approximately $\pm$ 2.6 standard deviations) and the 99.9% reference range (approximately $\pm$ 3.3 standard deviations), 82% and 98% of people will have all 20 tests within the reference range (0.99^{20} and 0.999^{20}, respectively). These facts can be useful when interpreting an isolated abnormal result.

For example, the reference range of alkaline phosphatase is 30–110 U/L. This covers two standard deviations below the mean and two above the mean. One standard deviation is therefore 20 U/L [$(110 - 30) \div 4$]. A result of 150 U/L is two standard deviations above the upper limit of the reference range and therefore four standard deviations above the mean. This is very unlikely to occur in a normal individual. However, the result may be normal if the quoted reference range is inappropriate. For example, in pregnancy and growing children alkaline phosphatase is produced by the placenta and bone. These are good examples of why it is important to consider whether the population reference range is appropriate for the individual being tested.

When deciding if a result is abnormal, look at related tests. Alkaline phosphatase is one of the liver function tests (others are bilirubin, gamma glutamyl transferase, alanine aminotransferase, aspartate aminotransferase and lactate dehydrogenase). Abnormalities in the other tests would suggest that the abnormal alkaline phosphatase could be the result of liver disease. An elevated alkaline phosphatase in isolation may indicate another problem, such as bone disease.

◑ Laboratory accuracy

We often know the within-laboratory, within-method variability as this is usually quoted by the laboratory. Modern laboratories provide remarkably consistent results for many analytes—typical coefficients of variation (see Table 4.3) are 1–6% for the components of multiple biochemical analysis, electrolytes, calcium and phosphorus and renal and liver function tests.

Table 4.3 Coefficient of variation

The coefficient of variation (CV) is calculated as: CV = standard deviation of the measured value ÷ mean value of the measurements × 100
Variability is different at different absolute values of the measurement and is usually quoted at a specific clinically relevant value. For example: CV for plasma sodium: 0.8% at 139 mmol/L CV for plasma bilirubin: 6.1% at 10 micromol/L
The coefficient of variation is one way of expressing the variability of biological measurements. Laboratories sometimes also refer to the imprecision of a measurement.

National quality control programs monitor the accuracy and imprecision of different methods used in different laboratories. One result has been that the differences between laboratories for individual methods are now usually a small component of the overall variability of measurements.

○ Why values vary within one individual

In addition to the variations caused by specimen collection and handling and the differences within and between laboratories and their methods, there is intra-individual variation. Assuming specimen collection and processing errors do not occur, the largest source of variability is within the individual. Values vary by age and sex and within the menstrual, diurnal and seasonal cycles. Intra-individual biological variability for different analytes can range from very large to moderate, for example, 8% for total cholesterol[2] versus 40% for microalbuminuria assessed by the albumin:creatinine ratio[3]. In addition, the longer the interval between tests, the greater the total intra-individual variability of the measure.

It is much more difficult for laboratories to provide information on the total intra-individual variability than for the within-laboratory, within-method variability, which is automatically generated by their quality control programs. However, it is the total variability within an individual which is important when interpreting results.

○ Are changes in results caused by intra-individual variability or the effects of treatment?

One trap is the phenomenon of regression to the mean.[4] Results within an apparently homogeneous group of patients are likely to lie within the 95% reference range for that measurement. If the same patients are re-tested at a different time, the pattern of the overall results will look much the same. In a normal distribution, values are bunched around the group mean and progressively 'thin out' further from the mean. However, individual results are likely to have changed, particularly those at the extremes.

The initial results at the extremes are the result of extreme random variability in one direction or the other. The same amount and direction of variability is unlikely to occur on the second measurement in the same individual. Subsequent measurements will therefore move closer to the middle (or regress to the mean). Results from other individuals who initially were closer to the mean may now lie closer to the extremes of the distribution.

This phenomenon can be exploited intentionally or unintentionally in trials that select and treat individuals with high values of a measurement to demonstrate that a treatment is effective. Regression to the mean is one reason why randomised placebo controlled prospective trials are the gold standard for assessing treatments.

A large difference between two measurements is more likely to be a signal of a true change than the result of the background noise of measurement variability. Similarly, the smaller the total intra-individual variability, the more likely a specific absolute change is a signal. The less likely the observed change is caused by variability, the surer one can be that the change is real.

These three elements are brought together in the concept of the least significant change. To be 80% confident the observed change is real, the change should exceed approximately twice the intra-individual coefficient of variation (CV_i) (Table 4.4). For example:

- A total cholesterol that decreases from 7.0 to 5.6 mmol/L after starting a statin is a 20% fall from the initial value. The CV_i for total cholesterol is 8% so the least significant change is approximately 16% ($2CV_i$). You can be 80% sure that the 20% change is real rather than apparent.
- A decrease in microalbuminuria from an albumin:creatinine ratio of 5.0 mg/mmol to 2.0 mg/mmol after starting an angiotensin converting enzyme (ACE) inhibitor is a 60% fall. The total CV_i of the albumin:creatinine ratio is 40% so the least significant change is approximately 80% ($2CV_i$). It is likely that this 60% change is apparent rather than real.

Table 4.4 When is a change significant?

Least significant change

1. The overall variability of the difference between two measurements is greater than the variability of the individual measurements: $\sqrt{2}\ CV_i$.

2. The more confident one wishes to be that the change in a measurement is a signal rather than noise, the greater the change needs to be relative to this: $\sqrt{2}\ CV_i \times z$. The z value is used to refer to normally distributed values and describes the distance of a particular value from the mean in numbers of standard deviations (SD). The greater the distance from the mean (the z value) the less likely a result has occurred by chance. z varies from 1.28 for 80% confidence to 2.6 for 99% confidence.

3. Generally an 80% confidence is used (z = 1.28):
   Least significant change = $\sqrt{2}\ CV_i \times 1.28 = 1.8\ CV_i$.
   This approximates to $2CV_i$.

Intra-individual coefficient of variation (CV_i)

For a list of intra-individual CV_i for different analytes, see reference 5.

Variability of the difference between two measurements

CV_{i1} = intra-individual coefficient of variation for the first measurement
CV_{i2} = intra-individual coefficient of variation for the second measurement
The variability of the difference between two measurements is $\sqrt{CV_{i1}^2 + CV_{i2}^2}$.
If $CV_{i1} = CV_{i2}$ (as measuring the same variable), then $CV_{i1}^2 + CV_{i2}^2 = 2CV_{i1}^2$, so the variability of difference is $\sqrt{2CV_{i1}^2} = \sqrt{2}\ \sqrt{CV_{i1}^2} = \sqrt{2}CV_{i1}$.

◐ The effects of treatment on measurements may be delayed

Laboratory results may take a long time to change after starting treatment. This may reflect pharmacokinetics, biology or a combination of the two.

The half-life of thyroxine in the body is approximately seven days. Testing after one week will only show half the expected total effect. (This may sometimes still be useful information.) By six weeks (six half-lives in this case) 98.4% of the effect will have occurred $[1 - (\frac{1}{2})^6]$.

When starting a thiazolidinedione (glitazone) the full effect on blood glucose requires a steady state of the drug (pharmacokinetic effect) but also requires the shift in fat metabolism that in turn causes the reduction in glucose (biologic effect). Finally, the glycated haemoglobin (HbA1c) reflects the average blood glucose over the preceding 4–6 weeks because of the slow turnover of the red cells (biologic and pharmacokinetic effects).[6] The combination of these factors means that testing after 1 week of treatment may show little change in the HbA1c and that 2–3 months may be needed to show the full effect of treatment.

Another glycated protein (albumin, which becomes fructosamine) has a much faster turnover. It therefore reflects the average glucose over a shorter period (2–3 weeks).

One can reduce the variability of the measurement change by reducing the variability of the baseline and final measurements (e.g. using the mean of two measurements for each). If both initial and final measurements were repeated the variability of the change would be reduced to CV_i (not $\sqrt{2}CV_i$).

Using the microalbuminuria example, with two measurements before and after the intervention, the least significant change would be 51% (1.28 × 40%). You could then be 80% sure that the 60% observed change was real and not apparent.

◐ Summary

When interpreting laboratory results it is important to know that the sample was collected and handled correctly. The appropriate reference range for the test should be used. Different laboratories may report different results on the same specimen.

When comparing results over time, use the same laboratory and method for testing. Consider the variability of results within the individual and the least significant change, that is, the amount of difference between measurements that is likely to be a real biological signal instead of resulting from the noise of biological variability within the individual and within the end measurement variability of the laboratory. As a rough rule, the least significant change is twice the intra-individual coefficient of variation ($2CV_i$).

If an important clinical decision depends on whether a change occurs with a particular treatment, consider making two (or more) measurements before and after starting treatment. This reduces the variability and the possibility of misinterpreting the regression to the mean of an initial high or low value. Monitoring trends with time involves more measurements and gives a more reliable indication of change than a single comparison at two points.

Remember, the more tests you do the more likely you are to get at least one false positive outside the laboratory reference range. Aim to limit the number of tests to those that are relevant to the clinical situation rather than requesting a screening battery.

When assessing the effects of treatment, consider how long the treatment will take before the therapeutic effect reaches a steady state (e.g. 4–6 half-lives of a drug) and how long the biological response will take before the measurement you make reaches a steady state. Trying to assess therapeutic effects before the response to treatment has reached a steady state can seriously underestimate the therapeutic effect.

References

1. Phillips P. and Beng C. Electrolytes—'fun with fluids'. *Check (Continuous Home Evaluation of Clinical Knowledge) program of self assessment. No. 323.* South Melbourne: Royal Australian College of General Practitioners, 1999.
2. Cooper G.R., Myers G.L., Smith S.J. and Schlant R.C. Blood lipid measurements. Variations and practical utility. *JAMA* 1992; 267: 1652–60.
3. Phillipou G. and Phillips P.J. Variability of urinary albumin excretion in patients with microalbuminuria. *Diabetes Care* 1994; 17: 425–7.
4. Irwig L., Glasziou P., Wilson A. and Macaskill P. Estimating an individual's true cholesterol level and response to intervention. *JAMA* 1991; 266: 1678–85.
5. *Desirable specifications for total error, imprecision and bias, derived from intra- and inter-individual biologic variation.* Updated 2010 Feb 15, www.westgard.com/biodatabase1.htm [cited Mar 3, 2010].
6. Phillipov G. and Phillips P.J. Components of total measurement error for haemoglobin A1c determination. *Clin Chem* 2001; 47: 1851–3.

5 Moving beyond sensitivity and specificity: using likelihood ratios to help interpret diagnostic tests

J. Attia

Synopsis

Properties of diagnostic tests have traditionally been described using sensitivity, specificity and positive and negative predictive values. These measures, however, reflect population characteristics and do not easily translate to individual patients. Likelihood ratios are a more practical way of making sense of diagnostic test results and have immediate clinical relevance. In general, a useful test provides a high positive likelihood ratio and a small negative likelihood ratio.

⦿ Introduction

In clinical practice physicians are often faced with interpreting the results of diagnostic tests. These results are not absolute. A negative test does not always rule out disease and some positive results can be false. As the prevalence of disease varies, the results of a test may have different implications; haematuria is more likely to be a sign of cancer in an elderly man than it is in a young woman.

⦿ Sensitivity and specificity

Clinical epidemiology has long focused on sensitivity and specificity as well as positive and negative predictive values as a way of measuring the diagnostic utility of a test.[1] The test is compared against a reference (gold) standard and the results are tabulated in a 2 × 2 table (Fig. 5.1). Sensitivity is the proportion of those with disease who test positive. In other words sensitivity is a measure of how well the test detects disease when it is really there; a sensitive test has few false negatives. Specificity is the proportion of those without disease who test negative. It measures how well the test rules out disease when it is really absent; a specific test has few false positives.

Although well established, sensitivity and specificity have some deficiencies in clinical use. This is mostly because sensitivity and specificity

Figure 5.1 Estimating the sensitivity and specificity of diagnostic tests

True diagnosis
'gold standard'

		Disease present	Disease absent	
	Positive	a True positive	b False positive	a + b
Test results	Negative	c False negative	d True negative	c + d
		a + c	b + d	

Sensitivity = a/(a + c)
Specificity = d/(b + d)

Positive predictive value = a/(a + b)
Negative predictive value = d/(c + d)

$$\text{Positive likelihood ratio} = \frac{a/(a + c)}{b/(b + d)} \qquad \text{Negative likelihood ratio} = \frac{c/(a + c)}{d/(b + d)}$$

are population measures, i.e. they summarise the characteristics of the test over a population.

How do we interpret results for an individual patient? What is the probability of disease in a 50-year-old male with suspected angina who has more than 1 mm of ST segment depression during an exercise stress test? What does a negative d-dimer test mean, in terms of the chance of having a deep vein thrombosis, for a 40-year-old female with a swollen calf? It is impossible for the clinician to know whether a positive result is a true positive or a false positive or whether a negative result is a true negative or a false negative.

○ Predictive values

What clinicians need is a measure that combines the true and false positives (or negatives) into one. The positive predictive value is such an attempt; it expresses the proportion of those with positive test results who truly have disease (Fig. 5.1). Another way of expressing this is to ask: given that a patient has tested positive what is the probability that they truly have disease?

However, this measure is critically dependent on the population chosen and the prevalence of disease. The lower the prevalence, the less well the test performs. The same caveats apply to the negative predictive value. This means that the positive predictive value and negative predictive value are not transferable from one patient to another or from one setting to another.

○ Likelihood ratios

Likelihood ratios are independent of disease prevalence. They may be understood using the following analogy. Assume that a patient tests positive on a diagnostic test. If this were a perfect test, it would mean that the patient would certainly have the disease (true positive; TP). The only thing that stops us from making this conclusion is that some patients without disease also test positive (false positive; FP). We therefore have to correct the TP rate by the FP rate; this is done mathematically by dividing one by the other (Fig. 5.1).

Algebraically, we can show that the positive likelihood ratio equals the probability of a positive test in those with disease divided by the probability of a positive test in those without disease.

$$\text{Positive likelihood ratio} = \text{TP rate} \ / \ \text{FP rate}$$
$$= (a/[a + c]) \ / \ (b/[b + d])$$
$$= \text{sensitivity} \ / \ (1 - \text{specificity}).$$

Likewise if a patient tests negative we are still worried about the likelihood of this being a false negative (FN) rather than a true negative (TN). This likelihood is given mathematically by the probability of a negative test in those with disease compared with the probability of a negative test in those without disease. The negative likelihood ratio equals the probability of a negative test in those with disease divided by the probability of a negative test in those without disease.

$$\text{Negative likelihood ratio} = \text{FN rate} \ / \ \text{TN rate}$$
$$= (c/[a + c]) \ / \ (d/[b + d])$$
$$= (1 - \text{sensitivity}) \ / \ \text{specificity}.$$

Likelihood ratios have a number of useful properties:
- Because they are based on a *ratio* of sensitivity and specificity they do not vary in different populations or settings.
- They can be used directly at the individual patient level.
- They allow the clinician to quantitate the probability of disease for any individual patient.

Interpreting likelihood ratios is intuitive: the larger the positive likelihood ratio, the greater the likelihood of disease; the smaller the negative likelihood ratio, the less the likelihood of disease.

To see how likelihood ratios work let us take the example of the 50-year-old male with the positive stress test. It is known that a more than 1 mm depression on exercise stress testing has a sensitivity and specificity of 65% and 89% respectively for coronary artery disease when compared to the reference standard of angiography.[2] This means that the positive likelihood ratio = 0.65/(1 − 0.89) = 5.9.

The *likelihood* of this patient having disease has increased by approximately six-fold given the positive test result. To translate this into a *probability* of disease one must use Bayes' theorem. Bayes' theorem states that the pretest *odds* of disease multiplied by the likelihood ratio yields the post-test *odds* of disease. Note that because of the theorem's mathematical properties the likelihood ratios must be used with odds rather than a percentage probability of disease. Bayes' nomogram is used to avoid the bother of first converting fractions to odds then multiplying by the odds ratio, getting the post-test odds, and converting back to a fraction (Fig. 5.2).[3] In the nomogram the pretest probability is located on the first axis and joined to the likelihood ratio on the second axis to read off the post-test probability on the third axis (alternatively, this can be done electronically using the 'stats calculator' on the website of the Centre for Evidence-Based Medicine Toronto).

For example, if we estimate from our clinical assessment that the 50-year-old male has a 40% chance of having coronary artery disease, we join 40% on the first axis with 6 on the second axis and read off the post-test probability of 80%, i.e. the patient has an 80% chance of having coronary artery disease given the positive test result.

Likewise, let us estimate that the 40-year-old woman has a 17% chance of having a deep vein thrombosis. A d-dimer test has a sensitivity of 89% and a specificity of 77%. This means that the negative likelihood ratio = (1 − 0.89)/0.77 = 0.14.

Using Bayes' nomogram and joining 17% with 0.14, we read off a post-test probability of approximately 3%. This means that after a negative test the woman has a 3% chance of having a deep vein thrombosis.

It is important to note that likelihood ratios always refer to the likelihood of having disease—the positive and negative designation simply refers to the test result—hence the interpretation of the post-test odds is always a likelihood of having disease.

These scenarios highlight some additional advantages of using likelihood ratios. They enable the clinician to talk quantitatively about the risk of disease, which may allow more informed decision making on the part of the patient. Likelihood ratios emphasise the reality that we are never 100% sure of the diagnosis. Rather than looking at diagnostic tests as yes or no answers to the question of whether a patient has disease, we realise that positive

Figure 5.2 Bayes' nomogram

Pre-test probability is located on the first axis and joined
to the appropriate likelihood ratio on the second axis.
The post-test probability is then read off the third axis.

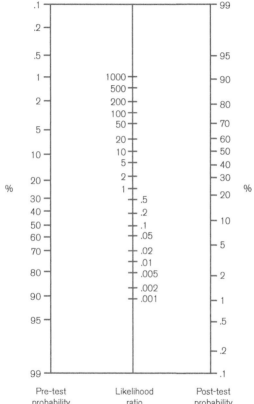

| Pre-test probability | Likelihood ratio | Post-test probability |

or negative results simply increase or decrease the likelihood of disease,
judged on the basis of our history and physical examination. Various items
of the history and examination can be seen as diagnostic tests and can have
likelihood ratios associated with them.

Although likelihood ratios are clinically very useful, a significant barrier to
using them in routine practice is the amount of time required to do literature
searching in order to identify the sensitivity and specificity of the tests.

Fortunately, as their use is increasing, authors have compiled likelihood ratios for common tests and clinical signs and symptoms.[4,5,6] Additionally, the online calculator referred to earlier allows users to enter the results of a diagnostic test study and automatically calculate the likelihood ratios, complete with 95% confidence intervals.

◗ Pretest probability

Bayes' nomogram requires an estimation of the probability of disease. There are two methods of estimating pretest probability:

- Use your clinical experience and 'gut feeling' following the history and examination to create a number. This is the most frequent method used, although studies show significant variation of estimates even between experienced clinicians[7].
- Apply clinical decision rules.

Clinical decision rules have been published for a small number of clinical problems. For example, based on three questions regarding the quality of chest pain, clinicians can estimate the pretest probability of coronary artery disease.[2] Likewise various signs and symptoms can be given a point score to arrive at a pretest probability of deep vein thrombosis (Table 5.1);[8] this is how the pretest probability of 17% was assigned in the scenario above. Unfortunately such decision rules are rare and difficult to find, although they have recently been compiled in a book[9] and a subscription-only electronic database[10].

Table 5.1 Clinical decision rule for deep vein thrombosis

Clinical feature	Score
Active cancer	1
Paralysis, paresis or recent plaster	1
Bedridden for more than three days or major surgery within four weeks	1
Localised tenderness	1
Entire leg swollen	1
Calf swelling more than 3 cm	1
Pitting oedema	1
Collateral superficial veins	1
Alternative diagnosis as likely as or greater than that of deep vein thrombosis	−2

The total score reflects the probability of having a deep vein thrombosis: ≤ 0 is low probability (3%), 1–2 is moderate (17%) and ≥ 3 is high (75%).

☉ Summary

Likelihood ratios are a useful and practical way of expressing the power of diagnostic tests in increasing or decreasing the likelihood of disease. Unlike sensitivity and specificity, which are population characteristics, likelihood ratios can be used at the individual patient level. Using likelihood ratios and Bayes' nomogram allows us to convert a pretest probability, based on an educated guess or a clinical decision rule, to a post-test probability.

References

1. Bauman A. The epidemiology of clinical tests. *Aust Prescr* 1990; 13: 62–4.
2. Diamond G.A. and Forrester J.S. Analysis of probability as an aid in the clinical diagnosis of coronary-artery disease. *NEJM* 1979; 300: 1350–8.
3. Fagan T.J. Nomogram for Bayes theorem. *NEJM* 1975; 293: 257.
4. Black E.R., Bordley D.R., Tape T.G and Panzer R.J., eds. *Diagnostic Strategies For Common Medical Problems.* 2nd ed. Philadelphia: American College of Physicians, 1999.
5. Guyatt G. and Rennie D., eds. *Users' Guides to the Medical Literature: Evidence-Based Clinical Practice.* Chicago: American Medical Association Press, 2002.
6. Simel D.L. and Rennie D., eds. *The Rational Clinical Examination; Evidence-based Clinical Diagnosis,* New York: McGraw-Hill, 2009.
7. Attia J., Nair K., Sibbritt D., Ewald B., Paget N., Wellard R. et al. Generating pretest probabilities: a neglected area in clinical decision-making. A study of the assessment of baseline risk estimates (SABRE). *MJA* 2004; 180: 449–54.
8. Wells P.S., Anderson D.R., Bormanis J., Guy F., Mitchell M., Gray L. et al. Value of assessment of pretest probability of deep-vein thrombosis in clinical management. *Lancet* 1997; 350: 1795–8.
9. Ebell M.H. *Evidence-Based Diagnosis: A Handbook Of Clinical Prediction Rules.* New York: Springer, 2001.
10. *Essential Evidence Plus.* www.essentialevidenceplus.com (accessed March 8, 2010).

QUICK FLICK

5

6 Point-of-care testing comes of age in Australia

M. Shephard

Synopsis

A wide range of point-of-care tests is available and being used in both hospital and community settings for acute and chronic illnesses. There have been significant improvements in device technology as well as advances in training methods, procedures to monitor analytical quality, and electronic capture and management of test results from a central location. Various point-of-care tests have been found to be non-inferior to laboratory testing for managing chronic conditions in general practice and Aboriginal medical services. Maintaining the analytical quality of devices and ensuring that staff are properly trained are critical elements in sustaining a high quality point-of-care testing service.

◑ Introduction

Point-of-care testing can be defined as pathology testing performed onsite during the patient consultation. It allows a rapid test result to be generated and used to make an immediate, informed clinical decision.

There have been significant technological and analytical advances in point-of-care testing devices and reagent manufacture. An increasing range of tests can now be performed on very small sample volumes in less than 10 minutes. The analytical performance of many point-of-care testing devices is equivalent to that of a laboratory and meets profession-derived analytical goals.[1,2]

◑ Clinical applications in different disease states

Point-of-care tests (both singly and in profile) are now available for acute and chronic situations and can be used, for example, in managing diabetes, prescribing warfarin, assessing electrolyte and acid-base disturbances and risk stratifying patients with suspected acute coronary syndrome. Table 6.1 lists examples of the more common biochemistry and haematology tests. Some tests, such as haemoglobin and international normalised ratio (INR), have both chronic and acute applications.

Table 6.1 Point-of-care tests for chronic and acute care

Parameters	Test
Chronic care	
Carbohydrate metabolism	Glucose
	Glycated haemoglobin
Lipids	Total cholesterol
	Triglyceride
	High-density lipoprotein cholesterol
	Low-density lipoprotein cholesterol (calculated)
Renal function	Urea
	Creatinine (estimated glomerular filtration rate)
	Urine albumin
	Urine albumin:creatinine ratio
Haematological/ coagulation	Haemoglobin
	INR
Liver function	Total protein
	Albumin
	Alanine aminotransferase
	Aspartate aminotransferase
	Gamma-glutamyl transpeptidase
	Alkaline phosphatase
	Bilirubin
Acute care	
Electrolytes	Sodium
	Potassium
	Chloride
	Total CO_2
	Anion gap
Arterial blood gas	pH
	Partial pressure CO_2
	Partial pressure O_2
	Saturation O_2
	Base excess

continues

Table 6.1 Point-of-care tests for chronic and acute care *continued*

Parameters	Test
Cardiac function	Troponin I
	Troponin T
	Creatine kinase myocardial band
	Myoglobin
	N-terminal pro B-type natriuretic peptide
	Brain natriuretic peptide
Miscellaneous	
	C-reactive protein
	Ionised calcium

○ Glycaemic control

HbA1c remains the gold standard pathology test for long-term monitoring of glycaemic control in patients with diabetes. Devices measure HbA1c using either immunoassay or boronate affinity chromatography methods.

There are numerous strip-based testing devices for glucose monitoring. These generally measure whole blood glucose rather than plasma glucose, although newer devices can report a plasma-equivalent glucose concentration.

○ Blood lipids

Measuring blood lipids is useful for cardiovascular disease risk assessment and for managing patients on lipid lowering therapy. Testing devices measure a full lipid profile on capillary or venous blood. However, they calculate the low-density lipoprotein (LDL) cholesterol using the Friedewald formula and cannot, as yet, determine LDL cholesterol directly as laboratories can now do.

○ Assessing renal function

Quantitative measurement of urine albumin or the urine albumin:creatinine ratio is a key component in the review of patients with diabetes. Plasma creatinine measurement is currently the subject of international standardisation, in which both laboratory and point-of-care testing methods are being aligned to an isotope dilution mass spectrometry reference method.

○ Warfarin monitoring

Point-of-care INR testing is becoming increasingly popular in general practice for monitoring patients on warfarin.[3] Results can be linked with computer decision support software that automatically recommends the patient's next dose.

◗ Acute care

In an acute situation, electrolytes (including the anion gap), blood gases and cardiac markers, notably troponin I or T, can be assessed. Some devices can measure these cardiac troponins down to the nanogram per millilitre range. Newer markers including brain natriuretic peptide (BNP) and N-terminal pro B-type natriuretic peptide (NT-proBNP) remain expensive and their clinical utility continues to be debated.

◗ Clinical applications in different healthcare settings

In Australia, point-of-care testing is being used in the community as well as in hospitals, particularly in rural and remote areas where access to laboratory services may be poor.

◗ Hospital environments

Point-of-care testing has an important role in the hospital setting, both in critical care and emergency departments as well as in wards and clinics run by the hospital. Within this environment, it is important that the laboratory is closely linked with remote sites in the hospital where point-of-care testing devices are located.

Most modern emergency and high dependency units have immediate onsite access to point-of-care instrumentation including blood gas analysers (which are now also known as critical care analysers), cardiac readers and devices for measuring drugs of abuse.

Traditionally, blood gas analysers used electrodes for analyte sensing. While capable of analysing batches of patient samples (that is, they were multi-use), they were subject to drift and therefore required regular calibration, manual monitoring with liquid quality control samples and rigorous preventative maintenance schedules (including replacement of membranes). These procedures were generally carried out by a scientist or technician from the hospital's laboratory.

However, significant advances in technology have resulted in the development of disposable multi-use and single-use cartridges for such analysers that contain all the sensors, reagents and waste storage required for measuring not only standard blood gas parameters (listed in Table 6.1) but also a wide variety of other tests. The modern-day critical care analyser thus offers measurement of blood gases; electrolytes such as sodium, potassium, chloride and ionised calcium; metabolites such as urea, creatinine, glucose and lactate; and up to five haemoglobin derivatives plus bilirubin by CO-oximetry.[4]

Given the variety of critical care analysers on the market today, the choice of an analyser is dependent on factors such as the suite of tests required, ease of use, costs of the capital purchase and ongoing consumables, and analyser size. Most critical care analysers are large, expensive, bench-top, point-of-care testing devices. The high costs of these devices need to be assessed against the benefits of reduced staff costs for maintenance and the convenience of having the measurement available at the point of care.[4]

Other technologically advanced features of the modern critical care analysers include: dedicated software to allow laboratory support staff to monitor the analyser remotely and initiate troubleshooting procedures, calibrations and quality control testing from a central point, as well as to download results to the laboratory or hospital information system (so-called connectivity capability); the ability of analysers to automatically suppress unreliable results, including those following repeated calibration or quality failure; password protection to restrict patient testing to trained operators only; and even the ability to automatically detect and then clear a sample clot, which would otherwise have the potential to cause significant analytical problems.[4] Quality procedures for monitoring analytical quality can now be fully automated (so-called Auto QC); quality control samples can be pre-programmed to occur at specified times throughout the day or night. In addition most critical care analysers have an array of further 'in-built' or 'on-board' quality checks that monitor the integrity of the device and its measurement and signal generating systems.

Drugs of abuse can be measured qualitatively using point-of-care testing devices in the emergency department. Tests that can measured in this way include illicit drugs such as amphetamines, methamphetamines, cocaine, opiates and tetrahydrocannabinol and prescription drugs including barbiturates, benzodiazepines, methadone and tricyclic antidepressants.

Many hospitals conduct routine diabetes or coagulation clinics where point-of-care testing for HbA1c and INR are widely used, while ward-based glucose testing represents a significant investment in most hospitals.

◗ Community environments

While the hospital setting is the traditional environment of point-of-care testing, it is now widely acknowledged that point-of-care testing is being increasingly devolved to the community setting. There are now a number of working examples of innovative community-based, point-of-care testing models that have improved clinical outcomes in both chronic and acute situations and are analytically sound (see box).

Models of community-based point-of-care testing

The national Quality Assurance for Aboriginal and Torres Strait Islander Medical Services (QAAMS) Program (www.qaams.org.au) provides HbA1c and urine albumin:creatinine ratio testing for diabetes management in over 100 indigenous medical services across Australia.[25]

Queensland Health's statewide i-STAT network provides portable analysers throughout Queensland. These measure blood gases, electrolytes and coagulation, haematological and cardiac markers in critical care situations.[14]

The Integrated Cardiovascular Clinical Network SA (iCCnet SA) operates in rural South Australia (www.iccnetsa.org.au).

○ Managing point-of-care testing

A systematic approach is needed to organise and manage a sustainable and clinically effective point-of-care testing service both in community and hospital settings.[5]

Physical requirements

Only a small area of dedicated bench space is generally required to conduct most point-of-care testing. Most devices require an AC power source although an increasing number of newer devices can also work off battery power. Storage of reagents and consumables is generally at room temperature or 4°C, depending on the individual test.

Clinical governance

There should be a clearly defined organisational structure with lines of accountability for each and every facet of a point-of-care testing service. As a minimum requirement, there should be a point-of-care testing director (usually a senior clinician), a point-of-care testing coordinator (experienced in the practice of point-of-care), a multidisciplinary point-of-care management committee (comprising representatives from all stakeholder groups involved with the point-of-care testing service) and onsite point-of-care device operators (who routinely perform point-of-care testing on patients).

Staff training

Training programs for staff who perform the tests (such as doctors, nurses and Aboriginal health workers) are required. The type and duration of training needed depends on the complexity of the device and the range of tests available, as well as the number of people being trained. For example, a training session for a simple device such as a glucose meter for a small number of nurse trainees in a hospital ward may take less than half a day, while regional training workshops for the community-based QAAMS program, the largest national point-of-care testing program for diabetes management, take two full days for 20–30 trainees. Initial and ongoing training with competency assessment and updates are crucial for a sustainable high quality point-of-care testing service. Web-based training is now available for some Australian models.[2,6]

Analytical quality

A management system incorporating quality control and quality assurance processes is needed to continually ensure that the analytical quality of point-of-care testing results is appropriate for patient care, whether testing is conducted in the community or the hospital environment.

The frequency of these checks depends on a number of factors including device complexity, size of the point-of-care network and volume of patient testing at each site. For example, in the QAAMS program for diabetes management, quality control and quality assurance testing are performed monthly.[2] Should an abnormal result be obtained that does not fit the patient's clinical picture, the treating practitioner should repeat the point-of-care test and send the sample to the laboratory for confirmation of the result.

To sustain a point-of-care testing service, it is important to have ongoing technical support from the manufacturer of the device.

Test results

As mentioned previously, a further recent technological advance has been the capacity to send results electronically from multiple point-of-care testing devices to a central management point and from there to a clinical or hospital information system. This improved connectivity has enhanced the ability to develop large-scale point-of-care testing networks and streamline the delivery of testing services. Many Australian diagnostic companies provide connectivity software for their testing devices.

◯ Is point-of-care testing effective?

There is a growing evidence base for the clinical, operational and economic effectiveness of point-of-care testing in hospitals and in the community.

Chronic care

For chronic care, there are published examples of how point-of-care testing can be an effective tool for improving control of chronic conditions either by reductions in HbA1c (for diabetes management) or increased time in therapeutic or target ranges (coagulation studies)[6,7].

Acute care

The ability to perform tests such as potassium levels and blood gases by point-of-care testing in under five minutes on an acutely ill patient can inform initial management. For example, being able to measure potassium levels in a patient presenting with severe vomiting or diabetic ketoacidosis in a remote health centre is particularly useful. Similarly the ability to rapidly stratify risk in patients with suspected acute coronary syndrome using supportive cardiac marker point-of-care testing can have benefits. These relate to reduced length of stay in emergency departments or reduced mortality through more rapid and effective risk stratification and treatment.[8,9]

General practice

A large randomised controlled trial of point-of-care testing in Australian general practice was commissioned by the Department of Health and Ageing.[10] As part of the trial, the effectiveness of point-of-care testing versus laboratory testing was assessed for managing chronic conditions in general practice. Data from 53 practices located in urban, rural and remote locations in Australia were analysed. Based on the primary outcome of the percentage of patients with test results in the target range, point-of-care tests for HbA1c, urine albumin, albumin:creatinine ratio, total cholesterol and triglycerides were non-inferior to laboratory testing, but INR and HDL cholesterol testing was inferior.[11,12]

○ Limitations of point-of-care testing

While point-of-care testing may appear simple and easy to adopt, it is critical that health professionals seek the support of their local laboratory or specialist point-of-care testing service provider to support and maintain their service. These services may assist when selecting a device and with training and quality surveillance. The capacity to sustain a point-of-care testing service in a remote health service setting is often limited by high rates of staff (device operator) turnover.[13]

At present there is no Medicare rebate for point-of-care tests in general practice (other than a small group of mainly qualitative tests such as a pregnancy test). This limits the potential uptake of point-of-care technology and means a thorough cost–benefit analysis is needed before making the decision to implement it.

○ Summary

General practice and particularly rural and remote medical services are increasingly using point-of-care testing. Technological advances in device and reagent manufacture have now ensured that this type of pathology testing can be performed safely and effectively. It is convenient and accessible for the patient and allows immediate decision making for the doctor. Nonetheless, in implementing point-of-care testing, a significant commitment to operator training (particularly in the face of high staff turnover rates in remote areas) and surveillance of analytical quality are paramount.

References

1. Shephard M. Analytical goals for point-of-care testing used for diabetes management in Australian health care settings outside the laboratory. *Point of Care: The Journal of Near-Patient Testing and Technology* 2006; 5: 177–85.

2. Shephard M.D.S. and Gill J.P. The analytical quality of point-of-care testing in the 'QAAMS' model for diabetes management in Australian Aboriginal medical services. *Clin Biochem Rev* 2006; 27: 185–90.

3. Claes N., Buntinx F., Vijgen J,. Arnout J., Vermylen J., Fieuws S. et al. The Belgian Improvement Study on Oral Anticoagulation Therapy: a randomized clinical trial. *Eur Heart J* 2005; 26: 2159–65.

4. Pearson S., Bennitt W., Halloran S.P., Thomas A. and Vandyken S. *Report 05091. Survey of Fourteen Blood Gas Analysers.* London: NHS Purchasing and Supply Agency, 2006. www.pasa.nhs.uk/cep [cited 2010 April 12].

5. Australasian Association of Clinical Biochemists (AACB). *Point of Care Testing Implementation Guide.* Mt Lawley, WA: AACB, 2008. www.aacb.asn.au/admin/?getfile=1442 [cited 2009 Oct 8].

6. Shephard M.D.S. Cultural and clinical effectiveness of the 'QAAMS' point-of-care testing model for diabetes management in Australian Aboriginal medical services. *Clin Biochem Rev* 2006; 27: 161–70.

7. Shephard M.D.S, Mazzachi B.C., Shephard A.K., McLaughlin K.J., Denner B. and Barnes G. The impact of point of care testing on diabetes services along Victoria's Mallee Track. Results of a community-based diabetes risk assessment and management program. *Rural Remote Health* 2005; 5: 371. www.rrh.org.au/publishedarticles/article_ print_371.pdf [cited 2009 Oct 8].

8. Singer A.J., Ardise J., Gulla J. and Cangro J. Point-of-care testing reduces length of stay in emergency department chest pain patients. *Ann Emerg Med* 2005; 45: 587–91.

9. Zarich S., Bradley K., Seymour J., Ghali W., Traboulsi A., Mayall I.D. et al. Impact of troponin T determinations on hospital resource utilization and costs in the evaluation of patients with suspected myocardial ischemia. *Am J Cardiol* 2001; 88: 732–6.

10. Laurence C., Gialamas A., Yelland L., Bubner T., Ryan P. and Willson K; the PoCT Trial Management Committee. A pragmatic cluster randomised controlled trial to evaluate the safety, clinical effectiveness, cost effectiveness and satisfaction with point of care testing in a general practice setting—rationale, design and baseline characteristics. *Trials* 2008; 9: 50.

11. Bubner T.K., Laurence C.O., Gialamas A., Yelland L.N., Ryan P., Willson K.J. et al. Effectiveness of point-of-care testing for therapeutic control of chronic conditions: results from the PoCT in General Practice Trial. *MJA* 2009; 190: 624–6.

12. Gialamas A., Yelland LN., Ryan P., Willson K., Laurence C.O., Bubner T.K. et al. Does point-of-care testing lead to the same or better adherence to medication? A randomised controlled trial: the PoCT in General Practice Trial. *MJA* 2009; 191: 487–91.

13. Shephard M.D., Mazzachi B.C., Watkinson L., Shephard A.K., Laurence C., Gialamas A. et al. Evaluation of a training program for device operators in the Australian Government's Point of Care Testing in General Practice Trial: issues and implications for rural and remote practices. *Rural Remote Health* 2009; 9: 1189.

14. Pathology initiatives help patients. *Health Matters* 2008; 13: 15. www.health.qld.gov.au/news/health_matters/2008/hm_September_08. pdf [cited 2009 Oct 8].

Further reading

Price C.P. and St John A., eds. Point-of-care testing for managers and policymakers: from rapid testing to better outcomes. Washington, DC: AACC Press, 2006.

7 Urine testing

J.F. Mahony

Introduction

Urine is tested to determine the presence or absence of urinary tract disease. Macroscopic examination, a dipstick test, microscopy and culture of appropriately collected fresh urine are the usual methods. Repeated fixed abnormalities may lead to a specific diagnosis. Normal urine is rare in patients with progressive renal disease; the exceptions are renovascular disease and interstitial nephritis. Table 7.1 shows some properties of normal urine.

Technical aspects: a standard method of urine collection

The midstream urine is best collected in the following sequence:

1. Wash hands.
2. Expose and wash the external genitalia with dilute soap solution and rinse with sterile water using pads or cotton-wool balls. *Do not use antiseptics*.
3. Pass a small amount of urine.
4. Collect the next aliquot into a wide-mouthed sterile container.
5. Cap and label.

- All urine should be examined fresh, preferably using an early morning or concentrated specimen.
- Routine urine testing should be avoided during menstruation. If deemed necessary on clinical grounds (e.g. septicaemia), a suprapubic specimen should be obtained for urinalysis, microscopy and culture.
- Each specimen should be collected as a midstream specimen.
- Examination of a centrifuged deposit (5 min at 3000 rpm) improves the detection of casts and crystals.
- There is considerable inter-laboratory variation in the reception, handling and reporting of urine tests.
- Mechanical means of counting cells and casts in urine have recently proved useful and will play a greater role in future.

Table 7.1 Normal urine

Property	Amount	Comments
SG	1.000–1.030	Depends on hydration; fixed SG > 1.010 indicates renal disease
pH	5–8	Usually acid in morning
Protein	0–trace	Especially in concentrated urine and alkaline urine
Protein:creatinine	< 30 mg/mmol	
Albumin:creatinine	Male < 2.5 mg/mmol Female < 3.5 mg/mmol	
Blood	0	Avoid menstrual urinalysis; a very sensitive test
Glucose	0	Positive in diabetes mellitus/renal glycosuria
Microalbumin	0	First sign of diabetic nephropathy
WCC	< 2000/mL	Consider sterile pyuria if negative culture
RBC	< 1000/mL	Consider myoglobinuria after a positive dipstick
Bacteria	< 10⁴/mL	Any are abnormal in suprapubic collections
Hyaline casts	+	In concentrated urine

○ Is the result abnormal?

One or more of the following abnormalities may be found in asymptomatic patients. Often the presence of two such abnormalities allows a confident diagnosis.

Macroscopic examination

Red urine may be due to the presence of blood, the consumption of beetroot or of rifampicin. Dark-brown urine may be due to porphyrins, old blood and alkaptonuria. Rarely, melanoma can cause black urine. Cloudy urine is usually due to phosphates and frothy urine to proteinuria. A milky appearance and high fat content can be due to chyluria, usually seen in filariasis and, less often, lymphatic obstruction.

Urinalysis

Proteinuria

Commercially available test strips are specific for albumin and microalbumin. They do not detect protein in normal urine or Bence-Jones proteins. False positives may occur and 'trace' findings can often be disregarded, for example, in concentrated urine. Proteinuria should be quantitated and confirmed with other tests (e.g. sulfonylsalicylic acid, which detects all proteins and not only albumin). In young people, postural (orthostatic) proteinuria should be excluded. Persistent proteinuria requires investigation.

Microalbuminuria

Commercial test strips are now available to detect and measure small amounts of albumin, at 20, 50 and 100 mg/L. Detecting microalbumin in patients with diabetes mellitus is critical in identifying those at risk of progressive diabetic nephropathy.

Albumin:creatinine ratio (ACR)

Historically, 24 hour urine collections for daily protein excretion have been used, with an upper normal limit of 250 mg/day, and these are still useful in the investigation of nephrotic syndrome. However, it is difficult to obtain accurate 24-hour collections and there is interest in measuring smaller amounts of albumin to detect renal disease. It has been found that the albumin:creatinine ratio in spot urine collections, preferably early morning specimens, accurately reflects degrees of albuminuria. The normal ranges for ACR are up to 2.5 mg/mmol in males and 3.5 mg/mmol in females. A figure between the upper limit of the reference range and 30 mg/mmol is regarded as microalbuminuria, regularly sought as the earliest sign of renal involvement in diabetes mellitus and in those with a GFR less than 60 mL/min/1.73 m^2. An ACR of 30 mg/mmol suggests proteinuria of 500 mg/24 h or more.

Haematuria

Dipsticks are quite sensitive. Positives should be confirmed microscopically and red cell casts sought in a centrifuged deposit. Even if the patient is asymptomatic, full investigation of renal function and urinary tracts is mandatory—some 80% of older patients will have urological causes, including carcinoma, prostatic hypertrophy in men and urethrotrigonitis in women. Usually, good quality renal ultrasound and cystoscopy are both necessary to exclude malignancy. Even if normal, careful follow-up for at least 2 years is advised. Myoglobin can also react with Haemostix, so this should be considered (and can be confirmed by immunological testing) when red cells are not seen microscopically; elevated serum muscle enzyme levels also implicate myoglobin.

Glycosuria
A finding of glycosuria on dipstick warrants investigation for diabetes mellitus or renal glycosuria.

Urinary pH
Urinary pH control is useful in some forms of management such as the prevention or dissolution of uric acid stones with an alkali, allopurinol and a high fluid intake. Diagnostically, persistently alkaline urine may indicate stones, renal tubular acidosis or infection due to *Proteus* sp. Persistently acidic urine may indicate gout.

Specific gravity (SG)
SG must be interpreted in the context of the timing of urine collection, state of hydration, recent fluid intake, recent intravenous pyelogram and so on. If the SG is 1.010 under varying conditions, advanced renal failure is likely. The SG allows a better interpretation of proteinuria; for instance, trace proteinuria with SG 1.030 (concentrated urine) is unlikely to be of any significance.

Microscopic examination of urine
White cells
Normal urine contains less than 2 000 leucocytes per mL. Pyuria is most often due to urinary tract infection; sterile pyuria may be found in analgesic nephropathy, calculus disease, gonococcal urethritis, tuberculosis, partially treated infection or, most often, poor urine collection technique. The presence of numerous epithelial cells also indicates poor collection technique. Persistent sterile pyuria is an indication for intravenous pyelography and further early morning collections for detection and culture of acid-fast bacilli.

Red cells
Red cells are rare in normal urine; more than 1 000 per mL or more than two per high power field are abnormal and require investigation. Urine collected during menstruation will regularly contain red cells, a false positive. Finding significant proteinuria or red cell casts in the same urine indicates a primary glomerular or systemic vascular lesion. Microscopic haematuria in the presence of pyuria is likely to be due to trigonitis or other lower urinary tract infection. The percentage of dysmorphic red cells, if greater than 80%, may help differentiate glomerular causes from lower tract causes of bleeding.

Casts
Casts are likely to be formed when urinary protein excretion is increased and/or the flow rate is low.

Hyaline casts

Hyaline casts are found in normal concentrated urine and require no further investigation.

White cell casts

White cell casts indicate that infection is present and likely to be of renal origin; in a male, or in a female with recurrent infection, further investigation is always justified.

Red cell casts

Red cell casts are significant in that glomerular injury due to glomerulonephritis, severe hypertension or vasculitis is responsible; further investigations aimed at determining the presence of an antigen (e.g. antistreptolysin O titre, DNA antibody-binding activity, hepatitis B surface antigen, hepatitis C antibody and so on) or activation of immune complexes (such as cryoglobulins and immunoglobulins) should precede renal biopsy.

Granular casts

Granular casts and haem casts probably have the same origin and significance as red cell casts.

Broad casts

Broad casts indicate the tubular atrophy and interstitial fibrosis of chronic renal failure but are uncommon. Serum electrolytes, creatinine and urea nitrogen will reveal the degree and consequences of renal impairment.

Crystals

Crystals are commonly seen in the urinary sediment, best found in warm (37°C) specimens, but are not often useful in detecting renal disorders. In asymptomatic individuals calcium oxalate crystals are found more often than uric acid or other crystals. Both calcium oxalate and uric acid crystals may be found in 'normals' with acid urine and a diet high in oxalates and purines (respectively) when the urine is concentrated; however, both may also be found in stone formers, and uric acid in gout or treated lymphomas. Cystine crystals are rare, being found in cystinuria and other related aminoacidurias.

Bacteriuria and cultures

Bacteria

Bacteria are never seen in fresh and properly collected normal urine. Their presence in fresh urine indicates significant urinary tract infection. Normal midstream urine contains less than 1 000 organisms per mL after culture; more than 10^5 per mL of a single organism usually indicates bacterial infection; and any organisms are significant in a suprapubic specimen in a child. Between 10^4 and 10^5 organisms per mL is regarded as equivocal, requiring a repeat test, but, if found in a clinical setting such as in-dwelling catheter, renal calculus or diabetes mellitus, infection is likely. Mixed cultures of two organisms may also be found in the these settings but are more often due to contamination from using a poor collection technique. One should be suspicious of a report of bacteriuria when pus cells are absent from the urine; the usual causes are poor collection technique (indicated by the presence of many epithelial cells) or prolonged delay in examining the urine after its collection. The test should be repeated with careful attention to the collection technique (see earlier) before initiating antibacterial therapy in an asymptomatic patient. Repeated cultures of the same organism suggest renal rather than lower urinary tract infection.

The organism identified by culture must also be considered. The usual pathogens are *E. coli*, other coliforms, *Streptococcus faecalis* and *Klebsiella*; however, *Proteus* and *Pseudomonas* spp. are also found, especially in patients with calculi. *Staphylococcus epidermidis* and *Staphylococcus aureus* are occasionally pathogenic. Well recognised contaminants include skin organisms such as *Staphylococcus epidermidis* and normal vaginal flora such as diphtheroids; on rare occasions such bacteria and pyuria are found in properly collected urine samples on two occasions and require treatment.

Drug sensitivities

Antibacterial agents which are well concentrated in urine are most often used, and sensitivities to sulfonamides, trimethoprim, nitrofurantoin, ampicillin, tetracycline, cephalosporins, norfloxacin and aminoglycoside antibiotics are usually reported. Such a range is necessary to allow for variations in the sensitivities of organisms to the drugs, patient allergy, age, pregnancy and renal impairment. Occasionally further drug sensitivities are required, particularly when infection is chronic, for example when there is an in-dwelling catheter.

Antibacterial activity

The presence of antibacterial activity will explain sterile pyuria or failure to show a positive culture in suspicious clinical circumstances.

Combinations

Proteinuria and haematuria

Proteinuria and haematuria are hallmarks of glomerulonephritis, especially when proteinuria is severe. However, both may be found in 'normals' after jogging or heavy exercise as well as in urinary tract infection, neoplasm and hypertension. Finding red cell casts makes lower tract pathology unlikely and investigation is directed towards renal parenchymal disease. The urine should be retested at least 48 hours later in people who go jogging.

Haematuria and white cells

Haematuria and infection are most likely due to urethrotrigonitis in women and prostatitis in men.

Red cells, white cells, casts

Red cells, white cells and casts of both and eosinophils are seen in interstitial nephritis, most commonly due to drugs including but not limited to methicillin and other penicillins, sulphonamides and proton pump inhibitors.

A sediment of red cells, white cells, red cell or granular casts, broad casts and lipiduria

These indicate a severe glomerular lesion with a nephrotic element and are most often seen in collagen disorders such as systemic lupus erythematosus or advanced glomerulonephritis.

Further reading

Gyory A.Z. et al. Clinical value of urine microscopy by normal and automated methods. *Lab Hematology* 1998; 4: 211–6.

Schroder F.H. Microscopic haematuria requires investigation. *BMJ* 1994; 309: 70–2.

Yamagata K. et al. A long-term follow-up study of asymptomatic haematuria and/or proteinuria in adults. *Clin Neph* 1996; 45: 281–8.

Part 2

Biochemistry Tests

8 Plasma sodium

T.H. Mathew

Synopsis

Disorders of sodium metabolism are common in a hospital setting but are also seen in general practice. There is always an explanation to be found for important deviations of the plasma sodium concentration from normal. The plasma sodium concentration itself cannot be used in isolation from the clinical setting. Determinating the patient's fluid status is paramount in formulating a management plan. In all but the most severe disturbances of sodium metabolism, restoration of the plasma sodium concentration to the normal range should be accomplished slowly over a few days. Rapid correction, particularly of hyponatraemia, should be avoided as it may cause permanent cerebral damage.

○ Introduction

A plasma sodium concentration is one of the most frequently performed chemical tests. The measurement represents a ratio determined equally by the amount of available sodium and water. The single most important fact to appreciate in assessing a plasma sodium result is that it cannot be used in isolation as an indicator of total body sodium excess or deficiency. The four basic disorders of water and sodium metabolism are:

1. hyponatraemia—a relative excess of water in relation to sodium
2. hypernatraemia—a relative deficit of water in relation to sodium
3. hypovolaemia—a reduction of extracellular fluid where total body sodium (salt) may be normal or reduced
4. oedema—a reflection of sodium excess and hypervolaemia.

In a hospital setting hyponatraemia is the commonest of these disorders but in general practice oedema is prevalent. Appropriate management is based on a thorough understanding of the relationship of sodium to water and the variables controlling these factors. Sodium is mainly found in the extracellular compartments of the body where its concentration is easily and quickly altered by changes in extracellular fluid volume (ECFV). The normal range of plasma sodium is 135–145 mmol/L.

�‌ Technical aspects

Plasma sodium is measured in the water phase of the plasma but is expressed in mmol/L of the whole plasma. Pseudohyponatraemia is said to be present when the plasma sodium measurement is below normal but can be corrected in the laboratory to normal by removing excess protein or lipid from the plasma compartment of the sample. This condition is seen in paraproteinaemias or severe hyperlipidaemia where the plasma sodium concentration may be less than 120 mmol/L yet the true plasma water sodium concentration is 145 mmol/L. A plasma osmolality is a quick and easy way of checking for pseudohyponatraemia when it is suspected. The measurement of plasma osmolality is unaffected by protein and lipids that occupy space in the plasma sample. The sodium concentration may be reduced a small amount through this same mechanism by elevated levels of urea, mannitol or glucose and in these situations the osmolality of the plasma will be raised. The sodium electrode on blood gas machines measures the sodium concentration in the water of the plasma directly and there is no problem of pseudohyponatraemia with this method, which offers another way to check the true sodium level if osmometry is not readily available.

◌ Physiological and clinical aspects

Once an abnormal plasma sodium result is to hand, the first step in management is to assess the ECFV. This can be satisfactorily accomplished at the bedside. An expanded ECFV should be suspected when there is dependent oedema, raised jugular venous pressure, pulmonary congestion and/or a third heart sound. A contracted ECFV (volume depletion) should be suspected when there is reduced tissue turgor, low jugular venous pressure, postural hypotension, tachycardia and/or poor perfusion of peripheral tissues. Serial body weights are most helpful in confirming the clinical assessment of the state of volume load. Even with experience this assessment may be difficult, particularly in the elderly patient. It is common to observe up to 5% change in body weight from the baseline without any clinical evidence of fluid overload or depletion. The chest X-ray is a useful aid when the clinical signs leave uncertainty.

Hyponatraemia

Hyponatraemia is seldom of clinical significance when the plasma sodium is above 125 mmol/L, despite the lower level of normal being set at

135 mmol/L. It is usually unnecessary to take urgent action till the level is less than 120 mmol/L. When the plasma sodium is 120–135 mmol/L, appropriate modification to oral water and sodium intake will lead to a gradual increase in the plasma sodium concentration.

An age over 70 years and a rapid rate of change of the sodium concentration increase the likelihood of symptoms from hyponatraemia. In a young healthy patient a drop in plasma sodium to less than 125 mmol/L over a few hours may result in a depressed sensorium and the possibility of seizures whereas a plasma sodium of less than 110 mmol/L may be well tolerated, even in the elderly, when the decline occurs gradually over some weeks.

Symptoms attributable to hyponatraemia include lethargy, anorexia, cramps and confusion. Signs may include altered sensorium, depressed deep tendon reflexes, hypothermia and seizures.

Table 8.1 summarises the three main mechanisms, effect on ECFV and causes and treatment of hyponatraemia. A notable cause, particularly in the elderly, is the combined use of thiazides with triamterene or amiloride. Severe hyponatraemia (down to less than 100 mmol/L) may develop as a new event even after many months of apparent tolerance of this combination.

Table 8.1 Hyponatraemia

Mechanism	ECFV	Causes	Treatment
Water retention	Mild increase (no oedema)	Excess water intake (intravenous fluids or compulsive water drinking) Inappropriate ADH secretion (CNS disturbance, tumours, drugs)	Water restriction
Sodium and water deficiency with a larger deficit in sodium	Decreased	Urine loss (diuretics, Addison's disease, sodium losing nephropathy) GIT loss Skin loss (sweating, burns)	Isotonic saline
Combined sodium and water excess with greater increase of water	Increased	Circulating volume increased (cardiac failure, renal failure) Circulating volume decreased (nephrotic syndrome, cirrhosis)	Diuretic (albumin infusion in severe hypoalbuminaemia)

Water retention

When hyponatraemia exists with a normal or mildly increased ECFV the diagnostic possibilities include drugs that stimulate antidiuretic hormone (ADH) or simulate its action. Examples of these are nicotine, carbamazepine, non-steroidal anti-inflammatory drugs and COX 2 inhibitors.

In hospital inpatients, following stress, pain, trauma or surgical operations, there is an increased secretion of ADH for a few days (even longer in some older patients). This leads to water retention if too much water is administered either as intravenous fluid (4% glucose and N/5 saline; 5% glucose) or orally. Care must be taken in such patients and electrolyte monitoring is necessary until they are convalescent. Women in the reproductive age seem to be particularly sensitive to cerebral damage from acute hyponatraemia in these circumstances.

Inappropriate secretion of ADH occurs in a number of conditions including carcinomas of the lung and the pancreas, pulmonary conditions (pneumonia, tuberculosis) and central nervous system disorders including stroke and infection. In about a third of people with these conditions the osmostat seems to be reset and in this group (usually with a serum sodium of 125–135 mmol/L) the hyponatraemia is stable and no treatment is indicated.

Dehydration with sodium loss in excess of water

The combination of clinical dehydration and hyponatraemia is diagnostic of excessive loss of sodium from the gut, skin or urine. When the site of loss is not obvious, loss from the urinary tract (such as from undiagnosed polycystic disease or reflux nephropathy) should be the prime suspect. Adrenal insufficiency should be suspected if renal imaging is normal.

Fluid overload with water retention in excess of sodium

The hyponatremic patient with oedema must have cardiac or renal failure, cirrhosis or nephrotic syndrome. With these latter two conditions the urine sodium will be low in the absence of exposure of the patient to diuretic therapy.

Hypernatraemia

Hypernatraemia is usually defined as a plasma sodium greater than 150 mmol/L. It is a less common condition than hyponatraemia. Renal concentrating defects do not of themselves usually result in hypernatraemia. It is necessary to add to these conditions a disturbance in the thirst mechanism or limited access to oral fluids. Hypernatraemia tends to be seen only in the young, the elderly and the sick. The thirst mechanism is very effective in preventing hypernatraemia, with oral intake frequently rising to about 10 L per 24 hours in conditions such as diabetes insipidus.

Table 8.2 summarises the mechanisms, effect on ECFV and causes and treatment of hypernatraemia.

The clinical signs and symptoms of hypernatraemia are mainly neurological and are due to shrinkage of the brain cells. In severe cases structural damage (tearing of vessels, venous sinus thrombosis) has been reported. An acute rise in plasma sodium concentration is of more concern than a slow and steady rise, with a considerable mortality being experienced when the sodium exceeds 160 mmol/L.

The earliest symptoms of hypernatraemia are restlessness, irritability and lethargy and the signs are tremor, twitching and ataxia. The elderly and the very young are more susceptible to a given level of hypernatraemia and the clinical changes are more severe when the rise occurs over a few hours or days.

A reading of more than 160 mmol/L is a medical emergency when accompanied by only minor symptoms and signs because the situation can deteriorate rapidly with the onset of seizures leading to death. A plasma sodium concentration of less than 150 mmol/L is seldom of concern though an attempt should be made to diagnose the cause and to take corrective action.

Table 8.2 Hypernatraemia

Mechanism	ECFV	Causes	Treatment
Sodium and water loss with water loss predominant	Decreased	Renal loss (osmotic diuresis) Extrarenal loss (excessive sweating, diarrhoea)	Hypotonic saline
Pure water loss	Normal or minimal decrease	Renal loss (nephrogenic or central diabetes insipidus) Extrarenal loss (respiratory, skin)	Water replenishment
Sodium intake excessive	Increased	Hypertonic input (intravenous, dialysis, oral intake) Primary aldosteronism Cushing's syndrome	Diuretics and water replenishment

Combined loss of sodium and water with water loss predominant

Body fluid loss that is hypotonic (sweating, polyuria) is usually associated with an intact thirst mechanism and therefore the tendency to hypernatraemia will be corrected by extra water intake. It is only when there is restricted access to water (such as when a person is elderly and bedridden) or if the thirst mechanism is impaired that hypernatraemia will occur.

An osmotic diuresis as a cause of hypernatraemia may be driven by glucose (particularly in uncontrolled diabetes with a drowsy non-ketotic hyperosmolar patient), urea (in recovering acute renal failure) or mannitol (such as in a forced diuresis protocol). The tube-feeding syndrome has disappeared as a cause of hypernatraemia due to the recognition that adequate water is essential in any enteral high-protein feeding regimen.

Water loss with no sodium loss

This condition is seen only when renal concentrating defects that affect water reabsorption are present. The cause may be central diabetes insipidus (where the production of ADH from the posterior pituitary is deficient) or renal (nephrogenic) diabetes insipidus. In the latter condition the response of the renal tubule to normal amounts of ADH is impaired. The causes of nephrogenic diabetes insipidus are numerous and include chronic kidney disease (analgesic nephropathy, medullary cystic disease), drugs (lithium, amphotericin, colchicine), electrolyte abnormalities (hypokalaemia, hypercalcaemia) and other causes (myeloma, amyloidosis).

The clinical signs will be mainly of hypernatraemia rather than fluid loss, for two-thirds of the water loss is borne by the intracellular compartment because the membrane is freely permeable to water. Thus the ECFV shows only minor signs of dehydration.

Excessive sodium intake

This infrequent cause of hypernatraemia results from the excessive administration of sodium-containing fluids (by any route) and manifests clinically as both fluid overload and hypernatraemia. The administration of normal saline as the sole intravenous fluid can lead to hypernatraemia, especially in patients with increased lung or skin water loss, as the kidneys are unable to produce a sufficiently hypertonic fluid to excrete the residual salt, urea and so on in the available water. Primary aldosteronism and to a lesser extent Cushing's syndrome cause a similar situation but are characterised by an 'escape' mechanism leading to only minor degrees of fluid overload and mild hypernatraemia.

QUICK FLICK **8**

○ Is the result abnormal?

The normal limits of plasma sodium are clearly defined at 135–145 mmol/L. The difficulty, as discussed throughout this chapter, is to decide which values outside these limits are clinically meaningful. The important aspects in deciding the meaning of an individual result and in determining a course of action are the clinical state of the patient, the rate of change of the plasma sodium concentration and, finally, the absolute reading. There is no fixed clinical response to a reading of, say, 122 mmol/L. In one patient simple correction to water intake is appropriate and in another urgent intravenous saline and other initiatives are indicated.

◎ What action is needed if the result is abnormal?

Hyponatraemia
The first step is to assess the state of the ECFV by clinical means. Table 8.1 summarises the diagnostic possibilities. Treatment depends on the cause and the clinical situation:

- In states of water retention, restriction of oral water intake will suffice.
- In overload states, diuretics combined with water restriction will correct both the fluid overload and the hyponatraemia.
- In volume depletion, therapy will consist of replenishment with sodium and water. This may often be accomplished orally but when the loss is from the gastrointestinal route, intravenous therapy is usually required. Replenishment should be with isotonic saline that will allow gradual correction of the hyponatraemia.

Rapid correction of hyponatraemia should be avoided unless the clinical situation is compelling. There is very little place for hypertonic saline (e.g. 3% saline), which may lead not only to fluid overload but also to cerebral disturbance that may be permanent. An appropriate program is one that leads to correction of the plasma sodium concentration to the normal range within 2–3 days.

Hypernatraemia
Again the first step is to assess the state of the ECFV by the bedside and to consider the clinical possibilities. Simple observations such as daily urine volumes and a urinary sodium will clarify the diagnosis. Therapy depends on the cause of hypernatraemia. When the diagnosis is predominant water loss, removal of the offending drug, correction of the electrolyte abnormality and administration of ADH may be helpful. Water replenishment will also hasten the return of the plasma sodium concentration to less than 150 mmol/L. When sodium administration has been excessive, diuretics combined with liberal water administration will be helpful. When the cause has been water loss combined with sodium loss, hypotonic saline is indicated.

The plan should be to return the plasma sodium concentration to near the normal range within a few days. An acceptable rule of thumb is to achieve 50% of the necessary correction in 24 hours, with the remaining 50% being accomplished over the next two days.

Summary

The management of plasma sodium abnormalities is basically logical and straightforward and is based on an understanding of normal sodium handling. The clinical possibilities to explain the various combinations of fluid state and sodium status are not great in number. The overriding consideration in formulating an appropriate management plan is to aim at correcting the sodium and fluid status over some days rather than hours. The approach outlined above is applicable and will solve the vast majority of sodium abnormalities presenting to the practitioner in or out of hospital.

QUICK FLICK 8

9 Serum potassium

G.S. Stokes and E.P. MacCarthy

Introduction

Hypokalaemia and hyperkalaemia are potentially lethal disorders, often iatrogenic, which can be handled readily once the underlying mechanism is identified. A finding of a low serum potassium concentration (< 3.0 mmol/L) or high serum potassium concentration (> 6.0 mmol/L) is an indication for urgent notification of the responsible doctor.

Technical aspects

As red blood cells are rich in potassium, high levels can result from stasis or haemolysis in vitro, or from prolonged tourniquet application.

Is the result abnormal?

Before any definitive action is taken it should be confirmed that the result, particularly in the case of hyperkalaemia, genuinely reflects the prevailing plasma potassium levels. Three common causes of artefactually high potassium values are contamination with potassium EDTA used in haematology tests, leakage of potassium from red cells due to storage/ transport on ice or refrigeration, and too long a period between collection and analysis (more likely when remote areas are the source). If an abnormal value is obtained a repeat sample should be taken without a tourniquet and centrifuged promptly. In hospital settings access to a blood gas machine with a potassium electrode allows quick checks to be done. Immediate evidence of dangerously abnormal levels may be found in an electrocardiograph. Some causes of abnormal potassium levels are shown in Table 9.1.

Table 9.1 Some causes of abnormal potassium levels

Causes of hypokalaemia	Causes of hyperkalaemia
Gastrointestinal	**Metabolic and renal**
Vomiting, gastric suction	Acidosis
Diarrhoea, purgative abuse	Renal failure
	Hypoaldosteronism
Metabolic and renal	Addison's disease
Renal tubular acidosis	
Liddle's syndrome	**Tissue damage**
Primary aldosteronism (Conn's syndrome)	Burns, massive trauma
Secondary aldosteronism (oedematous	Haemolysis
states, Bartter's syndrome, Gitelman's	
syndrome, hypertension)	**Drugs**
Glucocorticoid excess (Cushing's disease,	Spironolactone
ectopic ACTH, exogenous steroids)	Amiloride
Alkalosis	Triamterene
Periodic muscular paralysis	Potassium supplements
	ACE inhibitors
Drugs	Angiotensin II receptor antagonists
Carbenoxolone, licorice	Digitalis (excess)
Some diuretics (see text)	Suxamethonium
Insulin (excess)	
Corticosteroids	**Artefact**
	Red cell damage
	Thrombocytosis
	Storage/transport too cold

○ Is the abnormality iatrogenic?

In explaining abnormal serum potassium levels, costly investigation can often be avoided by early recognition of the role of drugs. Thiazide diuretics probably constitute the most common cause of mild hypokalaemia although it should be emphasised that most patients receiving these agents in conventional dosage, with or without potassium supplements, never become hypokalaemic. Chlorthalidone in high doses is more likely than the thiazides to produce hypokalaemia, and indapamide rather less. When frusemide is used to treat the anxious obese (a dubious indication) or women with 'cyclic oedema' the dosage may be increased surreptitiously by the patient, inducing potassium depletion. Potassium depletion is more prevalent, too, in patients treated with diuretics for chronic oedematous states. Patients on such treatment require regular measurement of their serum potassium. A large intake of licorice can also lower serum potassium levels.[1]

QUICK FLICK 9

Laxative abuse is another common cause of unexpected hypokalaemia. Whereas patients with infective or inflammatory bowel disease severe enough to cause potassium depletion will be symptomatic, individuals with a bowel fixation may regard their explosive, liquid motions as appropriate.

Although its causes are fewer than those of hypokalaemia, hyperkalaemia is of more immediate danger to the patient, with a high risk of a dangerous and possibly fatal outcome.

Hyperkalaemia can be precipitated by the use of potassium-sparing diuretics, such as amiloride, triamterene or spironolactone, in patients with chronic renal failure or those taking concurrent potassium supplements. Hyperkalaemia can occur in patients taking drugs which inhibit the renin-angiotensin system such as angiotensin converting enzyme (ACE) inhibitors or angiotensin II receptor antagonists and may occur also in patients with renal disease given non-steroidal anti-inflammatory or beta-adrenergic blocking drugs.

Hyperkalaemia will be provoked more readily in elderly or diabetic patients with hyporeninaemic hypoaldosteronism or in those treated for heart failure or hypertension with a spironolactone/ACE inhibitor combination.

◑ What action should be taken if hyperkalaemia is found?

Whatever the history may reveal in the way of suspect drugs, hyperkalaemia should be regarded as possibly indicative of renal impairment and this should be sought carefully. In a state of stable renal impairment hyperkalaemia can usually be controlled by correction of acidosis (using oral sodium bicarbonate provided the patient is not oliguric or fluid overloaded) and reduction of foods rich in potassium, together with the elimination of any precipitating factors such as dehydration or renal tract obstruction or infection. The presence of acidosis indicates severe renal failure and a patient presenting in this state requires thorough investigation and aggressive treatment. If renal function is normal, investigations should be carried out to eliminate adrenal insufficiency as the cause of hyperkalaemia.

◑ In cases of hypokalaemia, how can the route of potassium loss be definitely established?

If the history and physical examination have failed to identify this clearly, it is simple to establish whether the route of potassium loss is gastrointestinal or renal. The key test is measurement of serum potassium concentration in relation to the concurrent 24-h urinary excretion of potassium.[2] If the patient has been taking diuretics or potassium supplements, these are suspended 5 days before the test. In patients with extrarenal potassium loss, urinary potassium excretion will be appropriately low in compensation (less than 30 mmol/24 h) while hypokalaemia from renal tubular disease or adrenocortical overactivity or surreptitious diuretic or licorice ingestion will be accompanied by a urinary potassium excretion inappropriately high for the low plasma level (over 30 mmol/24 h for a plasma potassium of 3.5 mmol/L or less).

A further simple test which can support a diagnosis of surreptitious laxative abuse is titration of the urine with alkali to a pH of 10: appearance of a pink colouration in the urine at a pH between 8 and 10 suggests the presence of phenolphthalein, a common constituent of laxative preparations. Inspection of the colonic mucosa by sigmoidoscopy may reveal melanosis coli, in which there is black pigmentation due to chronic laxative abuse.

While not posing such an urgent problem as hyperkalaemia, uncorrected hypokalaemia may lead to muscle weakness and, occasionally, cardiac or respiratory arrest. It should be particularly remembered that in cardiac failure diuretics may induce hypokalaemia which dangerously sensitises the heart to digitalis drugs.

○ Summary

The first thing to think of with abnormal serum potassium concentration is whether or not it is drug induced. Systemic causes to consider are tissue trauma, gastrointestinal losses, renal failure and adrenal insufficiency.

References

1. Conn J.W., Rovner D.R. and Cohen E.L. Liquorice-induced pseudoaldosteronism. Hypertension, hypokalemia, aldosteronopenia, and suppressed plasma renin activity. *JAMA* 1968; 205: 492–6.
2. Kaplan N.M. Hypokalaemia in the hypertensive patient, with observations on the incidence of primary aldosteronism. *Ann Intern Med* 1967; 66: 1079–90.

10 Serum urea

T.H. Mathew

Synopsis

Serum urea is an end product of protein catabolism and, because it is mainly excreted by the kidney and is easily measured, was in past years a popular way to measure kidney function. However, because the serum concentration of urea is subject to many extrarenal variables it has been replaced by serum creatinine (and the estimation of glomerular filtration rate [GFR] derived from it) as the mainstay of day-to-day assessment of kidney function. Serum urea remains a useful tool in clinical management when used with insight, for it provides information not only about kidney function but also about the state of hydration, protein catabolic rate and nutritional status.

○ Introduction

A generation ago serum urea (then called blood urea, as the estimation was performed on whole blood), which is quick and simple to measure by hand, was the standard measure used clinically to estimate kidney function on a day-by-day basis. The serum urea concentration, however, depends on urine flow and is affected by a highly variable production rate (see below), making it an unsatisfactory tool for reliable assessment of kidney function. Serum creatinine has replaced serum urea as the most useful means of assessing kidney function. Urea clearance for assessing kidney function is seldom performed currently, having been supplanted by creatinine-based formulas that estimate GFR.

○ Technical aspects

Confusion may arise when the serum urea is expressed as serum or blood urea nitrogen (BUN). This means of expressing the serum urea, although widespread in North America, is rarely used in Australia. There is no advantage in expressing serum urea as BUN. It is sufficient to be aware that each molecule of urea (the molar mass of urea is 60 g) contains two molecules of nitrogen (the molar mass of two molecules of nitrogen is 28 g). Accordingly, the factor for converting urea mass units to those of urea nitrogen is 0.47 and for converting urea nitrogen to urea mass units the conversion factor is 2.1.

Urea is readily diffusible through most of the body tissues including red blood cells. Consequently, the intracellular level is the same as that found in plasma and haemolysis of blood samples or delay in processing does not affect the measurement.

○ Physiological aspects

Urea is produced exclusively by hepatic enzymes of the urea cycle and is the major nitrogen-containing metabolic product of protein catabolism in humans. The kidney is responsible for excreting more than 90% of urea, with losses through the skin and gastrointestinal tract accounting for the remainder. On an average protein diet urinary excretion of urea is 35–45 g (580–750 mmol)/day.

There is no evidence for active transport of urea by the kidney. It is freely filtered by the glomerulus and passively transported out of the proximal renal tubule into the interstitium under the influence of a concentration gradient established by water reabsorption. The small molecular weight, its ability to diffuse freely and its presence in generous amounts make urea a major factor contributing to the osmolar gradients generated in the kidney through the countercurrent mechanism. Under conditions of diuresis only 40% of the urea load is reabsorbed whereas in antidiuresis the amount reabsorbed increases to about 70%.

Urea measurements are used to help assess the adequacy of dialysis. Because urea moves readily across the dialysis membrane, the plasma level changes substantially through the course of the dialysis. Measurement pre- and post-dialysis (expressed as a reduction ratio) has become one of the accepted markers of adequacy of dialysis.

○ Factors affecting the serum urea without altering renal function

Reduced urine flow
A mild reduction in renal plasma flow results in reduced urine output without affecting the GFR. This same reduction may, however, significantly increase the serum urea without changing the serum creatinine concentration. Factors causing a reduced renal plasma flow include:
- mild volume depletion. Fluid loss from any cause or excessive use of diuretics (particularly in the elderly, when the signs may be subtle) is

a common cause of mild dehydration. Serial body weights are a useful guide to changes in hydration. A high index of suspicion and a careful clinical history are necessary to come to a correct clinical assessment.

- cardiac failure. The reduction in cardiac output in congestive cardiac failure leads to a reduced renal plasma flow and urine flow rate. An improvement in cardiac function in this setting will be accompanied by a restoration of renal plasma flow and a return of the serum urea concentration to baseline.

Altered urea production

Urea production is readily varied by altering the amount of protein available for metabolism and by drugs that affect the metabolic process. Examples of this are:

- gastrointestinal bleeding. Upper gastrointestinal bleeding will provide a protein 'meal' that may be substantial in size. The rise in serum urea often precedes the passage of melaena stools.
- dietary protein intake. Daily protein intake in normal health may vary greatly on a day-to-day basis and is a major factor in fluctuations in the serum urea concentration. The serum urea concentration may double in response to a change from a low to a high protein intake and when renal function is abnormal this change may be three- or four-fold.
- metabolic state. Urea production is markedly increased in the presence of hypercatabolism such as is seen with infection, burns or trauma or postoperatively. An increased serum urea concentration may be an early sign of unsuspected sepsis.
- drugs. Corticosteroids and tetracyclines (except doxycycline and minocycline) significantly increase protein catabolism and result in an increase in serum urea concentration. These agents must be used with great caution in renal failure, where further elevation of an already raised serum urea concentration may lead to a vicious cycle of vomiting, dehydration and uraemia. Conversely, androgens diminish urea production by inducing an anabolic state. These agents were used in the predialysis era to assist in the treatment of acute renal failure.
- liver disease. Urea production depends on the function of hepatic enzymes. In severe liver disease urea production may be affected, resulting in abnormally low levels, but in practice this is seen only in the late stages of liver failure.

Obstruction

Partial obstruction of the urinary tract that results in a reduction of urine flow to less than 2 mL/min creates a situation similar to that seen with dehydration. Here the reduced urine flow rate allows more time for increased tubular reabsorption, leading to a reduced excretion of urea and a consequent rise in the serum urea concentration without any change in the serum creatinine concentration.

○ The ratio of serum urea:serum creatinine

The main advantage of serum urea determinations lies in their comparison with serum creatinine concentration. This is sometimes expressed as a serum urea:serum creatinine ratio. While this means of expressing the results draws attention to some of the factors listed above, the ratio itself may be misleading, particularly when renal function is unstable or multiple clinical factors are evident. As a consequence the ratio does not have an established place in the clinical practice of most physicians.

○ Is the result abnormal?

The reference range for serum urea in most laboratories is 2.5–6.4 mmol/L. The neonatal range is 0.5–1.0 mmol/L lower than in adults, and in adults over 60 years of age the range may be marginally higher than in younger adults. The concentration of serum urea is slightly higher in males than in females.

○ What action is needed if the result is abnormal?

An abnormal serum urea should always be pursued until an explanation for the abnormality is evident. The first step is to determine the renal function (by serum creatinine measurement) and to compare the degree of elevation of urea and creatinine. If the elevation is comparable then one need look no further for an explanation of the elevated urea and should follow the course outlined in Chapter 11).

If the serum urea is increased out of proportion to renal function, then the list of non-renal factors affecting the serum urea (above) should be checked. These include symptoms of obstruction (e.g. voiding difficulties), volume depletion (to be suspected if renal function is normal and the patient is on diuretics), cardiac failure, gastrointestinal bleeding and drugs. Dietary protein intake should be assessed and if found to exceed more than 2 g/kg/day should be suspected as the likely cause. If a likely cause is found, corrective action should be taken and the serum urea checked again a few days later.

If a cause of an increased serum urea (out of proportion to renal function) is not clinically evident, a 24-h urine volume should be obtained. If the measured volume is below 1.5 L/day the effect of increasing fluid input to achieve a urine flow of more than 2.5 L/day should be determined. Obstruction should be excluded by ordering urinary tract imaging (initially ultrasound). Faeces should be tested for blood. While a hypercatabolic state is usually obvious it may be present in the absence of fever, overt trauma or inflammation. Once the cause is suspected corrective action should be taken with reassessment at a later date.

If the serum urea is lower than normal, once again comparison with renal function should be made. A low protein intake is frequently seen in vegetarians and manifests as a serum urea concentration below the normal range. The most common cause of a reduced serum urea is a state of volume expansion such as occurs in pregnancy or in the presence of the syndrome of inappropriate secretion of antidiuretic hormone. Another common cause is a low protein intake, usually in the context of anorexia from any cause. This is a particularly common cause in hospital inpatients, who may have inadequate food intake for many days. Other possibilities to exclude are severe liver disease, polyuria (particularly that seen with compulsive water drinking) or an anabolic state associated with the use of androgenic steroids. These factors can usually be identified by the bedside.

◗ Summary

The determination of serum urea concentration will continue to be clinically important. If serum urea measurements are used with insight then they can contribute significantly to clinical management decisions. The serum urea concentration or the urea clearance used on its own has no place in determining kidney function. Used in conjunction with an assessment of renal function the serum urea reflects the state of hydration and protein catabolic status and is a guide to adequate protein nutrition.

11 Assessing renal function*

B.J. Nankivell

Synopsis

The indications for and selection of the most appropriate tests of renal function depend on the clinical question being asked, the accuracy needed and the cost and inconvenience to the patient. Serum creatinine and estimated glomerular filtration rate (eGFR) yield reasonable estimations of renal function with minimal cost. Urinary creatinine clearance is more accurate only if the urine collection is complete and is also cumbersome. Isotopic measurement of GFR is the gold standard and can be used when greater accuracy is required or with patients at the extremes of muscle mass or poor renal function. GFR is conventionally corrected for body surface area to adjust for differences in body size, to determine normality and to imply renal disease at low values. Results should be interpreted against physiological influences on renal function such as pregnancy, blood pressure levels and hydration status.

○ Introduction

Critical assessment of renal function is used to evaluate the presence of chronic kidney disease (CKD), assess the degree of damage and monitor disease progression, as well as to calculate drug doses when renal excretion forms the dominant pathway of clearance (Table 11.1). The GFR is accepted as the best overall index of the many complex functions of the kidney. This chapter evaluates various methods of renal functional assessment and their application in clinical practice.

---

* This chapter represents a consolidation of the content of Chapters 9 and 10 of the second edition, updated by Dr Nankivell. (Editor)

Table 11.1 Indications for renal function testing

Test	Setting	Clinical indication
Serum creatinine or eGFR	Screening for renal disease	Hypertension Urine abnormalities Potential renal diseases (e.g. diabetes) Non-specific symptoms (e.g. tiredness)
	Monitoring renal function	Chronic renal disease Transplantation Drug toxicity (e.g. aminoglycosides)
eGFR or creatinine clearance	Initial evaluation of renal disease	Glomerulonephritis Proteinuria Chronic renal failure Chemotherapy dosing
	Monitoring renal disease	Chronic renal failure Glomerulonephritis
Isotopic GFR	Accurate GFR	Glomerulonephritis therapy monitoring
	Low levels of GFR	Dialysis commencement Chronic renal failure
	Altered muscle mass	Body builder Chemotherapy dose in wasted patient

◯ Renal function and GFR

Each kidney contains one million nephrons—the functional units—each of which comprises a glomerulus attached to a renal tubule. The glomerulus is a high-pressure filtration system composed of a specialised capillary network, optimised to generate an ultrafiltrate free from blood and albumin. This is the first step in forming urine.

GFR is the rate (volume per unit time expressed as mL/min) of ultrafiltrate formed by the glomeruli and is a direct measure of glomerular function. Any nephron damage with alteration in glomerular function affects the kidney's ability to clear metabolic substances and toxins from the blood. GFR correlates with underlying structural injury and reflects the severity of chronic kidney disease, becoming reduced well before symptoms of renal failure develop. Unfortunately it is not an ideal index, being difficult to measure directly—hence a number of surrogate markers and derived methods for estimating renal function have been developd for clinical practice.

Although the glomeruli determine the rate of glomerular filtration, damage to the renal tubules also predicts progressive renal failure. Renal tubules make up 95% of the renal mass, perform most of the metabolic work and modify the ultrafiltrate, transforming it into urine. They also control acid-base balance, sodium excretion, urine concentration or dilution, water balance, potassium excretion and small molecule (e.g. insulin) metabolism. Measurement of tubular function is difficult and impractical for daily clinical use, hence GFR is used as the primary method to evaluate the health of the kidneys.

○ Normal range for GFR

The GFR in any individual varies according to the body mass which in turn corresponds to the renal mass. Larger individuals have bigger kidneys and a correspondingly higher GFR appropriate for their size, and vice versa. The raw GFR (in mL/min) is conventionally corrected for body surface area (BSA, which correlates closely with renal mass) producing a 'normalised' value expressed as mL/min/1.73 m^2. Body surface area is calculated from a nomogram based on height and weight, and 1.73 m^2 approximates the average BSA for normal young men and women. The corrected GFR is 8% lower in women. In addition various physiological factors influence GFR including pregnancy, protein loading, variations in renal blood flow, dehydration and certain medications, and these should be considered in the interpretation of an individual GFR result (Table 11.2).

Values outside the normal range of corrected GFR suggest the presence of renal disease; low values suggest renal impairment but there may be increased GFR (e.g. from early diabetic hyperfiltration). The normal

Table 11.2 Conditions that influence GFR

Increased GFR	Pregnancy
	Acute dietary protein loading
	Increased muscle mass (e.g. body builder)
	Hypertension
	Hyperglycaemia (diabetes)
	Calcium channel blocker therapy
Decreased GFR	Renal hypoperfusion (shock, hypotension, dehydration, cardiac failure)
	Intrinsic renal disease (e.g. glomerulonephritis)
	NSAID therapy
	Sepsis

corrected GFR is given as 90–130 mL/min/1.73 m². Impaired renal function is conventionally defined as 30–89 mL/min/1.73 m² and renal failure is below 30 mL/min/1.73 m².

▷ Measurement of GFR by renal clearance

GFR cannot be directly measured in humans but can be estimated from urinary clearance of an 'ideal filtration marker', a substance (x) that is freely filtered by the glomerulus without either significant tubular reabsorption or secretion. The urinary clearance of x can be demonstrated mathematically to quantify GFR accurately and is given by the equation:

$$\text{Urinary clearance}(x) = U_x V / P_x$$

where U_x is the urinary concentration of an ideal filtration marker (x), V is the urine flow rate and P_x is the average plasma concentration of x.

▷ Methods to estimate GFR

GFR can be estimated from the serum level of a filtration marker (such as endogenously generated creatinine, urea or cystatin C molecules), the urinary clearance of these markers (e.g. creatinine clearance) or the plasma or urinary clearance of an exogenously administered agent (such as Tc^{99m} DTPA or the fructose polysaccharide inulin). Each method of GFR estimation has advantages and disadvantages in terms of accuracy, cost and inconvenience. Selection of the most appropriate test depends on the clinical question asked, the accuracy required and social and resource issues (Table 11.3).

Table 11.3 Assessment of renal function

Method	Accuracy	Cost	Convenience
Serum creatinine	**	$	***
Serum urea	*	$	***
Serum Cystatin C	***	$$	***
eGFR	***	$	***
Urinary creatinine clearance	** to ***	$$	*
Isotopic GFR	****	$$$$	*

▷ Serum creatinine

The serum creatinine concentration is the single most useful clinical measure of kidney function. It is commonly used to screen for renal disease or to investigate urinary sediment abnormalities, hypertension or even non-specific symptoms such as tiredness. Serum creatinine levels are also used to monitor progression of CKD and response to therapy, or to detect nephrotoxicity (from gentamicin or anti-cancer therapies) or rejection (in kidney transplantation). Serum urea can also estimate renal function but is less accurate because it varies markedly with dietary protein intake, catabolism or malnutrition, and also with the state of hydration.

○ **The balance concept**

The plasma concentration of a substance in a steady state depends on the balance of its input (either from endogenous production or exogenous intake) versus its rate of disappearance from the blood (by excretion or metabolism). When an ideal filtration marker is used (without hepatic metabolism or non-renal clearance) and when the input remains constant (e.g. by endogenous creatinine generation), the steady state plasma concentration is inversely proportional to GFR. Several days are usually required to achieve stable serum creatinine levels following acute changes in renal function, making all creatinine-based GFR estimates inaccurate while in flux.

The creatinine in blood is predominantly derived from conversion of creatine to creatinine in muscles. The individual daily generation rate is remarkably constant, varying by about 5%. Almost all the creatinine in blood is filtered by the glomerulus (small amounts are cleared by the bowel and tubular secretion), making it a clinically useful marker of GFR.

As nephrons are lost with progressive kidney disease, the glomerular filtering surface area and the GFR become reduced. The serum creatinine concentration increases in a non-linear inverse relationship with GFR, approximating a mathematical hyperbola (Fig. 11.1) If nephron numbers are halved, the serum creatinine doubles, although the absolute change depends on the starting level. For example, a rise in serum creatinine from 70 to 140 micromol/L represents the same 50% fractional loss of nephrons as an increase from 500 to 1 000 micromol/L. However, in absolute terms, the number of nephrons lost from an initially normal kidney with the smaller rise in serum creatinine is much greater.

Creatinine generation is proportional to an individual's total muscle mass. In those with smaller muscle mass, such as children, women, the elderly and patients with malnutrition or cancer, the serum creatinine levels are lower than expected (ranging from 35 to 50 micromol/L) for a given GFR, and there is a danger of overestimating true GFR. For example, a small elderly woman with a GFR as low as 20–30 mL/min may have a serum creatinine at the upper normal range. Low creatinine values also occur in early normal pregnancy, where true GFR increases by 35–50%. Conversely a muscular body builder or athlete may have a higher serum creatinine for a given GFR

Figure 11.1 Serum creatinine and GFR

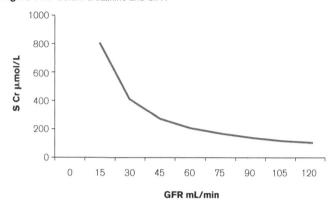

(which is usually normal or even increased) which leads to an underestimate of true GFR. These errors resulting from variations in body muscle mass can be overcome by an accurately measured creatinine clearance or by isotopic GFR (see below).

A small amount of creatinine also originates from dietary sources, where cooking converts a variable fraction of creatine from ingested meat to creatinine, which is absorbed in the gut and enters the blood. This ingested creatinine is usually clinically irrelevant except with unusually large meat intakes.

◯ Laboratory measurement

Measurement of serum creatinine varies substantially according to the method used, laboratory calibration and random variation. A modified kinetic Jaffe method using a colourimetric alkaline picrate assay is performed in most autoanalysers. The assay is precise and reproducible (the intra-laboratory variation is 3–5%) and generally accurate to within 10–20 micromol/L in the normal range, but less accurate at very high or low levels. The original Jaffe method, developed over a century ago, is subject to interference from non-creatinine chromogens such as bilirubin, acetoacetate or pharmaceuticals including cephalosporins (Table 11.4). Many different modifications have been developed to limit the errors that contribute to inter-laboratory variation and compromise the accuracy of the results obtained. Calibration using isotope dilution mass spectrometry (IDMS) as a traceable gold standard has been developed to limit these measurement errors and equipment manufacturers have gradually improved their reagents and technology.[1] Use of IDMS-validated methodology has resulted in a systematic shift to values on average about 6% lower than those from the older creatinine methods, necessitating a corresponding adjustment to the MDRD formula for eGFR calculation; all Australian laboratories now use these newer methods.

Alternatively, enzymatic creatinine measurement can avoid assay interference in particular situations (e.g. bilirubin in jaundice or acetoacetate in severe childhood dehydration or diabetic ketoacidosis). While it is more accurate and preferred in these patients, it is marginally less precise and reproducible on repeated measurement.

Endogenously produced creatinine is an imperfect filtration marker, with about 15–20% being secreted by the tubular cells and added to the creatinine filtered by the glomeruli. Tubular secretion thus causes an overestimation error in GFR, increasing with renal impairment. Some medications, such as trimethoprim and cimetidine, competitively inhibit the organic cation secretion pathways and reduce tubular creatinine secretion, decreasing urinary creatinine clearance and increasing serum creatinine levels. Their use can result in transient and reversible elevation of serum creatinine by 30–40 micromol/L, where GFR remains unaltered. These agents can be deliberately used to control the error from tubular secretion during a 24-h urinary collection, improving the accuracy of the GFR result. Although serum creatinine has wide confidence intervals for estimating absolute GFR, its simplicity, convenience, low cost, excellent laboratory measurement precision and modest normal biological variation make it particularly useful for monitoring variation in kidney function in individuals. A change of 30 micromol/L may be clinically significant. The broad normal reference range for serum creatinine is 50–120 micromol/L, varying somewhat by laboratory. Some have a lower reference range for females (40–90 micromol/L compared to 60–110 micromol/L for men). Laboratories are advised to report results in micromol/L.

○ Estimated GFR (eGFR)

Serum creatinine is highly dependent on a patient's age, sex and body size, and a number of corrections and formulae have been developed to correct for errors resulting from differences in muscle mass and creatinine generation. These calculations provide an estimated GFR (eGFR).[2] Some formulae yield an uncorrected GFR value (expressed as mL/min), whereas others provide a corrected GFR (as mL/min/1.73m²) which is useful for determining normality.

The most famous early formula is the Cockcroft-Gault formula which is simple to use and reasonably accurate (except in the elderly where it underestimates GFR). It is given as:

$$\text{Creatinine clearance (mL/min)} = (140 - \text{age [yrs]}) \times \text{weight [kg]} / \text{serum creatinine (micromol/L)}.$$

The default result is for females; multiply the result by 1.22 for males.

More recent additions are the MDRD formulae (there are several variations) which do not use a body mass estimate and present results normalised for BSA. Its disadvantages include its exponential factorial design (that requires a scientific calculator or a specific computer program). Earlier versions required a serum albumin, eliminated in later formulae with fewer variables. The simplest of the current series of MDRD formulae is an 'abbreviated' form needing only basic demographic information which can be used for automated eGFR reporting; for the current IDMS traceable creatinine assays the formula is:

$$\text{GFR (mL/min/1.73 m}^2) = 175 \times (\text{serum creatinine [micromol/L]} \div 88.4)^{-1.154} \times \text{age}^{-0.203}.$$

Multiply by 0.742 for a female and by 1.120 for African race (omitted in Australia).

Serum creatinine results were originally calculated as mg/dL, which is converted to micromol/L by division by 88.4. For the older non-IDMS-aligned creatinine assays the coefficient in this equation is 186. Current Australian and international guidelines recommend automatic reporting of the eGFR using the revised MDRD formula when serum creatinine is requested.[3] It is important to remember that these calculations are valid only when the creatinine level is stable.

Because the MDRD formula was derived from renal failure patients enrolled in a study of low protein diet and hypertension control, it is most accurate at lower GFR levels (better than the Cockcroft-Gault) and performs indifferently at higher GFR levels.[4] This is reflected in the original recommendation that higher eGFR results should be reported as > 60 mL/min/1.73m^2, which has subsequently increased to > 90 mL/min/1.73m^2 in some documents. MDRD underestimates GFR in many normal individuals, falsely classifying chronic kidney disease (CKD) and generating additional investigations.[5] In order to calculate drug excretion rates for in-hospital drug dosage for dose critical medications the Cockcroft-Gault formula can be used as an absolute GFR estimate (rather than the normalised value). In general practice the MDRD eGFR is also acceptable and demonstrates a comparable concordance.

Other newer GFR formulae provide better GFR estimates at normal serum creatinine ranges and include the CKD-EPI formula (more accurate than MDRD and designed for IDMS creatinines[6]) and the Mayo quadratic equation. Specific ethnic groups may also warrant their own formulae (employing an abbreviated 4-variable MDRD equation with a correction factor) as the original formulae were derived predominantly from mixed Caucasian and African American patients. Dedicated MDRD formulae for Chinese and Japanese patients are more accurate in these populations.

Children have the Schwartz formula, which uses height or length and is adjusted by a correction factor determined by categories such as age (pre-term, full term or child to 12 years of age), and the Counahan-Barratt formula.[7]

Overall, these methods are fair estimates of GFR but become inaccurate when body mass is significantly outside the normal range (e.g. with morbid obesity or severe malnutrition and disease). For the Cockcroft-Gault equation, a partial correction using the 'ideal' or lean body weight (instead of the measured weight) can improve this result, although an isotopic GFR or a 24-h urinary creatinine clearance provides a more accurate result.

○ Urinary creatinine clearance

Creatinine clearance involves a 24-h urine collection to measure creatinine excretion, which is divided by serum creatinine concentration. The same urine collection can be used to measure protein excretion as part of the initial evaluation of glomerulonephritis or chronic renal failure, to monitor disease progression or response to therapy, or to aid the timing of dialysis commencement.

Its major weakness is incomplete collection, when some urine is discarded into the toilet, which would underestimate true GFR. This is suspected by low urinary creatinine excretion (mmol/day) values or low urinary volumes. Some authorities have recommended alternative measures such as an eGFR (the MDRD formula is often a better measure in renal failure[5]) or an isotopic GFR. However, in a catheterised patient or in a hospital with careful collection, it can provide an accurate estimate of GFR. GFR can be overestimated in renal impairment because of tubular secretion of creatinine, potentially correctable by cimetidine therapy or by averaging urea and creatinine clearances (Table 11.4).

Table 11.4 Errors in measurement of creatinine

Condition	Creatinine clearance	Serum creatinine*
Assay inference		
Ketosis	Nil	↑
Hyperbilirubinaemia	Nil	↓
Cephalosporin	Nil	↑

continues

Table 11.4 Errors in measurement of creatinine *continued*

Condition	Creatinine clearance	Serum creatinine[#]
Inhibition of tubular secretion of creatinine		
Cimetidine/trimethoprim	*↓	↑
Alteration of creatine/creatinine load		
Eating cooked meat	↑	↑
Low protein diet	↓	↓
Body building	Nil	↑
Muscle wasting	Nil	↓
Renal disease	↓	↑

*Becomes more accurate at low levels of GFR when increased tubular secretion of creatinine is blocked
#Estimated by the Jaffe method

○ Serum cystatin C

Serum cystatin C is a low molecular protein produced by all nucleated cells and is eliminated primarily by renal excretion (85% by glomerular filtration). It is freely filtered at the glomerulus and not reabsorbed but completely catabolised by the tubular cells. Advantages include independence from muscle mass, and its enthusiasts claim superior sensitivity and accuracy compared with simple serum creatinine (it is broadly comparable to eGFR calculated from serum creatinine) but the assay is more expensive and difficult to perform.[8] Serum cystatin C results can be transformed into eGFR using several formulae, although none is currently recommended for clinical practice.

○ Isotopic GFR

Clearance of a radioactively labelled ideal filtration marker is the most accurate measurement of GFR, especially in patients with renal failure or abnormal muscle mass. The technique uses an ideal filtration marker chemically attached to an isotopic tracer that emits a minute but measurable radiation. Common markers used include Tc[99m] DTPA, Cr[51]EDTA and I[125] iothalamate ('cold' iothalamate measured biochemically can also be used). The tracer is given as a single intravenous injection followed by two plasma samples taken at 1 and 3 hours later. The plasma clearance of isotope is derived and GFR calculated. Isotopic GFR can be used for accurate interval monitoring of renal function over time, for donor kidney transplant assessment or in end-stage renal failure patients approaching dialysis. Due to its cost and inconvenience it is used sparingly.

○ Interpretation of results

GFR is the best overall measure of kidney function and correlates with outcome. GFR is used for the screening and definition of CKD, classification of severity by level and serial monitoring. CKD is conventionally defined as any kidney damage, regardless of cause, and/or a GFR level below 90 mL/min/1.73m². The lower limit of normal has previously been defined as 80 mL/min/1.73m², which is actually a more accurate threshold that has been derived from population studies of normal subjects. CKD is subcategorised into five stages by degree of loss of GFR (Table 11.5). Uraemic symptoms of lethargy, anorexia and itching often begin at CKD stage 4 (GFR of 15–29 mL/min/1.73 m²) and dialysis is considered at stage 5 (GFR < 15 mL/min/1.73 m²).

Table 11.5 Classification of chronic renal failure by severity

Stage	GFR range	Associations
CKD 1	Above 90 mL/min/1.73 m²	Evidence of kidney damage
CKD 2	60 to 89 mL/min/1.73 m²	Mild CKD
CKD 3	30 to 59 mL/min/1.73 m²	Moderate CKD
CKD 4	15 to 29 mL/min/1.73 m²	Severe CKD
CKD 5	Below 15 mL/min/1.73 m²	Kidney failure

Commencement of dialysis considered for GFR between 5 and 10 mL/min/1.73 m²

In clinical practice, a mildly elevated serum creatinine should prompt repeat testing (with eGFR) with good hydration. Reversible causes of renal dysfunction such as dehydration or use of diuretics, ACE inhibitors, non-steroidal anti-inflammatory drugs (NSAIDs, including COX-II selective inhibitors) and other nephrotoxins should be excluded, along with avoidance of meat and exogenous creatine. Further investigations could include renal imaging (for urinary obstruction), urine microscopy for casts, spot urine analysis for blood, protein or albumin (indicative of glomerulonephritis), a 24-h urinary protein excretion and creatinine clearance and finally a renal biopsy in certain circumstances.[9]

With healthy ageing, GFR is gradually lost at a rate of 0.3–0.75 mL/min/year beyond 40 years of age when assessed by creatinine clearance in ageing populations.[10] The serum creatinine often remains largely normal or is minimally elevated with ageing, despite true renal functional loss, because of muscle attrition. The Cockcroft-Gault formula also underestimates an elderly patient's GFR. The majority of healthy elderly subjects have a stable GFR above 100 mL/min if accurate inulin clearances are used as the gold standard. However, in grouped population studies of elderly individuals with associated comorbidity (including hypertension, vascular disease or heart failure), increased age correlated with lower GFR, reflecting a greater proportion with kidney disease. Hence, age-adjusted reference intervals for GFR are controversial. In practice the functional impairment commonly seen in elderly patients is often modest and generally of minor clinical concern, assuming there is no haematuria, proteinuria or other sign of renal injury.[11]

◗ Summary

GFR measurement is the major clinical tool available for day-to-day estimation of the excretory function of kidneys, which has functional and prognostic implications. GFR varies because of physiological factors such as pregnancy, hydration, medications and blood pressure level. Serum creatinine measurement (or an eGFR) is the cheapest and most convenient estimate of GFR, being derived from a single blood sample. Automatic reporting of eGFR provides a more accurate absolute measurement of renal function, aiding the diagnosis and categorisation of CKD. Interpretation of serum creatinine and eGFR values requires understanding the underlying physiology and potential errors from variations in muscle mass. Urinary creatinine clearance is more accurate only if complete, but is cumbersome. Isotopic GFR using intravenous nuclear tracers attached to an ideal filtration substance and two subsequent blood samples to derive plasma clearance is the most accurate overall test. It is useful when accuracy is needed, with poor renal function, at extremes of body mass and with catabolic states, but it is expensive and time consuming. GFR is corrected for body surface area to define normality, and abnormal values imply renal disease. The most appropriate test of renal function should be selected according to the indication, the required accuracy and the clinical situation.

References

1. Stevens L.A., Manzi J., Levey A.S., Chen J., Deysher A.E., Greene T. et al. Impact of creatinine calibration on performance of GFR estimating equations in a pooled individual data base. *Am J Kidney Dis* 2007; 50: 21–35.
2. Stevens L.A., Coresh J., Greene T. and Levey A.S. Assessing kidney function—measured and estimated glomerular filtration rate. *NEJM* 2006; 354: 2473–83.

3. Matthew T.H., Johnson D.W. and Jones G.R. Chronic kidney disease and automatic reporting of estimated glomerular filtration rate: revised recommendations. *MJA* 2007; 187: 459–63.

4. Levey A.S., Coresh J., Greene T., Stevens L.A., Zhang Y.L., Hendriksen S. et al. Using standardised serum creatinine values in the modification of diet in renal disease study equation for estimating glomerular filtration rate. *Ann Intern Med* 2006; 145: 247–54.

5. Poggio E.D., Wang X., Greene T., Van Lente F. and Hall P.M. Performance of the modification of diet in renal disease and Cockcroft-Gault equations in the estimation of GFR in health and in chronic kidney disease. *J Am Soc Nephrol* 2005; 16: 459–66.

6. Levey A.S., Stevens L.A., Schmid C.H., Zhang Y.L., Castro A.F. 3rd, Feldman H.I. et al. A new equation to estimate glomerular filtration rate. *Ann Intern Med* 2009; 150: 604–12.

7. Schwartz G.J. and Work D.F. Measurement and estimation of GFR in children and adolescents. *Clin J Am Soc Nephrol* 209; 4: 1832–43.

8. Tidman M., Sjostrom P. and Jones I. A comparison of GFR estimating formulae based on s-cystatin C and s-creatinine and a combination of the two. *Nephrol Dial Transplant* 2008; 23: 154–60.

9. Connnolly J.O. and Woolfson R.G. A critique of clinical guidelines for detection of individuals with chronic kidney disease. *Nephron Clin Pract* 2009; 111: c69–73.

10. Glassrock R.J. and Winearls C. Ageing and the glomerular filtration rate: truths and consequences. *Trans Am Clin Climatol Assoc* 2009; 120: 419–28.

11. Nguyen M.T., Maynard S.E. and Kimmel P.L. Misapplications of commonly used kidney equations: renal physiology in practice. *Clin J Am Soc Nephrol* 2009; 4: 528–34.

12 Interpreting arterial blood gases*

A.K. Verma and P. Roach

Synopsis

Arterial blood gas analysis is used to measure the pH and the partial pressures of oxygen and carbon dioxide in arterial blood. The investigation is relatively easy to perform and yields information that can guide the management of acute and chronic illnesses. This information indicates a patient's acid-base balance, the effectiveness of gas exchange and the state of ventilatory control. Interpretation of an arterial blood gas result should not be done without considering the clinical findings, because the results change as the body compensates for the underlying problem. Factors relating to sampling technique, specimen processing and environment may also influence the results.

○ Introduction

Arterial blood gas analysis is a common investigation in emergency departments and intensive care units for monitoring patients with acute respiratory failure. It also has some application in general practice, such as assessing the need for domiciliary oxygen therapy in patients with chronic obstructive pulmonary disease. An arterial blood gas result can help in the assessment of a patient's gas exchange, ventilatory control and acid-base balance. However, the investigation does not give a diagnosis and should not be used as a screening test. It is imperative that the results are considered in the context of the patient's symptoms.

While non-invasive monitoring of pulmonary function, such as pulse oximetry, is simple, effective and increasingly widely used, pulse oximetry is no substitute for arterial blood gas analysis. Pulse oximetry is solely a measure of oxygen saturation and gives no indication about blood pH, carbon dioxide or bicarbonate concentrations.

---

*   This chapter replaces Chapter 11 of the second edition. (Editor)

◑ **Arterial puncture**

Blood is usually withdrawn from the radial artery as it is easy to palpate and has a good collateral supply. The patient's arm is placed palm up on a flat surface, with the wrist dorsiflexed at 45°. A towel may be placed under the wrist for support. The puncture site should be cleaned with alcohol or iodine, and a local anaesthetic (such as 2% lignocaine) should be infiltrated. Local anaesthetic makes arterial puncture less painful for the patient and does not increase the difficulty of the procedure.[1] The radial artery should be palpated for a pulse, and a pre-heparinised syringe with a 23 or 25 gauge needle should be inserted at an angle just distal to the palpated pulse (Fig. 12.1). A small quantity of blood is sufficient. After the puncture, sterile gauze should be placed firmly over the site and direct pressure applied for several minutes to obtain haemostasis. If repeated arterial blood gas analysis is required, it is advisable to use a different site (such as the other radial artery) or insert an arterial line.

   To ensure accuracy, it is important to deliver the sample for analysis promptly. If there is any delay in processing the sample, the blood can be stored in an ice/water mixture for approximately 30 minutes with little effect on the accuracy of the results.

Figure 12.1 Performing an arterial puncture

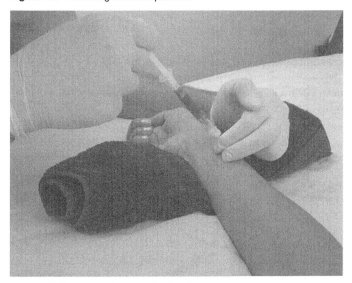

Reproduced with permission from Australian Prescriber

Complications of arterial puncture are infrequent. They include prolonged bleeding, infection, thrombosis and arteriospasm.

○ Interpreting a blood gas result

The automated analysers measure the pH and the partial pressures of oxygen (PaO_2) and carbon dioxide ($PaCO_2$) in arterial blood. Bicarbonate (HCO_3^-) is also calculated (Table 12.1).

Table 12.1 Interpreting a blood gas result

Reference ranges for arterial blood gases		
pH	7.35–7.45	
PaO_2	80–100* mmHg	10.6–13.3 kPa
$PaCO_2$	35–45 mmHg	4.7–6.0 kPa
HCO_3^-	22–26 mmol/L	
Base excess	−2 to +2 mmol/L	
Reference ranges for venous blood gases		
pH	7.32–7.43	
PvO_2	25–40 mmHg	
$PvCO_2$	41–50 mmHg	
HCO_3^-	23–27 mmol/L	

*Age and altitude dependent (see text)
Kilopascals: to convert pressures to kPa, divide mmHg by 7.5

These measurements should be considered with the patient's clinical features (Table 12.2).

Table 12.2 Correlating arterial blood gas results with clinical features

	Metabolic imbalances		Respiratory imbalances	
	Metabolic acidosis	Metabolic alkalosis	Respiratory acidosis	Respiratory alkalosis
pH	↓	↑	↓	↑
$PaCO_2$	N (uncompensated) ↓ (compensated)	N (uncompensated) ↑ (compensated)	↑	↓

	Metabolic imbalances		Respiratory imbalances	
	Metabolic acidosis	Metabolic alkalosis	Respiratory acidosis	Respiratory alkalosis
HCO_3^-	↓	↑	N (uncompensated) ↑ (compensated)	N (uncompensated) ↓ (compensated)
Base excess	↓	↑	N/↑	N/↓
Clinical features	Kussmaul-type breathing (deeper, faster respiration), shock, coma	Paraesthesia, tetany, weakness	Acute: air hunger, disorientation Chronic: hypoventilation, hypoxia, cyanosis	Acute: hyperventilation, paraesthesia, lightheadedness Chronic: hyperventilation, latent tetany
Common causes	With raised anion gap: diabetic ketoacidosis, lactic acidosis, poisons (e.g. ethylene glycol), drug overdoses (paracetamol, aspirin, isoniazid, alcohol) With normal anion gap: diarrhoea, secretory adenomas, ammonium chloride poisoning, interstitial nephritis, renal tubular acidosis, acetazolamide administration	Vomiting, prolonged therapy with potassium-wasting diuretics or steroids, Cushing's disease, ingestion/ overdose of sodium bicarbonate (e.g. antacids)	Hypoventilation: chronic lung disease with CO_2 retention (e.g. chronic obstructive pulmonary disease), respiratory depression from drugs (e.g. opioids, sedatives), severe asthma, pulmonary oedema	Hyperventilation: anxiety, pain, febrile illness, hypoxia, pulmonary embolism, pregnancy, sepsis

N = within normal range; ↑ = increased; ↓ = decreased

○ pH

The pH determines the presence of acidaemia or alkalaemia. If the body has compensated for the disorder, the pH may be in the normal range.

○ PaCO₂

The $PaCO_2$ reflects the state of alveolar ventilation. An elevated $PaCO_2$ reflects alveolar hypoventilation, whereas a decreased $PaCO_2$ reflects alveolar hyperventilation. Acute changes in $PaCO_2$ will alter the pH. As a general rule, a low pH with a high $PaCO_2$ suggests a respiratory acidosis, while a low pH with a low $PaCO_2$ suggests a metabolic acidosis.

There is a delayed response of $PaCO_2$ to an acute change. Increases in $PaCO_2$ occur relatively slowly, as the body's overall CO_2 stores are very large (approximately 20 L) and the volume of CO_2 generated by metabolism (200 mL/min) makes little overall difference. For instance, during a breath-hold, the $PaCO_2$ rises at a rate of only 2–3 mmHg per minute, hence patients with a very high $PaCO_2$ usually have a longstanding disorder. Accordingly, even when treated the $PaCO_2$ may take a long time to return to normal.

○ PaO₂

The state of arterial blood oxygenation is determined by the PaO_2. This reflects gas exchange in the lungs, and normally the PaO_2 decreases with age. This is due to decreased elastic recoil in the lungs in the elderly, resulting in a greater ventilation–perfusion mismatch. The expected PaO_2 when breathing air at sea level can be calculated with the equation $PaO_2 = 100 - (age \times 0.25)$. Consequently, a PaO_2 of 75 mmHg, which may be of concern in a young person, is usually unremarkable in an 85-year-old.

A PaO_2 that is less than expected indicates hypoxaemia. This can result from hypoventilation or a mismatch of ventilation and perfusion. If alveolar ventilation is adequate (that is, $PaCO_2$ is normal), then the hypoxaemia is almost certainly caused by a ventilation–perfusion disturbance. The nature of the hypoxaemia can be further assessed by the difference between the alveolar and arterial oxygen tensions.

○ The alveolar–arterial oxygen tension difference

If an arterial blood gas result shows hypoxaemia (low PaO_2) and inadequate alveolar ventilation (high $PaCO_2$), it must be determined whether the hypoxaemia is related to hypoventilation, or is secondary to a disturbance in ventilation–perfusion, or both. This is assessed by calculating the difference between the alveolar (PAO_2) and arterial (PaO_2) oxygen tensions (Table 12.3).

Table 12.3 The alveolar–arterial oxygen gradient

$P(A-a)O_2 = PAO_2 - PaO_2$	
PaO_2	= arterial oxygen tension
PAO_2	= alveolar oxygen tension
PAO_2	= $FiO_2(P_B - P_{H_2O}) - 1.2(PaCO_2)$
FiO_2	= oxygen fraction in inspired air
P_B	= barometric pressure (760 mmHg at sea level)
P_{H2O}	= water vapour tension (47 mmHg at 37°C)

The normal value is < 15 mmHg.

The alveolar–arterial difference, or gradient, can be estimated only if the oxygen fraction of inspired air (FiO_2, usually 0.21 on room air), barometric pressure and water vapour pressure are known. A normal reference range is 5–15 mmHg. The difference [$P(A-a)O_2$] increases with age, cigarette smoking and increasing FiO_2. An expected $P(A-a)O_2$ can be calculated using the formula $P(A-a)O_2 = 3 + (0.21 \times age)$.

All causes of hypoxaemia, apart from hypoventilation, increase the alveolar–arterial difference. In a patient breathing room air, a $P(A-a)O_2$ greater than 15 mmHg suggests a ventilation–perfusion mismatch related to disease of the airways, lung parenchyma or pulmonary vasculature. However, the result is non-specific in defining the actual pathology and again the patient's clinical features are essential for diagnosis.

○ Bicarbonate

Bicarbonate is a weak base that is regulated by the kidneys as part of acid-base homeostasis. The HCO_3^- measured in arterial blood reflects the metabolic component of arterial blood. Together, CO_2 and HCO_3^- act as metabolic and respiratory buffers respectively. They are related via the equation:

$$H_2O + CO_2 \leftrightarrow H_2CO_3 \leftrightarrow HCO_3^- + H^+$$

○ Compensatory changes

For any disturbance of gas tensions in arterial blood, a compensatory system exists to maintain homeostasis. In a metabolic disorder, where HCO_3^- may be retained or excreted by the kidneys, respiratory compensation can occur almost immediately to alter the rate and depth of ventilation to retain or remove CO_2. This occurs due to the exquisite sensitivity of chemoreceptors in the medulla to carbonic acid (H_2CO_3) or H^+. Renal compensation in response to a respiratory disorder takes much longer, sometimes between three and five days, to retain or remove HCO_3^- as required.

As a general rule, when compensation is present the arterial blood gas result shows two imbalances—derangement of both HCO_3^- and $PaCO_2$. A clue to which imbalance is the primary disturbance is obtained from the pH. If pH is leaning toward acidosis or alkalosis, then the parameter that matches the pH trend (that is, is increased or decreased corresponding to pH) is the primary problem and the other is due to compensation.

The base excess

The metabolic component of the acid-base balance is reflected in the base excess. This is a calculated value derived from blood pH and $PaCO_2$. It is defined as the amount of acid required to restore a litre of blood to its normal pH at a $PaCO_2$ of 40 mmHg. The base excess increases in metabolic alkalosis and decreases (or becomes more negative) in metabolic acidosis, but its utility in interpreting blood gas results is controversial.

While the base excess may give some idea of the metabolic nature of a disorder, it may also confuse the interpretation. The alkalaemia or acidaemia may be primary or secondary to respiratory acidosis or alkalosis. The base excess does not take into account the appropriateness of the metabolic response for any given disorder, thus limiting its utility when interpreting results.

Anion gap

The anion gap assists with the diagnosis of metabolic acidosis (Table 12.4). This difference between the concentrations of measured anions and cations increases with dehydration and decreases with hypoalbuminaemia. The gap also widens if there is an increase in the concentration of unmeasured anions such as ketones and lactate.

Table 12.4 The anion gap concept

- The anion gap is an artificial concept that may indicate the cause of a metabolic acidosis.
- It represents the disparity between the major measured plasma cations (sodium and potassium) and the anions (chloride and bicarbonate).
- When calculating the anion gap, potassium is often omitted from the calculation thus:

$$Gap = Na^+ - (Cl^- + HCO_3^-)$$

- The anion gap is normally between 8 and 16 mmol/L.
- A raised anion gap indicates an increased concentration of lactate, ketones or renal acids and is seen in starvation and uraemia.
- A raised anion gap is seen in overdoses of paracetamol, salicylates, methanol or ethylene glycol.
- A normal anion gap is seen if a metabolic acidosis is due to diarrhoea or urinary loss of bicarbonate.

○ Factors influencing blood gas results

A number of sampling and environmental factors may affect the result of the analysis. Delayed processing of the sample may yield a falsely low PaO_2, as the delay allows leucocytes to consume oxygen. This can be avoided by prompt transport of the sample on ice.

Air bubbles introduced when performing the arterial puncture can also cause a falsely high PaO_2 and a falsely low $PaCO_2$.[2] This can be avoided by gently removing air bubbles within the specimen immediately after collection without agitating the sample.

Body temperature can also affect arterial blood gas tensions. This is relevant in febrile or hypothermic patients, so body temperature should be recorded at the time of collection.[3]

○ Mixed acid-base disorders

It is possible to have a mixed respiratory and metabolic disorder that makes interpretation of an arterial blood gas result difficult. As a general rule, when a normal pH is accompanied by an abnormal $PaCO_2$ or HCO_3^- then a mixed metabolic–respiratory disorder exists. Table 12.5 provides some common clinical examples of mixed respiratory and metabolic disturbances, and Figures 12.2 and 12.3 are algorithms for the consideration of primary and mixed acid-base disorders.[4]

Table 12.5 Examples of mixed acid-base disorders

Mixed metabolic/ respiratory disturbance	Example
Respiratory acidosis and metabolic acidosis	A patient with acute pulmonary oedema after an acute myocardial infarct
	Mechanism: poor cardiac circulation (causing a lactic acidosis/metabolic acidosis) with concurrent poor alveolar ventilation (due to pulmonary oedema) causing CO_2 retention and a concomitant respiratory acidosis

continues

Table 12.5 Examples of mixed acid-base disorders *continued*

Mixed metabolic/respiratory disturbance	Example
Respiratory alkalosis and metabolic alkalosis	A patient with hepatic cirrhosis who is given diuretics Mechanism: patients with hepatic cirrhosis can develop hepatopulmonary syndrome where the major symptom is dyspnoea (causing a respiratory alkalosis), while diuretics can cause a decrease in blood volume, which stimulates the renin-angiotensin-aldosterone system, increasing the exchange between Na^+ and K^+ or H^+ at the distal tubule, resulting in an increase in bicarbonate concentration and a metabolic alkalosis
Respiratory acidosis and metabolic alkalosis	A patient with longstanding chronic obstructive pulmonary disease who is given diuretics for concomitant heart failure Mechanism: longstanding air flow limitation may cause chronic hypercapnia and respiratory acidosis via impaired CO_2 excretion, while diuretics can cause a decrease in blood volume, which stimulates the renin-angiotensin-aldosterone system, increasing the exchange between Na^+ and K^+ or H^+ at the distal tubule, resulting in an increase in bicarbonate concentration and a metabolic alkalosis
Respiratory alkalosis and metabolic acidosis	A patient with chronic renal failure who begins to hyperventilate secondary to anxiety Mechanism: chronic renal failure causes a metabolic acidosis by uraemia and failure to excrete acids while the respiratory alkalosis results from blowing off excess CO_2 due to alveolar hyperventilation
Metabolic acidosis and metabolic alkalosis	A patient with chronic renal failure who suffers from severe intractable vomiting Mechanism: chronic renal failure causes a metabolic acidosis by uraemia and failure to excrete acids while a concurrent metabolic alkalosis results from the depletion in the body stores of H^+ and Cl^- through vomiting

Figure 12.2 Interpreting acidaemia on an arterial blood gas result

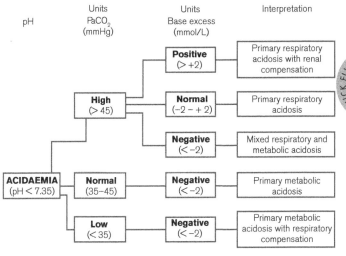

Image adapted with permission[4]

Figure 12.3 Interpreting alkalaemia on an arterial blood gas result

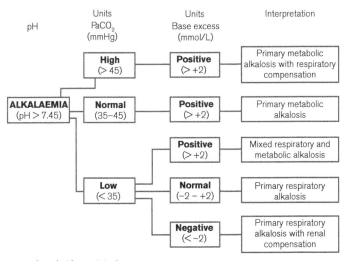

Image adapted with permission[4]

◗ Limitations of blood gas analysis

The blood gas analysis cannot yield a specific diagnosis. A patient with asthma may have similar values to another patient with pneumonia. Alternatively, a patient with chronic obstructive pulmonary disease and respiratory failure may have similar results to a patient with pulmonary oedema.

The analysis does not reflect the degree to which an abnormality actually affects a patient. A low PaO_2 does not necessarily indicate tissue hypoxia, nor does a normal PaO_2 indicate adequate tissue oxygenation. Oxygen utilisation is influenced by other factors such as regional blood flow, haemoglobin affinity for oxygen and cardiac output.

Blood gas analysis cannot be used as a screening test for early pulmonary disease. Severe disease may be present before significant changes are seen in blood gases.

◗ Venous blood gases

It is easier to obtain a venous sample than an arterial sample. In some situations analysis of venous blood can provide enough information to assist in clinical decisions. In general, the pH, CO_2 and HCO_3^- values are similar in venous and arterial blood (see Table 12.1). The main difference is the partial pressure of oxygen in venous blood is less than half that of arterial blood. Venous blood should not therefore be used to assess oxygenation.

◗ Summary

Measuring arterial blood gases can be a useful adjunct to the assessment of patients with either acute or chronic diseases. The results show if the patient is acidaemic or alkalaemic and whether the cause is likely to have a respiratory or metabolic component. The $PaCO_2$ reflects alveolar ventilation and the PaO_2 reflects the oxygenation of arterial blood. When combined with a patient's clinical features, blood gas analysis can facilitate diagnosis and management.

References

1. Lightowler J.V. and Elliot M.W. Local anaesthetic infiltration prior to arterial puncture for blood gas analysis: a survey of current practice and a randomised double blind placebo controlled trial. *J R Coll Physicians Lond* 1997; 31: 645–6.
2. Harsten A., Berg B., Inerot S. and Muth L. Importance of correct handling of samples for the results of blood gas analysis. *Acta Anaesthesiol Scand* 1998; 32: 365–8.

3. Williams A.J. ABC of oxygen: assessing and interpreting arterial blood gases and acid-base balance. *BMJ* 1998; 317: 1213–6.
4. Drage S. and Wilkinson D. Acid base balance. *Pharmacology* 2001; 13: 3. World Anaesthesia, World Federation of Societies of Anaesthesiologists. World Anaesthesia Online www.nda.ox.ac.uk/wfsa/html/u13/u1312_03. htm [cited May 19, 2010].

Further reading

Martin L. *All You Really Need To Know To Interpret Arterial Blood Gases.* 2nd ed. Philadelphia, PA: Lippincott Williams & Wilkins, 1999.

13 Calcium and vitamin D*

J.D. Wark and C.J. Yates

○ Calcium

○ Introduction

The approach to an abnormal plasma calcium result differs according to whether the plasma calcium was measured because of specific symptoms or signs, or whether the abnormal result was an incidental finding, for example during multiphasic screening.

This chapter will be confined to a consideration of the incidental detection of an abnormal plasma calcium.

Is the result abnormal?

Apart from the possibility of laboratory error, falsely elevated values can be due to haemoconcentration associated with the use of a tourniquet. In addition, in patients with abnormal plasma protein concentrations, the total calcium concentration will be affected, but not the ionised fraction, and appropriate corrections should be made.[1] Marginal abnormalities should be confirmed by repeated tests. The quoted 'reference range' is calculated in most laboratories to include 95% of normal individuals so even a confirmed and corrected value slightly outside the normal range need not indicate disease. Direct measurement of ionised, dialysable or ultrafiltrable calcium avoids problems associated with protein binding and is being used more frequently. Some laboratories provide a 'calculated' ionised calcium that agrees well with directly-measured ionised calcium.

Causes and effects of hypercalcaemia

The major causes of hypercalcaemia are listed in Table 13.1. In hospital practice malignancy is the most common cause but in asymptomatic patients primary hyperparathyroidism is much more frequent.[2] Clinical assessment should be directed particularly towards eliciting (1) symptoms

---

*   This represents a substantial update and expansion of the original article on calcium written by
    Professor R.G. Larkins in 1997. (Editor)

of hypercalcaemia and its consequences, such as thirst, polyuria, constipation and renal colic, and (2) symptoms and signs of the cause of hypercalcaemia. Particular attention should be paid to ingestion of thiazides and antacids containing calcium and sodium bicarbonate and to symptoms suggestive of malignancy. A lack of evidence of other causes of hypercalcaemia suggests hyperparathyroidism.

Table 13.1 Some causes of hypercalcaemia

1. Primary hyperparathyroidism
2. Malignant disease
   - with bone involvement, e.g. metastatic carcinoma of the breast
   - without bone involvement, e.g. squamous cell carcinoma of the lung, carcinoma of the kidney
   - haematological malignancy, e.g. multiple myeloma, lymphoma
3. Sarcoidosis
4. Vitamin D intoxication (including calcitriol therapy)
5. Milk alkali syndrome
6. Immobilisation (other causes should be excluded)
7. Thyrotoxicosis
8. Thiazide diuretics (typically the hypercalcaemia is transient)
9. Familial hypocalciuric hypercalcaemia

A positive family history of hypercalcaemia raises the possibility of multiple endocrine neoplasia with hyperparathyroidism and of familial hypocalciuric hypercalcaemia. Both these conditions are transmitted as Mendelian-dominant characteristics.

What further tests are required?
The diagnosis of primary hyperparathyroidism is supported by a low plasma phosphate, a raised plasma chloride and a low-normal plasma bicarbonate. Raised plasma parathyroid hormone (PTH) provides strong evidence for the diagnosis if renal function is normal. X-rays of the hands may reveal the characteristic subperiosteal erosions of hyperparathyroidism and other skeletal X-rays may reveal bone cysts in hyperparathyroidism or evidence of metastases in malignant hypercalcaemia. Bone scanning may reveal metastases. X-ray of the abdomen may reveal renal or ureteric calculi or nephrocalcinosis in patients with hyperparathyroidism or sarcoidosis and further imaging may be indicated to exclude carcinoma of the kidney if microscopic haematuria is present.

Serum angiotensin converting enzyme (ACE) levels are commonly raised in patients with hypercalcaemia due to sarcoidosis. Serum

25-hydroxyvitamin D (25OHD) levels are elevated in patients with vitamin D intoxication due to ergocalciferol (vitamin D_2) or cholecalciferol (vitamin D_3) but not if calcitriol is the cause (see below). Plasma parathyroid hormone-related peptide (PTHrP) is elevated in many patients with malignant hypercalcaemia but currently there is very limited access to this measurement.[3]

Management of hypercalcaemia

Patients with serum calcium values of 3.0 mmol/L or less do not usually require urgent treatment. If a cause of hypercalcaemia apart from primary hyperparathyroidism is found, this is treated on its merits. There is now reasonable agreement concerning the correct management of asymptomatic patients with presumptive primary hyperparathyroidism.[4] Indications for parathyroid surgery include serum calcium greater than 2.85 mmol/L, creatinine clearance less than 60 mL/min, osteoporosis and age less than 50 years. While the condition may be associated with progressive bone loss and the risk of renal impairment, renal calculi, hypercalcaemic crises, peptic ulcers and pancreatitis, in many patients mild, asymptomatic primary hyperparathyroidism follows a benign course.[5–7] In elderly patients without specific indications for surgical intervention—such as renal calculi, renal impairment, bone disease, pancreatitis, peptic ulceration or severe hypercalcaemia (greater than 2.85 mmol/L)—observation including at least annual measurement of serum calcium and creatinine plus bone density testing every one or two years is a reasonable approach. In relatively frail patients with biochemically mild primary hyperparathyroidism and low bone mineral density, long-term oral bisphosphonates may help the low bone density state.[8] Medical therapy with the calcimimetic drug cinacalcet is also an option in cases where surgery is problematic.[9] In patients where neck exploration is decided upon, an experienced surgeon is usually able to find and correct the parathyroid abnormality. Radiology, ultrasound or ^{99m}Tc-sestamibi isotope scanning may be helpful in preoperative localisation of the adenoma. For summary, see Figure 13.1.

The treatment of severe hypercalcaemia is urgent and requires replacement of fluid and electrolyte deficits together with specific drug therapy to lower the serum calcium level.[10] Intravenous bisphosphonates (zoledronic acid, pamidronate) have simplified the management of severe hypercalcaemia.

Causes and effects of hypocalcaemia

The main causes of hypocalcaemia are shown in Table 13.2. Postsurgical hypoparathyroidism is the most common cause in asymptomatic adults. In younger patients idiopathic hypoparathyroidism (probably autoimmune

Figure 13.1 Hypercalcaemia–management

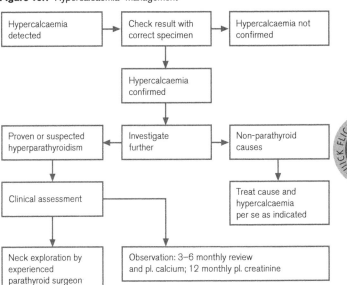

Table 13.2 Some causes of hypocalcaemia

Hypoparathyroidism–idiopathic, postsurgical, pseudohypoparathyroidism
Malabsorptive and nutritional vitamin D deficiency (osteomalacia and rickets; see main text)
Chronic renal disease
Hypomagnesaemia

in origin) is the most common cause and it may be associated with other autoimmune endocrine deficiency diseases and with mucocutaneous candidiasis. Vitamin D deficiency may present with hypocalcaemia at any age, although osteomalacia or rickets can also occur with a normal plasma calcium (see below).

Symptoms and signs of hypocalcaemia should be sought. They include paraesthesiae and carpal or pedal spasm, nail changes, cataracts and epilepsy. It may be possible to provoke carpal spasm by inflating the blood pressure cuff to greater than systolic pressure (Trousseau's sign) and a facial twitch may be elicited by tapping over the facial nerve (Chvostek's sign).

A history of thyroidectomy or a neck scar should be noted, and symptoms and signs of renal impairment and malabsorption should be sought. A family history of hypocalcaemia may be present in pseudohypoparathyroidism, which may be diagnosed by the characteristic skeletal features.

What further tests are required?

Plasma phosphate tends to be high in hypoparathyroidism and chronic renal failure and low in nutritional and malabsorptive osteomalacia and rickets. Skeletal alkaline phosphatase is usually raised in osteomalacia or rickets and renal failure. Plasma PTH is undetectable or inappropriately low in hypoparathyroidism but raised in hypocalcaemia due to chronic renal failure, osteomalacia, rickets and pseudohypoparathyroidism. Renal function should be checked and malabsorption excluded. Plasma 25-OHD levels are very low in patients with hypocalcaemia associated with malabsorption or nutritional osteomalacia or rickets, and skeletal survey may show osteopenia and possibly pseudofractures. Especially in malnourished patients or those with malabsorption, the plasma magnesium level should be measured because severe hypomagnesaemia is often associated with resistant hypocalcaemia.

Management of hypocalcaemia

Even if asymptomatic, hypocalcaemia associated with hypoparathyroidism or pseudohypoparathyroidism probably justifies treatment with calcitriol and oral calcium because of the risks of cataracts and epilepsy if left untreated.[10] The treatment must be monitored carefully with plasma calcium determination at least three monthly to avoid hypercalcaemia (Fig. 13.2). The target in treating hypoparathyroidism is to maintain the plasma calcium concentration in the lower normal range but avoid symptoms of hypocalcaemia. Avoidance of hypercalciuria is important to minimise the risk of renal calcium deposition.

In patients with hypocalcaemia associated with vitamin D deficiency, osteomalacia or rickets due to malabsorption or nutritional causes, the most appropriate form of vitamin D replacement to use is ergocalciferol or cholecalciferol (see below).

◐ Summary: abnormalities of serum calcium

Routine screening leads to abnormal plasma calcium results in about 5% of the community.[11] The abnormality may represent a laboratory error, an extreme of a normal distribution, a benign condition which from the subject's point of view would better have been undetected, a significant but untreatable underlying disease or a significant and treatable disorder. The relatively benign natural history of primary hyperparathyroidism makes it likely that only a small percentage of cases fall into the last category.

Figure 13.2 Hypocalcaemia–management

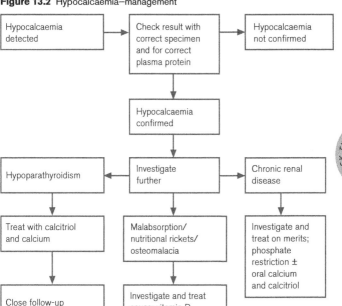

With the incidental finding of hypercalcaemia, the extent and direction of investigation and the final management decided upon should be based on the individual situation. Enthusiasm to get to the bottom of the problem and to obtain biochemical normalisation should be tempered in the subject who did not present complaining of the calcium abnormality, and in most cases it is not certain that it will do them any harm. In true hypocalcaemia a significant cause will be found in most cases and treatment generally is indicated to prevent complications.

◌ Vitamin D

◌ Introduction

Vitamin D influences calcium levels through direct effects on the gastrointestinal tract, bone and parathyroid hormone. While vitamin D toxicity is rare, vitamin D insufficiency is a significant problem within Australia and globally.[12,13] 25OHD is the product of hepatic hydroxylation of vitamin D that is either made in the skin or ingested in the diet. Although not the biologically active form, 25OHD is the major circulating form of vitamin D and is the best indicator of overall vitamin D status. Renal production of 1,25-dihydroxyvitamin D [1,25(OH)$_2$D] is the primary source of circulating levels of this highly active metabolite and is tightly regulated by factors including the hormone itself and PTH. Despite being highly active, serum 1,25(OH)$_2$D is not an appropriate indicator of vitamin D status due to its short plasma half-life, low levels and tight compensatory regulation that tends to maintain appropriate levels even in the presence of vitamin D deficiency or excess.

Measurement of circulating vitamin D metabolites

Mass spectrometry techniques are considered to be the gold standard for measuring 25OHD but are time consuming and require expensive equipment; therefore, less precise immunoassays and occasionally protein binding assays are used for clinical samples.[14] Competitive protein binding assays use plasma vitamin D binding protein to bind 25OHD. However, due to laboratories' having different preparations of binding protein, results can vary significantly.[15] As it employs antibodies, immunoassay compares more favourably with the gold standard.[16] Early protein binding assays and radioimmunoassays recognised 25OHD$_2$ and 25OHD$_3$ equally well, but 24,25(OH)$_2$D and other vitamin D metabolites were also recognised to the same extent resulting in a 10–20% overestimation of 25OHD.[14] A more recent immunoassay has 100% specificity for 25OHD$_3$ but only 75% specificity for 25OHD$_2$. However, the ability of some immunoassays to detect 25OHD$_2$ adequately has been questioned.

Vitamin D deficiency
What is abnormal?

There is no universally-agreed definition of vitamin D deficiency. However, most agree that an adequate level of 25OHD for bone health and probably for a number of other health indices is between 50 and 80 nmol/L. Previously the normal range had been determined by the 25OHD level associated with maximal PTH suppression, but several recent randomised controlled trials in older populations (over 60–65 years) have enabled the additional use of falls and fracture endpoints to draw conclusions. The threshold for PTH suppression clusters around 25OHD levels of 32–50 nmol/L and 68–75 nmol/L depending on the analytical process used.[17] Meanwhile, optimal reduction in the risk of falls, non-vertebral fractures and hip fractures requires vitamin D replacement to at least 60, 66 and 74 nmol/L, respectively.[18,19] Consequently, the International Osteoporosis Foundation recommends a target of 75 nmol/L for older populations and many laboratories report insufficient levels between 50–75 nmol/L with deficiency being less than 50 nmol/L.[20,21] In practical terms, 25OHD assays generally have suboptimal accuracy and precision, so a cut-off of 60 nmol/L for adequacy in the general population is reasonable based on currently available information.

Causes and effects of vitamin D deficiency

The major causes of vitamin D deficiency are listed in Table 13.3. Reduced sunlight exposure is an important cause of vitamin D deficiency, particularly in residential care and in community-dwelling groups who avoid sun exposure of their skin.[21] Sequelae include secondary hyperparathyroidism, osteoporosis, reduced muscle strength, falls, osteomalacia, rickets and hypocalcaemia (which may be precipitated by bisphosphonate administration). Although causal relationships have not been demonstrated, vitamin D deficiency has also been associated with insulin resistance, cardiovascular disease, some cancers (e.g. colon) and disorders involving the immune system (e.g. multiple sclerosis, type I diabetes, some infections).[22]

Table 13.3 Major causes of vitamin D deficiency[12,13]

Ageing
Dark skin pigmentation/sunscreen use
Limited outdoor activities
Concealing clothing (e.g. burqa)
Latitude further from the equator
Major illness
Season (winter)
Nephrotic syndrome
Obesity
Liver failure/cholestasis/biliary obstruction
Inadequate dietary intake
Atmospheric pollution
Malabsorption
Drugs (rifampicin, barbiturates, possibly phenytoin)

What further tests are required?

Vitamin D deficiency correlates with low or low-normal serum calcium and phosphate levels, normal or elevated alkaline phosphatase (of bone origin) and elevated PTH. Symptoms of malabsorption should prompt investigation for gastrointestinal disease and abnormal liver function tests may indicate hepatobiliary disease. Possible radiographic findings include osteopenia, cortical thinning and pseudofractures (in osteomalacia), and expanded epiphyseal growth plates and a rachitic rosary (in children with rickets).[10] Dual energy X-ray absorptiometry (DEXA) scans may reveal osteopenia or osteoporosis.

Management of vitamin D deficiency

In patients with vitamin D deficiency due to malabsorption or nutritional causes the most appropriate form of vitamin D replacement to use is vitamin D_2 or vitamin D_3, as there is a wide margin between therapeutic and toxic doses in these conditions.[10,21] Vitamin D replacement regimens vary according to 25OHD level, body mass index, sun exposure and physician. However, supplementation of 3 000 to 5 000 IU vitamin D_3 daily for 6 to 12 weeks is generally recommended to treat nutritional vitamin D deficiency.[21] Unless the underlying cause for vitamin D deficiency can be reversed, maintenance supplementation with 1 000 or 2 000 IU/day also is indicated. Larger dose preparations are not readily available in Australia. There is limited access to 50 000 IU tablets, which can be administered once monthly. Recent research has cast doubt on the efficacy and safety of annual 'megadosing' so this regimen cannot be recommended currently.[23] The estimated average vitamin D requirement for older adults to achieve a target of 75 nmol/L is 800–1 000 IU vitamin D_3 per day.[20]

Other nutritional deficits should be addressed and calcium supplements generally are indicated, at least until osteomalacia or rickets is healed.

Vitamin D toxicity

What is abnormal?

Lifeguards with high sun exposure have reported 25OHD levels up to 312 nmol/L without adverse effects. However, levels over 374 nmol/L due to ingestion of excessively high doses of vitamin D have caused intoxication.[14]

Causes and effects of vitamin D intoxication

No clinical or biochemical evidence of toxicity has been noted with doses of vitamin D_3 up to 4 000 IU/day.[24] However, risk is much greater with calcitriol administration (for renal osteodystrophy, hypoparathyroidism or osteoporosis) and with unregulated 1-hydroxylation of 25OHD by macrophages in granulomatous disorders (e.g. sarcoidosis, tuberculosis).[25] Symptoms are predominantly attributable to hypercalcaemia and include nausea, dehydration and lethargy, although increased falls and fractures were also evident in a recent study of annual 500 000 IU oral vitamin D_3 administration.[23] Long-term adverse effects also include nephrolithiasis and nephrocalcinosis associated with hypercalciuria.

What further tests are required?

Serum 25OHD is elevated in most patients with vitamin D_2 or D_3 intoxication; however, only $1,25(OH)_2D$ is raised in toxicity from calcitriol administration or granulomatous disorders. Vitamin D intoxication is associated with hypercalciuria and often renal impairment and hyperphosphataemia. With hypercalcaemia due to sarcoidosis, ACE levels are commonly raised.

Management of vitamin D intoxication

Vitamin D and calcium administration should be ceased immediately. Replacement of fluid and electrolyte deficits should be undertaken as needed. If calcitriol administration has caused vitamin D toxicity, cessation of therapy and withdrawal of concurrent calcium supplementation usually improves symptoms within 2 days. Hypercalcaemia due to elevated $1,25(OH)_2D$ in granulomatous disorders should be treated with prednisolone 15–30 mg/d. Because of the extensive fat deposition, intoxication due to high dose vitamin D_2 or D_3 may follow a protracted course and severe cases may require oral glucocorticoid therapy.[10]

One should be aware also that vitamin A is present in many over-the-counter vitamin D supplements and with overdosing may contribute to hypercalcaemia/hypercalciuria. Therefore, vitamin A intoxication may also need to be addressed.

○ Summary: vitamin D

At least 30% of Australian adults and many Australian children have vitamin D deficiency.[26] There are well-recognised groups in our community at high risk for vitamin D deficiency (e.g. frail elderly people and dark skinned people, especially those with restricted sun exposure). Given the potential associated complications, the presence of risk factors for vitamin D deficiency should prompt testing of 25OHD levels. Therapy should target 75 nmol/L in the elderly and those at risk for falls and low-trauma fractures, and requires individual consideration of 25OHD levels, body mass index and sun exposure. Re-testing 3 months later will guide ongoing management and avoid vitamin D intoxication. A target level of at least 50 or 60 nmol/L can be recommended in the rest of the community.

References

1. Parfitt A.M. Investigation of disorders of the parathyroid glands. *Clin Endocrinol Metab* 1974; 3: 451–74.

2. Aitken R.E., Bartley P.C., Bryant S.J. and Lloyd H.M. The effect of multiphasic biochemical screening on the diagnosis of primary hyperparathyroidism. *Aust N Z J Med* 1975; 5: 224–6.

3. Wysolmerski J.J. and Broadus A.E. Hypercalcemia of malignancy: the central role of parathyroid hormone-related protein. *Annu Rev Med* 1994; 45: 189–200.

4. Bilezikian J.P., Khan A.A. and Potts J.T. Jr. Third International Workshop on the Management of Asymptomatic Primary Hyperthyroidism. Guidelines for the management of asymptomatic primary hyperparathyroidism: summary statement from the third international workshop. *J Clin Endocrinol Metab* 2009; 94: 335–9.

5. Rubinoff H., McCarthy N. and Hiatt R.A. Hypercalcemia: long-term follow-up with matched controls. *J Chronic Dis* 1983; 36: 859–68.

6. Silverberg S.J., Shane E., Jacobs T.P., Siris E. and Bilezikian J.P. A 10-year prospective study of primary hyperparathyroidism with or without parathyroid surgery. *NEJM* 1999; 341: 1249–55.

7. Rao D.S., Wilson R.J., Kleerekoper M. and Parfitt A.M. Lack of biochemical progression or continuation of accelerated bone loss in mild asymptomatic primary hyperparathyroidism: evidence for biphasic disease course. *J Clin Endocrinol Metab* 1988; 67: 1294–8.

8. Khan A.A., Bilezikian J.P., Kung A.W.C. et al. Alendronate in primary hyperparathyroidism: a double-blind, randomized, placebo-controlled trial. *J Clin Endocrinol Metab* 2004;89: 3319–25.

9. Peacock M., Bolognese M.A., Borofsky M. et al. Cinacalcet treatment of primary hyperparathyroidism: biochemical and bone densitometric outcomes in a five-year study. *J Clin Endocrinol Metab* 2009; 94: 4860–7.

10. *Therapeutic Guidelines: Endocrinology.* 4th ed. Therapeutic Guidelines Limited, 2009.

11. Proceedings of the NIH consensus development conference on diagnosis and management of asymptomatic primary hyperparathyroidism. *J Bone Miner Res* 1991; 6: 9–13.

12. Holick M.F. Vitamin D deficiency. *NEJM* 2007; 357: 266–81.

13. Mithal A., Wahl D.A., Bonjour J.P. et al. Global vitamin D status and determinants of hypovitaminosis D. *Osteoporos Int* 2009; 20: 1807–20.

14. Holick M.F. Vitamin D status: measurement, interpretation, and clinical application. *Ann of Epidemiol* 2009; 19: 73–8.

15. Binkley N., Krueger D., Cowgill C.S. et al. Assay variation confounds the diagnosis of hypovitaminosis D: A call for standardization. *J Clin Endocr Metab* 2004; 89: 3152–7.

16. Hollis B.W., Kamerud J.Q., Selvaag S.R., Lorenz J.D. and Napoli J.L. Determination of vitamin-D status by radioimmunoassay with an I-125 labeled tracer. *Clin Chem* 1993; 39: 529–33.

17. Durazo-Arvizu R.A., Dawson-Hughes B., Sempos C.T. et al. Three-phase model harmonizes estimates of the maximal suppression of parathyroid hormone by 25-hydroxyvitamin D in persons 65 years of age and older. *J Nutr* 2010; 140: 595–9.

18. Bischoff-Ferrari H.A., Dawson-Hughes B., Staehelin HB. et al. Fall prevention with supplemental and active forms of vitamin D: a meta-analysis of randomised controlled trials. *BMJ* 2009; 339.

19. Bischoff-Ferrari H.A., Willett W.C., Wong J.B., Giovannucci E., Dietrich T. and Dawson-Hughes B. Fracture prevention with vitamin D supplementation—a meta-analysis of randomized controlled trials. *JAMA* 2005; 293: 2257–64.

20. Dawon-Hughes B., Mithal A., Bonjour J.P. et al. IOF position statement: vitamin D recommendations for older adults. *Osteopor Int* 2010.

21. Working Group of the ANZBMS, ESA and Osteoporosis Australia. Vitamin D and adult bone health in Australia and New Zealand: a position statement. *MJA* 2005; 182: 281–5.

22. Adams J.S. and Hewison M. Update in vitamin D. *J Clin Endocr Metab* 2010; 95: 471–8.

23. Sanders K.M., Stuart A.L., Williamson E.J. et al. Annual high-dose oral vitamin D and falls and fractures in older women a randomized controlled trial. *JAMA* 2010; 303: 1815–22.

24. Vieth R., Chan P.C.R. and MacFarlane G.D. Efficacy and safety of vitamin D-3 intake exceeding the lowest observed adverse effect level. *Am J Clin Nutr* 2001; 73: 288–94.

25. Vieth R. Vitamin D toxicity, policy, and science. *J Bone Miner Res* 2007; 22: V64–8.

26. Pasco J.A., Henry M.J., Nicholson G.C., Sanders K.M. and Kotowicz M.A. Vitamin D status of women in the Geelong Osteoporosis Study: association with diet and casual exposure to sunlight. *MJA* 2001; 175: 401–5.

14 Magnesium: the forgotten electrolyte

J. Wu and A. Carter

Synopsis

Magnesium is important for the proper functioning of various metabolic pathways and ion channels, so disturbances in magnesium concentration can cause clinical problems. Hypomagnesaemia has many renal and extrarenal causes whereas hypermagnesaemia is usually due to renal insufficiency. Magnesium should be monitored in conditions such as arrhythmia and when other electrolytes are abnormal.

○ Introduction

Magnesium is the fourth most abundant cation in the body and the second most abundant intracellular cation after potassium. Dietary sources of magnesium include whole grain cereals, green leafy vegetables, legumes, soybeans, nuts, dried fruit, animal protein and seafood.[1,2,3] The minimum recommended daily intake of magnesium for adults is 0.25 mmol (6 mg)/kg body weight.[4]

The total body magnesium of an adult male is approximately 1 mol (24 g).[1] Approximately 66% is distributed in bone, 33% in muscle and soft tissues, and less than 1% in blood. In blood, 55% of the magnesium is free (ionised) and physiologically active, 30% is bound to proteins (primarily albumin) and 15% is complexed to anions.[5]

○ Magnesium homeostasis

Under normal conditions the body maintains constant circulating concentrations of magnesium in the blood. Homeostasis depends on the balance between intestinal absorption and renal excretion, with kidney tubules having primary control.[4]

The main site of absorption is the small intestine, with smaller amounts absorbed in the colon.[4] Absorption can range from 24% of ingested magnesium in magnesium replete states to 76% in deficient states. Approximately 1 mmol is lost in gastrointestinal secretions daily.[1]

The kidney's handling of magnesium is more complicated. There is a circadian excretory rhythm with more magnesium excretion occurring at night.[3,6] Ionised and complexed magnesium are freely filtered at the glomerulus (70% of circulating magnesium). To maintain homeostasis, the nephrons normally reabsorb more than 96% of the filtered magnesium.[1,4] The amount reabsorbed can vary, however, from less than 30% to 99.5% depending on the individual's magnesium balance.[1,7]

Most reabsorption occurs in the thick ascending limb of the loop of Henle where 65–75% of filtered magnesium is reabsorbed passively down an electrochemical gradient which is actively maintained.[1,4] The amount reabsorbed is inversely related to tubular flow. Situations that abolish the positive luminal charge (e.g. loop diuretics, hypercalcaemia) will reduce the reabsorption of magnesium. The reabsorption of magnesium and calcium parallel each other in this segment, but the hormonal regulation of magnesium homeostasis is incompletely understood.[1]

⟡ Function

Magnesium is involved in over 300 enzymatic reactions. It is needed in energy metabolism, glucose utilisation, protein synthesis, fatty acid synthesis and breakdown, muscle contraction, all ATPase functions, for almost all hormonal reactions and in the maintenance of cellular ionic balance.[2]

Magnesium is needed for the proper functioning of the Na^+/K^+ ATPase pump, so a deficiency causes an increase in intracellular sodium and allows potassium to leak out of cells.[2] Loss of intracellular potassium also occurs in the renal tubules.[1] This can lead to a hypokalaemia that responds only to magnesium replacement.[2]

Magnesium also affects calcium homeostasis through two mechanisms. First, many calcium channels are dependent on magnesium. When the intracellular magnesium concentration is high, calcium transport into the cell and from the sarcoplasmic reticulum is inhibited. In magnesium deficiency the inverse occurs and consequently the intracellular concentration of calcium rises.[2] Second, magnesium is needed for the release and action of parathyroid hormone.[2] Magnesium's relationship with calcium means that patients with hypomagnesaemia may have a low plasma calcium that remains refractory to calcium supplementation until the magnesium deficiency is corrected.[2]

◌ Laboratory tests

Most laboratories measure total magnesium; measurement of ionised magnesium is not standard practice. The normal range for total magnesium is 0.7–1.0 mmol/L. Caution should be taken in interpreting results from patients who have low total magnesium and low albumin, as they may have normal concentrations of ionised magnesium. Blood levels may not reflect total body stores.[5] One reason for this is that in acidosis magnesium shifts from the intracellular to the extracellular space, whereas in alkalosis the reverse occurs.[2] This can cause a dilemma particularly in determining the presence or absence of hypomagnesaemia.

◌ Hypomagnesaemia

Due to magnesium's wide-ranging functions, magnesium deficiency may be the cause of numerous serious pathologies.[1,2,3,8,9]

As total blood magnesium concentrations do not always reflect total body stores, a high index of suspicion is needed particularly in patients at high risk of magnesium deficiency (see Table 14.1). Magnesium is often not included in routine electrolyte testing, so it is important that clinicians remember to order and monitor it. Changes in magnesium concentrations for an individual might be significant, even if they remain within the normal range.[2] Occasionally the magnesium-loading test is required to confirm magnesium deficiency.[2,4] However, this test requires the patient to have normal renal function.[10]

Causes

The causes of hypomagnesaemia are extrarenal or renal (Table 14.1). A 24-h urine collection can be used to determine the presence or absence of renal magnesium wasting. In the presence of hypomagnesaemia, a 24-h urine total magnesium less than 0.5 mmol is evidence of an intact renal response to hypomagnesaemia. A value greater than 1.0 mmol indicates abnormal renal wasting. Alternatively, the fractional excretion of magnesium (FE_{Mg}) on a random urine specimen can be used. In the presence of hypomagnesaemia, an FE_{Mg} less than 2% indicates an appropriate response to hypomagnesaemia while an FE_{Mg} greater than 2% indicates renal wasting.[1]

Extrarenal causes

Conditions that cause malabsorption may lead to decreased gastrointestinal absorption of magnesium. These conditions include inflammatory bowel disease, chronic pancreatitis and alcohol abuse. In alcohol abuse, increased urinary magnesium wasting may also contribute to hypomagnesaemia. Proton pump inhibitors are suspected to cause hypomagnesaemia by disrupting the active absorption of magnesium within the small intestine.[11,12] As magnesium

Table 14.1 Causes of hypomagnesaemia*

Extrarenal causes		Renal causes	
Gastrointestinal	Diarrhoea Steatorrhoea Alcoholism Inflammatory bowel disease Vomiting Short bowel syndrome Sprue Chronic pancreatitis Parenteral nutrition Gastric suction	Drugs	Aminoglycoside toxicity Pentamidine toxicity Amphotericin B toxicity Thiazide and loop diuretics Calcineurin inhibitors (e.g. cyclosporin, tacrolimus) Foscarnet Cisplatin Alcohol Cetuximab[13]
Drugs	Proton pump inhibitors[11,12]	Loop of Henle	Hypercalcaemia
Skin	Burns Toxic epidermal necrolysis	Increased tubular flow	Osmotic diuresis
Intracellular shift	'Hungry bone' syndrome Refeeding syndrome[16]	Congenital renal magnesium wasting	

*Adapted from reference 1

is present in gastric secretions, vomiting and nasogastric suction are recognised (rare) causes of hypomagnesaemia. Skin loss of magnesium can be significant in burns patients. 'Hungry bone' syndrome ,which can occur following parathyroidectomy, can also drop blood calcium, magnesium and potassium concentrations.[1] The refeeding syndrome can induce low magnesium levels due to intracellular shift of magnesium.[16]

Renal causes

There are several rare congenital magnesium wasting syndromes of which Gitelman's syndrome is a better known example. Research into these conditions over the last few years has identified renal ion channels and transporters, thus increasing our understanding of renal magnesium handling.[13–15]

Drugs can cause renal wasting of magnesium. They either cause tubular toxicity (e.g. amphotericin B, aminoglycosides) or block renal reabsorption (e.g. loop diuretics).[1]

Hypercalcaemia can block renal reabsorption of magnesium, resulting in hypomagnesaemia. However, when hypercalcaemia is due to hyperparathyroidism, patients are usually normomagnesaemic because parathyroid hormone stimulates magnesium reabsorption.[1]

Effects

Hypomagnesaemia can cause hypokalaemia and hypocalcaemia. It is also associated with hyponatraemia and hypophosphataemia.[1]

Magnesium's usual role in the sodium-potassium ATPase pump and calcium-blocking activity is impaired by hypomagnesaemia, leading to membrane destabilisation and hyperexcitability.[8] Patients can develop Trousseau's and Chvostek's signs even in the presence of a normal ionised serum calcium concentration.[1] With severe hypomagnesaemia, patients can have tetany and seizures (Table 14.2).

The effect on the myocardium is an increase in atrial and ventricular arrhythmias. Some ventricular arrhythmias caused by hypomagnesaemia only respond to treatment with magnesium.[1]

Table 14.2 Clinical findings associated with altered magnesium concentrations*†

Total magnesium concentration (mmol/L)	Findings
< 0.5	Tetany Seizures Arrhythmias
0.5–0.7	Neuromuscular irritability
0.7–1.0	**Normal range**
1.0–2.1	Typically asymptomatic
2.1–2.9	Lethargy Drowsiness Flushing Nausea and vomiting Diminished deep tendon reflexes
2.9–5.0	Somnolence Loss of deep tendon reflexes Hypotension ECG changes Bradycardia

Total magnesium concentration (mmol/L)	Findings
>5.0	Complete heart block
	Cardiac arrest
	Apnoea
	Paralysis
	Coma

* Adapted from reference 1.
† When magnesium concentrations are altered, also check calcium and potassium.

Treatment

An attempt should be made to identify the underlying cause for the hypomagnesaemia. In asymptomatic hypomagnesaemic or magnesium-deficient patients, oral magnesium supplements are used. Recommended dosages vary. Commonly, magnesium aspartate (1.65 mmol magnesium ion per tablet) is prescribed at 2–4 tablets per day, given in divided doses.[17] As higher doses have a laxative effect, dosage will be limited by diarrhoea.[2,4]

Symptomatic or severe (< 0.4 mmol/L) hypomagnesaemia should be treated with intravenous magnesium, as correcting magnesium deficiency takes six times longer with oral supplementation—six weeks versus seven days.[9] Intravenous magnesium sulfate is the formulation commonly used. One 5 mL ampoule of magnesium sulfate contains 10 mmol of magnesium ions. 10–20 mmol of magnesium ions can be given in 100 mL of 0.9% sodium chloride over 1–2 hours. Sulfate anions, however, may bind calcium and aggravate existing hypocalcaemia. Calcium should thus be administered as well.[17,18] Patients with renal insufficiency should have their doses decreased appropriately, be monitored closely for decreased deep tendon reflexes, and have their magnesium concentrations checked regularly.[1,8]

○ Hypermagnesaemia

Causes

The most common causes of hypermagnesaemia are renal insufficiency and increased intake (Table 14.3). Severe hypermagnesaemia in the setting of renal insufficiency alone is, however, rare, unless the patient has increased magnesium intake as well.[7,16]

Table 14.3 Causes of hypermagnesaemia*

Decreased renal excretion		Renal insufficiency Familial hypocalciuric hypercalcaemia
		Lithium ingestion[9]
Excess magnesium intake	Parenteral	Dosing error
		Treatment of specific conditions e.g. eclampsia, torsades de pointes
	Oral	Damage to the intestinal epithelium may increase magnesium absorption
		Magnesium-containing antacids
		Epsom salts ($MgSO_4$) and other magnesium-containing cathartics
		Magnesium-containing enemas
		Aspiration
Other		Theophylline toxicity
		Hypothyroidism[16]
		Acute rhabdomyolysis[8]
		Addison's disease[16]

*Adapted from reference 1

Effects

Magnesium can block synaptic transmission of nerve impulses, causing loss of deep tendon reflexes. More severe toxicity can cause flaccid paralysis and apnoea. The effect on smooth muscle results in ileus and urinary retention. Through its effect on calcium and potassium channels, hypermagnesaemia can cause bradycardia and hypotension (Table 14.2). Hypermagnesaemia can also cause hypocalcaemia, possibly by inhibiting the release of parathyroid hormone. Hyperkalaemia has also been associated with hypermagnesaemia.[1]

Treatment

Hypermagnesaemia can be prevented by not using magnesium-containing antacids or cathartics in patients with renal insufficiency. Patients with normal renal function will usually recover after the infusion or oral intake of magnesium-containing compounds stops. Intravenous calcium can be used as an antidote for hypotension and respiratory depression. In patients with severe renal dysfunction, dialysis may be required.[1]

◯ Summary

Disturbances in magnesium homeostasis can lead to serious conditions some of which are only amenable to treatment with magnesium. Doctors must remember to measure magnesium especially in patients who are at risk. Patients with hypocalcaemia and hypokalaemia who are magnesium deficient should be treated with magnesium. Hypermagnesaemia can be prevented by not using magnesium-containing compounds in patients with renal insufficiency.

References

1. Topf J.M. and Murray P.T. Hypomagnesemia and hypermagnesemia. *Rev Endoc Metab Disord* 2003; 4: 195–206.

2. Gums J.G. Magnesium in cardiovascular and other disorders. *Am J Health-Syst Pharm* 2004; 61: 1569–76.

3. Fox C., Ramsoomair D. and Carter C. Magnesium: its proven and potential clinical significance. *South Med J* 2001; 94: 1195–201.

4. Schlingmann K.P., Konrad M. and Seyberth H. Genetics of hereditary disorders of magnesium homeostasis. *Pediatr Nephrol* 2004; 19: 13–25.

5. Moe S.M. Disorders of calcium, phosphorus, and magnesium. *Am J Kidney Dis* 2005; 45: 213–18.

6. Whang R., Hampton E.M. and Whang D.D. Magnesium homeostasis and clinical disorders of magnesium deficiency. *Ann Pharmacother* 1994; 28: 220–6.

7. Navarro-Gonzalez J.F., Mora-Fernandez C. and Garcia-Perez J. Clinical implications of disordered magnesium homeostasis in chronic renal failure and dialysis. *Semin Dial* 2009; 22: 37–44.

8. Tso E.L. and Barish R.A. Magnesium: clinical considerations. *J Emerg Med* 1992; 10: 735–45.

9. Tietz N.W., Burtis C.A., Ashwood E.R. and Bruns D.E., eds. *Tietz Textbook of Clinical Chemistry and Molecular Diagnostics.* St Louis, MO: Elsevier Saunders, 2006.

10. Arnaud M.J. Update on the assessment of magnesium status. *Brit J Nutr* 2008; 99: S24–36.

11. Broeren M.A.C., Geerdink E.A.M., Vader H.L. and van der Wall Bake A.W.L. Hypomagnesemia induced by several proton pump inhibitors. *Ann Intern Med* 2009; 151: 755–6.

12. Cundy T. and Dissanavake A. Severe hypomagnesaemia in long-term users of proton-pump inhibitors. *Clin Endocrinol (Oxf)* 2008; 69: 33–41.

13. Knoers N.V.A.M. Inherited forms of renal hypomagnesaemia: an update. *Pediatr Nephrol* 2009; 24: 697–705.

14. Todd A.R., Hoenderop J.G. and Bindels R.J. Molecular determinants of magnesium homeostasis: insights from human disease. *J Am Soc Nephrol* 2008; 19: 1451–8.

15. Xi O., Hoenderop J.G. and Bindels R.J.M. Regulation of magnesium reabsorption in DCT. *Euro J Physiol 2009*; 458: 89–98.

16. Musso C.G. Magnesium metabolism in health and disease. *Int Urol Nephrol* 2009; 41: 35–62.

17. Fluid and Electrolyte Guidelines Working Party, Safe Medication Practice Unit. *Prescribing Intravenous Fluids And Electrolytes*. 3rd edn. Queensland Health, 2008. [Available on request from Queensland Health]

18. Bringhurst F.R., Demay M.B., Krane S.M. and Kronenberg H.M. Bone and mineral metabolism in health and disease. In: Kasper D.L., Braunwald E., Fauci A.S., Hauser S.L., Longo D.L. and Jameson J.L., eds. *Harrison's Principles Of Internal Medicine*. 16th edn. New York: McGraw-Hill; 2005. Chapter 331.

15 Hyperuricaemia

B.T. Emmerson

Synopsis

When an elevated serum urate concentration is found the cause needs to be sought. Both genetic and environmental factors will contribute. In practice the major significant risk from hyperuricaemia is the development of gouty arthritis.

Introduction

In the apparently normal population the distribution of serum urate concentrations is skewed towards higher values as it includes many subjects who are asymptomatic at the time but who later develop gout. Even the 95% population range includes many who will later develop gout. It is therefore difficult to define the upper limit of the 'normal' serum urate. Pragmatically, the best value to choose is the point at which there is minimal overlap between the curves of the distribution of the serum urate concentration range in the healthy population compared with that in a population with gout. This overlap occurs at a value of approximately 0.42 mmol/L in males and 0.36 mmol/L in females. Approximately 7% of the apparently normal male population have serum urate concentrations greater than these values. These values are internationally accepted and provide useful bases for interpreting the clinical significance of hyperuricaemia. As gout can occur in patients whose uric acid concentration is within the reference range, microscopic examination and culture of aspirated joint fluid may be necessary to distinguish between gout, pseudogout and septic arthritis.

The serum urate rises in normal males at puberty by approximately 0.06 mmol/L and in normal females at the menopause by a similar amount. The annual risk of acute gout in a patient with a serum urate concentration of 0.54 mmol/L is approximately 5% or 1 in 20. This risk does not justify the treatment of asymptomatic hyperuricaemia although it would do so in someone who had already suffered acute attacks of gout. This reassurance does not necessarily carry over to patients with persistent hyperuricaemia greater than 0.6 mmol/L.

◘ Technical aspects

Current autoanalyser techniques for measuring the serum urate concentration in both serum and urine can be regarded as being reliable for all clinical purposes.

◘ Physiological aspects

Hyperuricaemia results from an imbalance between the production and excretion of urate. Urate is principally produced by de novo nucleoprotein production and metabolism, from dietary purine consumption and by the degradation of ATP within the body at a rate faster than can be reutilised. Two-thirds of the urate that is produced is excreted in the urine and one-third is eliminated in intestinal secretions by a passive process.

Elimination of urate by the kidney is determined by the renal clearance of urate, which is principally under genetic control (Table 15.1). There is, however, a wide range in the normal urate clearance (4–14 mL/min) and this reflects the wide variation in the ability of apparently normal subjects to eliminate urate by the renal route. A number of different racial groups in the Pacific area appear to have inherited a reduced ability to excrete urate, as reflected by a reduced urate clearance. Renal excretion of urate is also modified by a variety of conditions including the presence of renal disease, the consumption of drugs that retain urate (such as thiazide diuretics or low dose salicylate therapy), hypertension, the effect of lactate, ketones or angiotensin on the kidney tubule, and any factors which cause plasma volume contraction or a urine volume of less than 1 mL/min. Hyperuricaemia can also result from an increase in the production of urate, particularly when it is not matched by an increase in renal excretion. Thus a high purine diet (particularly one containing much flesh or nuclear material) will contribute as will the consumption of alcoholic beverages. This occurs first because the alcohol is metabolised to lactate, which acts to reduce the renal excretion of urate; second, because it increases ATP degradation to AMP and the purine bases; and third because of the purines which originate in yeast and which are contained in beer. Obesity is also associated with both increased production and reduced excretion of urate and is a common contributor to hyperuricaemia. The common pattern in this country of regular beer consumption associated with obesity, hypertriglyceridaemia and the insulin resistance syndrome is also frequently associated with the development of hyperuricaemia and gout.

Table 15.1 Common causes of sustained hyperuricaemia

1. Inherited reduction in urate excretion	
Low urate clearance in an otherwise normal kidney	
2. Acquired reduction in urate excretion	
Drugs	Thiazide diuretics Low dose salicylate
Metabolites	Lactate Ketones Angiotensin Vasopressin
Renal	Plasma volume contraction Hypertension Reduced urine flow rate ($<$ 1 mL/min)
3. Acquired increase in urate production	
High purine (nucleoprotein) intake, especially meat and seafood	
Regular alcohol consumption, especially beer and spirits	
Obesity and hypertriglyceridaemia with insulin resistance	
Tissue hypoxia due to systemic disease	
Myeloproliferative disorders	
Tumour lysis syndrome (acute nucleoprotein degradation following cytotoxic chemotherapy)	

QUICK FLICK 15

Many of the factors contributing to hyperuricaemia can be corrected when identified and this can lead to a fall in the serum urate concentration to within the normal range. However, this approach does require considerable motivation on the part of the patient. Any weight loss should be gradual. Weight loss should never be sufficient to induce ketosis as this would reduce the renal excretion of urate and aggravate the hyperuricaemia.

◑ Is the result abnormal?

If the cause of the hyperuricaemia is not apparent from the history and examination of the patient, it can be investigated by measuring the fall in the serum and urine urate concentrations after 1 week of dietary purine restriction. This will give an indication of the contribution of the patient's diet to the hyperuricaemia and allow the urate clearance to be calculated as well as the 24-h urinary urate excretion on a low purine diet. If this value is greater than 4 mmol/24 h on a low purine diet, the presence of excessive production of urate and the need to use xanthine oxidase inhibiting drugs are suggested.

◯ What action is needed if the result is abnormal?

The cause of hyperuricaemia can be determined either from the history and examination alone or by the investigations already suggested. Many of these causes can be corrected. If recurrent gout is present, however, and the patient feels that prevention of further attacks is justified by regular medication, then therapy with urate-lowering drugs is desirable. The goal should be to have a serum urate persistently below 0.36 mmol/L and the dose of drug given (either a xanthine oxidase inhibitor or a uricosuric agent) should be adjusted to achieve this goal. The initiation of such therapy in a patient with gout may precipitate an acute attack of gouty arthritis. This risk may be reduced by the concomitant administration of prophylactic colchicine (0.5 mg once or twice a day) or NSAIDs until there has been no gout for 6–12 months.

◯ Summary

The principal complications of hyperuricaemia are gout and renal colic. Simple clinical and laboratory assessment can usually identify factors contributing to the hyperuricaemia and attention can then be paid to their correction. If this is insufficient and gout remains a problem, urate-lowering drugs can be given on a regular basis and this should prevent future adverse effects. Asymptomatic hyperuricaemia should be regarded as an associated disorder, the cause of which should be sought and corrected where possible. It should rarely be treated with medication.

Further reading

Emmerson B.T. *Getting Rid of Gout—A Guide to Management and Prevention*. 2nd edN. Melbourne: Oxford University Press, 2003.

Emmerson B.T. The management of gout. *NEJM* 1996; 334: 445–51.

Emmerson B.T. Hyperuricaemia and gout. In: Noe D.A. and Rock R.C., eds. *Laboratory Medicine—The Detection and Interpretation of Clinical Laboratory Studies*. Philadelphia: Williams & Wilkins, 1994.

Emmerson B.T. Identification of the causes of persistent hyperuricaemia. *Lancet* 1991; 337: 1461–3.

McGill NW. Management of gout: beyond allopurinol. *Intern Med J* 2010; 40: 545–53.

16 Liver function tests

L.W. Powell, M.L. Bassett and W.G.E. Cooksley

◗ Introduction

An almost bewildering array of liver function tests is available for assessing the patient with suspected liver disease. Many of these are currently included in standard biochemical screens and clinicians are faced with an increasing number of abnormal tests to interpret. This review is designed to help the clinician assess, in particular, abnormal first-line screening tests and to determine when more expensive and specialised second-line biochemical or radiological and scanning procedures are required.

◗ Liver function tests

Liver function tests often included in biochemical profiles include total bilirubin, conjugated bilirubin, alkaline phosphatase, alanine transaminase, aspartate transaminase, gamma glutamyl transpeptidase (GGT), serum albumin and serum globulin.

The term 'liver function tests' is really a misnomer as few of these investigations really assess liver function; most are based on some property of the damaged hepatocyte or bile canaliculus. Nowadays, with increasing use of liver transplantation there is a need to assess liver function. Thus hepatologists usually distinguish between tests of hepatocyte damage (transaminases) or, in the case of biliary tract disorders, tests of cholestasis (serum alkaline phosphatase, GGT) and tests of synthetic function which include serum albumin and the measurement of prothrombin time. Many of the tests lack specificity. For example, elevated serum bilirubin or enzyme levels are encountered not infrequently in patients without primary liver disease (e.g. those with infection, trauma and cardiac failure). The difficulty arises in determining the probability of the presence of underlying liver disease and in the need to pursue the abnormal result further.

A rational and accurate interpretation of liver function tests requires a minimum knowledge of the relevant physiology and biochemistry. A discussion of this is outside the scope of the present chapter and interested readers are referred to standard texts.[1] However, several points warrant particular emphasis.

⊙ Is the result abnormal?

Serum bilirubin

In patients with normal enzymes and an unexplained elevation of serum total bilirubin, both conjugated and unconjugated fractions should be measured. This is important in the early detection of disorders associated with predominantly unconjugated hyperbilirubinaemia (e.g. Gilbert's syndrome, haemolysis) and in differentiating them from hepatobiliary diseases. This distinction may avoid much unnecessary investigation and anxiety on the part of both patient and doctor. Bilirubin in the urine occurs only when the serum conjugated bilirubin is raised and always indicates hepatobiliary disease.

Serum transaminases

Serum alanine aminotransferase (ALT)

This aminotransferase enzyme is present in high concentration in the hepatocyte. The highest serum ALT levels are found in acute viral hepatitis, drug hepatitis (e.g. paracetamol overdose) and ischaemic hepatic necrosis, when levels are frequently in excess of 1 000 U/L. However, there is only a crude quantitative correlation between serum levels and the extent of liver necrosis, and the height of the elevation is not a useful index of either severity or prognosis. A persistently elevated ALT level 6 months after an attack of viral hepatitis suggests chronic hepatitis and is an indication for further investigation, including liver biopsy. Lesser degrees of transaminase elevation are seen in many hepatobiliary diseases such as alcohol-related and drug hepatitis, chronic active hepatitis, intrahepatic and extrahepatic cholestasis, and hepatic neoplasms.

This enzyme is more specific for liver and is now routinely included in multiple biochemical analyses. As a result of studies in Asia, America and Europe in selected blood donors and in health insurance studies it has been suggested that the reference range should be lower, possibly < 30 IU for males and < 19 IU for females. There is no clear cut-off and arguments against using these figures relate to unnecessary anxiety and investigation as well as medicolegal implications. Laboratories therefore vary in their reference range. ALT is widely used in the management of patients with chronic hepatitis B and C. The level is usually higher than the aspartate aminotransaminase (AST) with one important exception: acute alcoholic hepatitis where the ALT:AST ratio may be 1 or less. In milder forms of liver injury the ALT level may be abnormal when the AST is still within the normal range. As patients progress from chronic hepatitis to cirrhosis the AST is often elevated but it is not as reliable as a decreasing platelet count.

Serum aspartate aminotransaminase (AST)

This aminotransferase enzyme is present in high concentration in the hepatocyte but is also present in the heart, skeletal muscle and kidney. Thus elevated serum levels are encountered frequently in ischaemic heart disease and with muscle injury (e.g. after intramuscular injections and rhabdomyolysis).

Serum alkaline phosphatase (AP)

This enzyme arises primarily from liver, bone and placenta. Hepatic alkaline phosphatase is associated with the biliary canalicular microvilli. Marked elevations are characteristic of intrahepatic cholestasis and extrahepatic obstruction although lesser elevations occur in many types of liver diseases. Alkaline phosphatase of bony origin may be distinguished from hepatic alkaline phosphatase by measuring serum 5'nucleotidase (5NT) which is specific for liver disease but, if the GGT is also elevated, it is likely that the alkaline phosphatase originates from the hepatobiliary system. Most laboratories can also identify hepatic and bone isoenzymes of alkaline phosphatase.

Serum gamma glutamyl transpeptidase (GGT)

GGT is found mainly in liver, kidney and muscle. It is a microsomal enzyme and increased serum levels occur following microsomal induction, particularly by alcohol, herbal remedies and drugs as well as microsomal injury from any cause. The main clinical applications of GGT levels are as a sensitive index of early liver disease or of continued heavy drinking in alcoholism.

Serum albumin

Albumin is synthesised exclusively by the liver. A low serum albumin may reflect chronic impairment of albumin synthesis by the liver although other causes such as shifts in albumin or fluid between compartments also alter serum albumin. A low serum albumin due to liver disease usually indicates a chronic disease process. In contrast the prothrombin time will be prolonged at an earlier stage of liver failure because of the shorter half-life of the coagulation factors synthesised by the liver, especially factor VII. The liver is the major site of synthesis of many coagulation factors. In addition vitamin K malabsorption (e.g. complicating severe or prolonged cholestasis) will reduce the synthesis of the vitamin K dependent factors, II, VII, IX and X. Thus, serum albumin and prothrombin time can be regarded as useful tests of liver function. Serum immunoglobulins are not tests of liver function but the levels are often elevated in liver disease, particularly in chronic autoimmune liver diseases.

○ What action is needed if the result is abnormal?

There are two situations that may be encountered clinically.

The serum bilirubin level is elevated but the enzyme levels are normal

In this situation one should recheck the history with a few specific questions. Does the patient suffer from non-hepatic illness (e.g. cardiac failure) which may affect hepatic handling of bilirubin? Is there a family history of haemolytic disease (e.g. thalassaemia) or of congenital disorders (e.g. Gilbert's syndrome)? Is the elevated serum bilirubin level predominantly conjugated or unconjugated?

It is worth noting that significant liver disease is rarely present if elevation of the serum bilirubin is the only persistent abnormality.

The serum enzymes are elevated with or without elevation of the serum bilirubin level

In this situation an appropriate procedure is as follows:

1. Consider the possibility of non-alcoholic fatty liver disease (NAFLD) or non-alcoholic steatohepatitis (NASH), now the commonest cause of elevated serum transaminase levels in our community. Associated conditions are obesity, elevated body mass index, diabetes and hyperlipidaemia.

2. Check the history for features suggesting acute or chronic viral hepatitis (recent travel, history of needle sharing—often years previously in the case of hepatitis C—and an ethnic background that may suggest hepatitis B) and for exposure to drugs (prescription, over-the-counter and alternative therapy), especially excessive alcohol intake. Some patients develop hepatic damage when taking as little as 40 g of ethanol (approximately four drinks per day), especially women, although most patients with alcoholic liver disease consume at least 100 g ethanol daily (approximately 10 standard drinks per day). Although it is common knowledge that heavy drinkers frequently underestimate their alcohol intake it is surprising how often alcoholic liver disease is overlooked as a diagnosis. Similarly as more and more medications are introduced it becomes increasingly difficult to predict hepatotoxicity and the medical practitioner needs to have available a comprehensive list of the side effects of all medications. Hepatotoxicity due to medications usually appears within the first 3 months of commencement of the medication, but there are some notable exceptions (e.g. methotrexate). If in doubt, the suspected drug should be stopped, particularly if alternative therapy is available.

3. Repeat the test on a further occasion to confirm the presence of a persistent abnormality before proceeding further.

4. Look for other conditions that may cause abnormal liver function tests, such as obesity, cardiac failure, chronic infections, thyrotoxicosis, diabetes mellitus, inflammatory bowel disease, coeliac disease, connective tissue diseases, haematological malignancies and disseminated malignancy. Arrange appropriate investigations depending on the degree of clinical suspicion.

5. If persistent and unexplained elevation is present, further (second- or third-line) investigations are indicated to determine the aetiology of the disorder. At this stage the clinician should make a conscious distinction between hepatocellular or cholestatic liver disease although in many cases, particularly with medication-induced liver injury, a mixed hepatocellular-cholestatic picture is present.

Hepatocellular or mixed hepatocellular-cholestatic pattern

If the abnormalities point to hepatocellular or mixed hepatocellular/cholestatic disease, the most helpful definitive investigation is liver biopsy. An ultrasound examination of the liver should be performed first to look for evidence of malignancy (primary or secondary), increased echogenicity (suggestive but not diagnostic of fatty infiltration) and evidence of cirrhosis and portal hypertension. Complementary tests that are helpful in determining aetiology, and in some cases may give a firm diagnosis without the need for liver biopsy, include:

- serology for hepatitis A, B and C, Epstein-Barr virus and cytomegalovirus
- tissue autoantibodies (antinuclear, smooth muscle and mitochondrial antibodies)
- transferrin saturation (ratio of serum iron to TIBC) and serum ferritin levels and, if these are abnormal, HFE mutations (C282Y and H63D) for haemochromatosis
- fasting triglyceride and glucose levels
- serum copper and ceruloplasmin levels
- serum alpha-1 antitrypsin levels
- serum alpha-fetoprotein (for primary hepatocellular carcinoma)
- tests for acute hepatitis—IgM antibodies against hepatitis A virus and hepatitis B virus (antiHBc). Measuring antibodies against hepatitis C virus (ELISA) and looking for the virus itself (PCR for HCV RNA) are helpful. HBsAg should also be checked.
- tests for chronic hepatitis—HBsAg and IgG antibodies against hepatitis B virus (antiHBc) and hepatitis C. If HBsAg is detected, HBeAg and HBV DNA should be measured. Antibodies against HDV and HEV will be carried out in appropriate circumstances.
- preimmunisation status—IgG antibodies against HAV and HBV.

16

QUICK FLICK

Cholestatic pattern

If the abnormalities point to a cholestatic disease process (predominant elevation of the serum AP with or without elevated conjugated bilirubin) one must distinguish between mechanical obstruction of the bile ducts and intrahepatic cholestasis. Ultrasound examination of the liver and biliary tree is the initial investigation of choice. Computerised tomography is useful in the assessment of possible tumours (e.g. pancreas, primary and secondary hepatic). If dilated bile ducts are demonstrated, one should proceed to more definitive radiological investigations such as cholangiography (either magnetic resonance imaging [MRI] or MRCP). Endoscopic retrograde cholangiopancreatography (ERCP) or percutaneous cholangiopancreatography to demonstrate the cause and site of the obstruction have largely been replaced by MRCP unless a therapeutic procedure is intended. If ultrasound examination does not confirm the presence of dilated bile ducts, percutaneous needle biopsy of the liver is usually recommended. In primary sclerosing cholangitis the bile ducts may not be dilated on ultrasound but MRCP may avoid the need for cholangiography.

Summary

Few areas of clinical medicine illustrate better the need for a thorough history and careful clinical examination than the investigation of suspected hepatobiliary disease. Although sophisticated tests such as ERCP, MRCP and liver biopsy often enable a precise diagnosis, their inappropriate use without proper integration with the clinical findings may result in unnecessary expense and misdiagnoses. It is also important to advise patients that investigation of hepatobiliary disease may involve a small amount of risk, particularly if either liver biopsy or ERCP is required. These investigations should be performed by experienced medical practitioners after other measures have failed to give a firm diagnosis and with full discussion of the benefits and possible complications. Despite the potential for complications, they are extremely useful investigations when used appropriately.

Reference

Fauci A.S., Braunwald E., Kasper D.L., Hauser S.L., Longo D.L. and Jameson J.L., eds. *Harrison's Principles of Internal Medicine*. 17th edn. New York: McGraw-Hill, 2008.

17 Interpretation and significance of a high blood cholesterol

A.M. Dart, C. Reid, G.L. Jennings, R.A.J. Conyers, E.M. Nicholls and H.G. Schneider

Synopsis

The interpretation of blood cholesterol measurements requires an understanding of the magnitude and causes of their biological and analytical variability. Recommendations for limiting such variability include blood sampling under standard conditions and using laboratories performing acceptably in national quality assurance programs. Even with these precautions, management decisions should only be made on the mean results of at least two samples, differing by no more than 0.75 mmol/L.

◐ Introduction

It is important for physicians to be aware of possible pitfalls in the interpretation of cholesterol (and triglyceride) measurements and to appreciate the causes of variability and the ways in which these may be minimised. This chapter will cover the measurement of total cholesterol, HDL cholesterol and triglycerides. *Interpretation of a high cholesterol concentration in the presence of a high triglyceride concentration (> 5.0 mmol/L) can be difficult.* In such circumstances it is usually best to reconsider the significance of cholesterol values after triglyceride values have been lowered.

Since in routine, rather than research, laboratories measurements are made of total cholesterol, high-density lipoprotein (HDL) cholesterol and triglyceride, reference will be made to these, although it must be realised that the pathologically relevant fraction is low-density lipoprotein (LDL) cholesterol. This is generally computed by the Friedewald equation as:

$$\text{LDL cholesterol} = \text{total cholesterol} - \text{HDL} - \text{triglycerides}/2.2$$

◗ **Technical aspects**

Total cholesterol

Analytical problems in total cholesterol measurement stem from two aspects of all laboratory measurements:

1. Precision—this relates to the variability of repeated measurements of the same sample using the same method. Precision or, more correctly, imprecision is reported as the coefficient of variation (CV). This is calculated as standard deviation/mean × 100 and is a measure of the dispersion of results about their mean. For cholesterol measurements a CV of ±5% is currently achievable and a goal of ±3% or better is desirable.

2. Bias—this relates to the divergence between the value assigned to a sample by the method in use and the 'true value' or 'gold standard' value determined by some other generally accepted reference method. Bias in routine clinical measurement of total cholesterol should not exceed 5%.

The effects of different levels of precision and bias are shown in Figure 17.1 and relate to the measurement of a single serum sample with a true total cholesterol concentration of 6 mmol/L. If such a sample is analysed 100 times in a laboratory with a bias of +5% and a CV of ±5%, then 95 of these estimations will be between 5.7 and 6.9 mmol/L. In the remaining five analyses the result would likely be outside these limits. In a laboratory with a bias of –5% (not shown), the corresponding 95% confidence limits would be 5.1 and 6.3 mmol/L. In all these instances any contribution from biological variability is ignored.

Routine cholesterol measurement utilises the enzymatic conversion of cholesterol with the formation of hydrogen peroxide, which can be determined by an associated photometric change. Calibrators are required to convert the measurement of physical change (e.g. optical density change) to cholesterol concentration. Once calibrated, the performance of an assay can be monitored by using a quality control (QC) sample. The Royal College of Pathologists of Australasia (RCPA) and the Australian Association of Clinical Biochemists have established the RCPA Quality Assurance Program (RCPA-AQAP). The QC sample produced for this program is analysed by a direct chemical method. Participating laboratories receive frozen aliquots and report their findings back to AQAP. In turn, the participating laboratories are informed of their performance as well as that of other participating laboratories.

Figure 17.1 The effects of different levels of precision (CV) and bias on the measurement of total cholesterol of serum with a true cholesterol concentration of 6 mmol/L

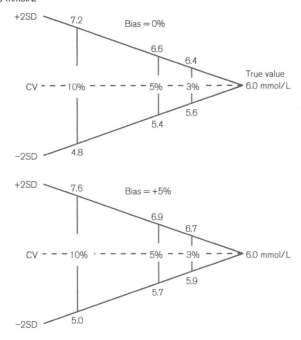

HDL cholesterol

While HDL was previously measured after precipitation of other lipoprotein fractions and the manual step added another possibility of error, the most common methods are now non-separation methods. They use reagents that inhibit the reaction of non–HDL cholesterol and therefore measure preferentially the HDL fraction of cholesterol. The consequence has been a better precision of the assays (regular CVs of 3–4% can now be expected). Very high triglyceride levels do interfere and can falsely elevate the measured HDL level. However, biological variability is now the major cause of variation in results and has been reported to be around 10%. Consequently, small changes in HDL (10–15%) should be noted but not over-interpreted.

Triglycerides

Most methods for triglyceride measurement rely on the conversion of triglyceride to free glycerol, which is subsequently determined. Free glycerol is, however, present in blood and available methods vary as to whether or not 'glycerol blanking' occurs (i.e. the estimation of free glycerol before triglyceride hydrolysis).

◑ **Physiological aspects**

Cholesterol
Even if samples were always measured with complete (100%) accuracy (see above), variation would be found on measuring repeat samples from the same subject. Several factors contribute to this variability, which is present despite overnight fasting or abstinence from food for several hours.

Posture
Blood samples taken in the standing position have higher cholesterol concentrations than those taken with the patients recumbent. Samples should be taken after several minutes' seated or supine rest.

Venous/capillary blood samples
Prolonged venous stasis leads to elevated cholesterol concentrations and should be avoided. Capillary and venous blood cholesterol concentration can differ and therefore a consistent approach should be used.

Diurnal variation
Total cholesterol values vary both diurnally and seasonally. Lowest values are found in the early morning and highest in the evening.

Plasma/serum
Anticoagulants in collecting tubes influence cholesterol measurements to a variable degree. Serum samples are generally preferred.

Physical state
Chronic illness may depress cholesterol levels. In particular, values taken during convalescence after myocardial infarction are depressed. Measurements within 24 hours of admission or 3 months postinfarction are recommended.

Drug therapy
Both prescribed and self-administered drugs may modify cholesterol levels, although triglyceride levels are usually more affected. Interpretation of blood lipid results should be made with knowledge of a current drug history (including alcohol).

Triglycerides

Serum triglyceride values show the greatest variability of all the commonly measured lipid parameters, in large part due to a large biological variation. Accurate triglyceride levels depend on prolonged fasting and are sensitive to weight change and many medications (e.g. diuretics, alcohol and oral contraceptives). A variety of hormones increase lipolysis and therefore free glycerol levels. In addition, levels may be raised in diabetes and liver failure. Long-term biological variability in the order of 10% has also been noted.

○ Uncertainty of measurement

An important question for the treating clinician is whether a change in the measured analyte is a real change or possibly caused by the imprecision of the measurement. In an effort to clarify this issue laboratories will be asked to report their 'uncertainty of measurement'. In the first instance the uncertainty of measurement will take into account only the internal variability of the method and not the bias. For lipid assays laboratories will be reporting the long-term variability of their internal quality-control materials and reporting the mean ±1.96 CV%. Based on the biological variation the desirable analytical CV is less than half the biological CV and this is likely to be achievable for lipids, indicating the maturity of the technologies used.

○ Is the result abnormal/positive?

The concept of abnormal or positive does not apply in any absolute sense to measurements of cholesterol and triglyceride. Rather, values of these parameters need to be considered in the light of the overall clinical picture, principally to assess the risk of macrovascular (particularly coronary) disease and to decide whether specific therapeutic agents are required.

The guidelines for treatment in a particular situation are available from several bodies, most notably the National Heart Foundation and the Pharmaceutical Benefits Scheme (PBS).[1,2]

○ What action is needed if result is abnormal/positive?

Initial therapy for values identified as inappropriately high for the particular clinical circumstances should generally first be treated by dietary modifications. Drug therapy should be instituted only when it is clear that dietary approaches are inadequate to achieve the required lipid levels. In addition, care needs to be taken to ensure that any such elevation is not secondary to some other underlying metabolic process. Thus, for example, an increase in cholesterol may be a manifestation of hypothyroidism, and elevated triglycerides or mixed hyperlipidaemia is commonly found in diabetes, alcohol excess and renal failure.

Once it is clear that specific pharmacological therapy is required, the appropriate choice depends on the nature of the lipid abnormality present.

Hypercholesterolaemia

This is now most commonly treated with a statin drug. Additional and/or alternative agents include bile acid binding resins (cholestyramine, colestipol). Fibrates are more useful at treating mixed hyperlipidaemia. Nicotinic acid is rather infrequently used due to an extensive side effect profile. (See Chapter 18 for further information.)

Hypertriglyceridaemia and mixed hyperlipidaemia

Fish oils are particularly successful in treating high triglyceride levels but have little effect on cholesterol. Fibrates are an effective treatment in mixed hyperlipidaemia, as is nicotinic acid. At present there is no specific treatment available to elevate HDL cholesterol and preliminary trials with experimental drugs have not resulted in improved outcomes. However, most cholesterol-lowering agents, such as statins, do produce a modest (approximately 10%) elevation.

◯ Summary

The technical and biological variations in lipid measurements, together with the fact that their reduction is rarely urgently required (possible exceptions may include severely elevated triglycerides associated with pancreatitis), mean that it is appropriate to obtain at least two and possibly more baseline measurements under standardised conditions before instituting pharmacological therapy. At the present time there is extremely good medication available to lower total (LDL) cholesterol and effective treatment for mixed hyperlipidaemia and hypertriglyceridaemia. Treatment for low HDL is inadequate. This will probably change in the next few years although further trials will still be required to establish that elevation of a low HDL is indeed therapeutically effective.

References

1. National Heart Foundation. *Lipid Management Guidelines (2001)* And *The Lipid Position Statement (2005)*.
2. Australian Government Department of Health and Ageing. *Schedule of Pharmaceutical Benefits*. Canberra: Australian Government Department of Health and Ageing, 2010.

18 Managing hyperlipidaemia: criteria for investigating lipids

P. Nestel

◇ Key principles

Major clinical trials reported in the last decade have established new principles.

◇ Lipid risk factors

The key conclusion from major secondary intervention trials (4S,[1] LIPID,[2] TNT,[3] which included those with chronic kidney disease, Heart Protection Study[4]) is that the reduction in clinical coronary heart disease (CHD) events—for example, mortality and recurrent infarction—is proportional to low-density lipoprotein (LDL) lowering *even when initial levels are normal*. Similar findings emerged from two earlier primary prevention trials (WOSCOPS,[5] AFCAPS[6]). A recent very large placebo controlled RCT called Jupiter showed that rosuvastatin significantly and strikingly reduced cardiovascular events prospectively even in subjects with LDL levels in the low normal range, although the effect was modified by the concentration of hs-CRP.[7] Lowering triglycerides and raising high-density lipoprotein (HDL) cholesterol have recently also been shown to reduce CHD events (VA-HIT[8]). The latter trial, in which LDL levels were normal, shows that triglycerides are an independent risk factor and further increase the risk in combination with low HDL or high LDL; this is supported by much epidemiological data. In the TNT[3] study with atorvastatin, a low HDL concentration remained a significant risk factor even among those in whom LDL was reduced substantially. Reductions of 25–30% in LDL cholesterol reduce first or further events by 30–35%. Recently further trials have demonstrated the benefits of LDL lowering with statins in diabetes (CARDS[9]), in the elderly (PROSPER[10]) and after acute coronary syndromes (PROVE IT[11]), with the latter also illustrating the concept 'the lower the LDL the better the outcome'.

◇ The concept of absolute risk

Full assessment and management of dyslipidaemia (abnormal plasma lipids) requires *full evaluation of other risk factors*. If raised cholesterol is an isolated factor then treatment should not be as vigorous as when there are multiple factors, especially if CHD is present.

Absolute risk is the probability that a subject will have an adverse cardiovascular event within either 5 or 10 years. There are algorithms that provide this information. In general a 10–15% risk over the following 5 years is considered high risk and regarded as a signal for medical intervention. High-risk groups include:

- people with existing clinical cardiovascular disease. If intervention with statins is not inappropriate, these patients do not require prior lipid assessment.
- people with diabetes, such as were studied in CARDS[8]. These appear to be in a similar high risk category but there is as yet no certainty about patients with early uncomplicated diabetes.
- individuals with multiple metabolic abnormalities including hypertension, raised LDL, low HDL and smoking, in whom the calculated risk places them in a high risk category. Age and maleness compound the risk calculation.

Recent research suggests that people with chronic kidney disease, a strong family history of premature cardiovascular disease and possibly the metabolic syndrome associated with abdominal obesity are also at high risk.

Lower risk categories include individuals with one or two less severe abnormalities that do not lead to a 15% risk.

The following multiples of risk are *approximations* derived from several prospective studies:

- existing CHD—five times the risk
- diabetes—four times the risk in women, less in men
- hypertension and associated left ventricular pathology—each doubles the risk
- family history of CHD under the age of 65—doubles the risk
- smoking—doubles the risk
- low HDL cholesterol, *itself a powerful independent risk factor*—doubles the risk
- other lifestyle factors (obesity, physical inactivity) and new factors such as homocysteinaemia—raise the risk by less certain multiples.

Charts of absolute or total risk are available from health organisations, pharmaceutical companies and the internet and are valuable in assessing the need for drugs and in motivating patients.

Additional biomarkers that indicate high risk are being suggested at an increasing rate. The best-validated is hs-CRP, as demonstrated in the Jupiter trial.[7]

◐ Critical importance of CHD

Identifying high-risk patients and treating them strenuously, even when plasma lipids appear normal, *represents the most cost-effective strategy for reducing further events*.

◐ Target for LDL lowering

Trial data from high-risk patients and *in those with existing CHD* suggest that *the target for LDL that had until recently been < 2.6 mmol/L and was then lowered to < 2 mmol/L might be lowered to < 1.8 mmol/L*. There are targets also for triglycerides and for HDL cholesterol but these have not been substantiated in sufficient clinical trials. However, levels of triglycerides > 2 mmol/L and HDL cholesterol < 1 mmol/L are undesirable, especially when raised levels of both are present in two common dyslipidaemic phenotypes, a situation shown by VA-HIT[8] to carry increased risk. However, raising HDL can be difficult since its regulation is strongly genetic. Moderately raised triglyceride levels in individuals with normal LDL and HDL levels mostly do not require treatment with drugs, which is often due to overweight or excess ethanol consumption.

◐ Benefits for most population groups

Recent trials have established benefit for menopausal women that is as great as for men and benefit for the elderly beyond their seventies. Given the powerful effect of age on CHD incidence, lipid lowering may accomplish more and be more cost effective in older people. Statins also benefit children over 8 years, with apparent safety, but should be limited to those with high LDL levels due to familial hypercholesterolaemia and treatment should preferably be initiated in specialist clinics[12].

◐ Comprehensive clinical benefits

Stroke, complications related to peripheral artery disease and most cardiological procedural interventions are also significantly improved with lipid lowering (although the evidence with stroke is less compelling to date). Importantly, atheromatous plaques may become stabilised more readily through depletion of their lipid. Statins and possibly fibrates have multiple effects on atherogenic processes beyond lipid lowering that include anti-inflammatory, anti-thrombogenic and vascular dilatory effects.

◐ Comprehensive screening

All healthy adults—possibly to the age of 80—should be screened for dyslipidaemia at intervals that depend on the total risk profile.

◑ Which lipids?

Adequate information to manage most patients is obtained through current practice: fasting plasma total cholesterol and triglyceride and HDL cholesterol. Calculation of LDL cholesterol is essential and generally included in the report. *Ratios of HDL to LDL or to total cholesterol have limited practical value other than in non-fasting plasmas and are therefore more applicable to population studies.*

◑ Understanding the principles of managing dyslipidaemias

Profile of dyslipidaemias

The five major dyslipidaemias of consequence are:

1. polygenic hypercholesterolaemia, where suboptimal regulation of cholesterol or LDL metabolism predisposes the individual to a lifestyle-induced rise in plasma lipids. Inappropriate eating habits and being overweight are common and often major causes. Initial management should therefore always include an adequate (3 month) period of properly explained dietary and other lifestyle changes. Drug intervention can usually be postponed for longer periods with safety.

2. mixed or combined hyperlipidaemia, which is analogous to the scenario above but also involves abnormal regulation of triglyceride or very low density lipoprotein (VLDL) metabolism. Being overweight and dietary causes, including alcohol excess, are very common and should be managed first.

3. familial hypercholesterolaemia (FH), which generally has higher LDL levels than are found in 1 or 2 and in which the risk for clinical CHD is also greater, demanding more vigorous intervention especially in women after the menopause and in men after the age of about 35 years (the risk being relatively low in young people and premenopausally unless LDL is very high or the woman is a heavy smoker). Although dietary changes can produce some LDL cholesterol reduction, cholesterol levels above 8 mmol/L should be lowered pharmacologically as soon as the high value is confirmed, especially in the presence of other risk factors.

4. familial combined hyperlipoproteinaemia, which is commoner than 3 and is one of the common dyslipidaemias in younger people with CHD. Both cholesterol (LDL) and triglyceride (VLDL and remnants of chylomicrons) are raised and HDL cholesterol is mostly low. The lipid profile can fluctuate: sometimes LDL predominates and sometimes VLDL (triglyceride), generally reflecting changes in environmental factors (weight gain and so on).

5. high triglyceride/low HDL cholesterol phenotype, which is seen increasingly as part of the overweight/insulin resistance or metabolic syndrome. Although the LDL concentration is mostly normal and can even be low, the type of LDL particle, small and dense, may be more atherogenic.

○ Do lipoproteins matter?

The common dyslipidaemias have one thing in common: the abnormalities are in the regulation of the lipoproteins that characterise them.

Further, the body deals with the complex interactions of all lipoproteins while our tests focus on individual lipids and underestimate the many interrelated processes that give rise to abnormal values. Does that matter? *Unexpected responses and failure to lower lipids adequately often reflect the changing balance in lipoprotein regulation that follows therapy.* For instance, LDL (or total cholesterol) may rise when combined hyperlipoproteinaemia is treated with a fibrate, or HDL cholesterol will not rise as expected. The nature and severity of the disordered regulation (mostly due to genetic factors) will determine the response to treatment; two identical lipid profiles may respond quite differently. So don't necessarily suspect the patient!

○ Identification of secondary causes of dyslipidaemia

Diabetes mellitus and insulin resistance associated with being overweight are probably the commonest primary disorders causing secondary dyslipidaemia, mostly the high-triglyceride, low-HDL phenotype. Renal disease poses few diagnostic problems but hypothyroidism, especially in older women, is often overlooked. Mild hypertriglyceridaemia in women on HRT is probably of little consequence.

Lipoprotein (a) (Lp(a)) has been recognised as a potential atherogenic lipoprotein if raised, especially when associated with high LDL cholesterol. It is mainly genetically determined and worth testing when other risk factors are clearly normal. It responds to very few drugs but notably to oestrogens after menopause. The protein apoE that is present in triglyceride-rich lipoproteins has several genotypes, one of which is apoE$_2$, giving rise to a form of combined hyperlipoproteinaemia known as type 3 which is highly atherogenic but usually responsive to statins and fibrates.

○ The role of genes

Virtually all dyslipidaemias have genetic, generally polygenic, influence. The probable balance of environmental to genetic factors should be ascertained from the family history, clinical stigmata of familial hypercholesterolaemia

QUICK FLICK 18

(FH)—eccentric corneal arcus, thickened Achilles tendons) and often from the severity of the dyslipidaemia. FH is the only common monogenic dyslipidaemia. However, the genetic contribution to moderate 'grass-roots' high LDL is at least 25% and some believe it is greater; for HDL cholesterol it is at least 50%. *The extent of the genetic contribution will influence the ease with which treatment succeeds.*

Isolated low HDL cholesterol is mostly genetic. In the absence of a satisfactory drug that raises HDL substantially, the principle is to lower LDL cholesterol to target levels.

Whom to test?

This is no longer as contentious as it once was, since all adults should be tested. However, *in certain categories of patient it is virtually mandatory*:

- people with existing CHD and/or with other vascular atheromatous disorders, although statin therapy is indicated irrespective of lipid values
- people with multiple risk factors
- people with a strong family history of raised lipids or premature CHD
- people with diabetes, in whom dyslipidaemia is very common
- people with renal disease, in whom dyslipidaemia contributes to adverse cardiovascular outcomes.

Other categories are better managed if their lipid profile is known—for instance, menopausal women, people with abdominal obesity and people who drink alcohol excessively.

Why is absolute risk important?

Calculations of absolute risk are based on prospective trials such as Framingham and therefore include risk factors that have been studied. Unmodifiable factors include family history, age and gender; modifiable factors include plasma lipids, blood pressure and smoking status. From these are calculated the probable risk of a clinical event from CHD over the following 5–10 years. This usually focuses a patient's attention. The probability is high for an older person with several risk factors. For a young person aged 20, even the presence of moderate FH, in the absence of other factors carries a relatively low risk that may not justify immediate pharmacological intervention.

Implementing principles of treatment

This is not a guide to detailed therapy, which has been fully covered recently.[15] Several of the above principles are, however, worth re-emphasising:

- Establish the nature of the lipid disorder.
- Assess the total risk.
- Determine the target for LDL cholesterol, triglyceride and HDL cholesterol from the Pharmaceutical Benefits Scheme (PBS) guidelines for lipid lowering[13] or the slightly more aggressive *NHF Lipid Management Guidelines*.[14]
- Maximise non-pharmacological interventions first and throughout treatment. Weight loss of a few kilograms improves the responsiveness to drugs.
- If absolute risk remains high, initiate drug therapy at levels of lipids shown in the guidelines.
- Aim to have patients reach target levels.
- Strive to have the patient maintain compliance.
- Consider ancillary treatments such as aspirin (in severely dyslipidaemic older patients), an antioxidant (like vitamin E) and fish oil, which has recently been shown to be effective in a secondary prevention trial[16]. Folate, which is cheap and safe, may soon be added to reduce homocystine levels.
- Test relatives of all dyslipidaemic patients.

◯ **Comments on pharmacotherapy**

- The advent of statins has greatly eased management, primarily of hypercholesterolaemia and of combined hyperlipidaemia when excess LDL predominates. Statins have different active duration periods. If myalgia occurs (painful muscles only) or creatine kinase (CK) rises moderately without myopathy then small doses of a statin taken as infrequently as second daily may result in a good response with minimal discomfort
- Fibrate is the drug of choice in phenotypes in which triglycerides predominate. Of the two available fibrates, gemfibrozil and fenofibrate, fenofibrate is preferred because it is more active, especially with respect to raising HDL, and is also far safer when combination with a statin is necessary.
- Combining statins with fenofibrate has not been as problematic as originally envisaged and is mostly effective in combined dyslipidaemia. However, the statin dose should be low initially and raised cautiously.
- Fish oils added to a fibrate for lowering triglyceride levels can be effective.
- Adding small amounts of a bile acid-sequestering resin to a statin is useful for reaching LDL cholesterol targets.
- Nicotinic acid is an excellent drug, especially for intractable combined hyperlipidaemia and for severe hypertriglyceridaemia. Some patients tolerate the side effect of flushing by taking aspirin simultaneously.

An extended-release form of nicotinic acid (extended release Niaspan) with a higher content per tablet than is currently available is available in several countries including the USA. ER Niaspan together with an anti-flushing agent laropiprant is currently being trialled. It should prove to be very useful in raising the HDL concentration and generally in patients with severe combined dyslipidaemia. An inhibitor of cholesterol absorption, ezetimibe, is now available. It lowers LDL cholesterol by about 18% when taken alone but together with a statin the effect becomes even greater due to synergy between the drugs. There are activators of the transcription factor PPARα that moderately lower triglycerides and raise HDL.

- Other exciting drugs are in late stage trial. One is an inhibitor of cholesterol ester transfer protein (CETP) which raises HDL cholesterol substantially while also lowering LDL. Although the first such drug, torcetrapib, had an unfortunate adverse effect unrelated to its effect on lipids, several newer compounds are in late stages of trial and appear not to share this problem.

References

1. Pedersen T.A., Olsson A.G., Faergeman O. et al. Lipoprotein changes and reduction in the incidence of major coronary heart disease events in the 4S study. *Circulation* 1998; 97: 1453–60.

2. LIPID Study Group. Long-term intervention with pravastatin in ischemic coronary disease (LIPID) study. *NEJM* 1998; 339: 1349–57.

3. Shepherd J., Kastelein J.P., Bittner V. et al. Intensive lipid lowering with atorvastatin in patients with coronary heart disease and chronic kidney disease. *JAMA* 2008; 51: 1448–54.

4. Heart Protection Study Collaborative Group. MRC/BHF heart protection study of cholesterol lowering with simvastatin in 20 536 high risk individuals: a randomised placebo-controlled trial. *Lancet* 2002; 360: 7–22.

5. West of Scotland Primary Prevention Study Group. Influence of pravastatin and plasma lipids on clinical events in the WOSCOPS study. *Circulation* 1998; 97: 1440–5.

6. Gotto A.M., Whitney E., Stein E.A. et al. Relation between baseline and on-treatment lipid parameters and first acute major coronary events in the Air Force/Texas Coronary Atherosclerosis Prevention Study (AFCAPS/TexCAPS). *Circulation* 2000; 201: 477–84.

7. Ridker P.M., Danielson E., Fonseca F.A.H. et al. Rosuvastatin to prevent vascular events in men and women with elevated C-reactive protein. *NEJM* 2008; 359: 2195–2207.

8. Rubins H.B., Robins S.J., Collins D. et al. Gemfibrozil for the secondary prevention of coronary heart disease in men with low levels of high density lipoprotein cholesterol. *NEJM* 1999; 341:410–18.

9. Colhoun H.M., Beveridge D.J., Durrington P.N. et al. Primary prevention of cardiovascular disease with atorvastatin in type 2 diabetes in the Collaborative Atorvastatin Diabetes Study (CARDS): multicentre randomised placebo-controlled trial. *Lancet* 2004; 364: 685–96.

10. Shepherd J., Blauw G.J., Murphy M.B. et al. Pravastatin in elderly individuals at risk of vascular disease (PROSPER): a randomised controlled trial. *Lancet* 2002; 360: 1623–30.

11. Nissen S.E., Tuzcu E.M., Schoenhagen P. et al. Effect of intensive compared with moderate lipid-lowering therapy on progression of coronary atherosclerosis. *JAMA* 2004; 291: 1071–80.

12. Wiegman A., Hutten B.A., de Groot E. et al. Efficacy and safety of statin therapy in children with familial hypercholesterolemia. *JAMA* 2004; 292: 331–7.

13. *Schedule of Pharmaceutical Benefits* 2005. Canberra ACT: Australian Government Department of Health and Ageing, 2005.

14. National Heart Foundation. *Lipid Management Guidelines (2001)* and *The Lipid Position Statement (2005)*.

15. Nestel P.J, O'Brien R. and Nelson M. Management of dyslipidaemia. *Austr Fam Physician* 2008; 37: 521–7.

16. Yokoyama M., Origasa M., Matsuzaki M. et al. Effects of eicosapentaenoic acid on major coronary events in hypercholesterolaemic patients (JELIS): a randomised open-label, blinded end point analysis. *Lancet* 2007; 369: 1090–8.

19 New cardiac markers

P.E. Hickman and J.M. Potter

Synopsis

The use of cardiac troponins in the diagnosis of the acute coronary syndrome (ACS) has changed our understanding of coronary artery disease. Cardiac troponins are slowly released from necrosing myocardium, so they are detectable in blood for several days. This prolongs the opportunity for identifying an infarction. Cardiac troponins have therefore significantly reduced the diagnostic role of creatine kinase-MB (CK-MB) isoenzyme. Although there is only one assay for cardiac troponin T (cTnT), confusion can arise because there are different non-standardised laboratory assays for cardiac troponin I (cTnI). However, the clinically important issue is the detection of troponin rather than its absolute concentration.

Of other new markers, C-reactive protein (CRP) may have a role in risk stratification but is not currently recommended for routine clinical use. In the context of the future diagnosis of other cardiac conditions, the neuroendocrine hormone B-type natriuretic peptide (BNP) may have a role in diagnosing and monitoring cardiac failure.

◯ Introduction

The cardiac troponins have provided an important new insight into the pathophysiology of the ACS and stimulated new approaches to the management of ischaemic heart disease. They have been so significant in defining myocardial injury that the current Universal Definition of Acute Myocardial Infarction uses the presence of troponin as a central diagnostic criterion.[1]

Other markers are also being studied. These include BNP (a potential cardiac marker for cardiac failure) and high sensitivity C-reactive protein (hs-CRP, as a predictor of future ischaemic heart disease). Many other markers have been proposed, including ischaemia-modified albumin, myeloperoxidase, growth differentiation factor-15 and proteomics.

However, a clear-cut clinical application for these markers remains to be demonstrated.[2]

○ Creatine kinase-MB isoenzyme (CK-MB)

Creatine kinase-MB is a cardio-selective marker but unlike cardiac troponin it is not unique to cardiac tissue. Its use is plagued by false positive and false negative results and it is no longer recommended for investigating possible myocardial infarction.[3]

○ Cardiac troponin T and cardiac troponin I

The troponins are part of the actomyosin contractile apparatus of muscle cells. Structurally unique forms of TnT and TnI are found in cardiac tissue, enabling the development of immunoassays that recognise only the cardiac forms of these two proteins. In most clinical situations both cTnT and cTnI seem to offer similarly useful clinical information.

While most of the troponin is contained within the contractile apparatus a small amount, approximately 5%, is found free within the cytoplasm. When a cardiac myocyte dies the troponin in the cytoplasm is immediately released into the circulation and this is followed by a steady continuing release of troponin from the structural elements of the cell.

Despite extended searching, there is currently no evidence that the cardiac troponins may be produced by tissues other than myocardium. However, the presence of cardiac troponin, while indicating that cardiac injury has occurred, provides no information as to the mechanism of injury. Cardiac troponin concentrations may rise in conditions unrelated to ischaemic damage such as pericarditis, trauma and sepsis.[4] While such rises are related to the severity of the intercurrent illness and are associated with greater morbidity and mortality, they provide no useful information about the likelihood of future ischaemic cardiac disease.[5]

When associated with coronary artery ischaemia even very low concentrations of cardiac troponin predict an adverse outcome.[6] The pathophysiological mechanism for the great majority of cases of the ACS is the presence of an unstable coronary plaque, with release of micro-emboli causing focal myocardial necrosis and release of cardiac troponin. The increased mortality is a reflection of the later separation of a large thrombus from the unstable plaque.[7] This improved understanding of the mechanism of the ACS has led to the current Universal Definition which requires a rise in cardiac troponin to above the 99th population percentile and to a concentration corresponding to a coefficient of variation (CV) < 10% to support a diagnosis of acute myocardial infarction.[1] Very recent information using the new highly sensitive troponin assays (see next paragraph) showed that a substantial proportion of patients enrolled in the GUSTO IV trial and at increased risk of myocardial infarction had troponin concentrations below that corresponding to a 10% CV. A further problem is that so-called healthy populations used to define parameters for troponin in health are often poorly defined and may contain persons with subclinical disease.

A recent development has arisen that may require a rethink about the significance of detectable troponin in blood. New high-sensitivity assays for both cTnI and cTnT have been used for clinical investigation and the cTnT assay has been commercially released. These assays suggest that the majority of normal, healthy persons have detectable cardiac troponin present in blood.[8,9] This finding, together with information which suggests that cardiac myocytes may turn over in healthy persons, suggests that as troponin assays improve and the limit of detection continues to fall, troponin may be found in the blood of all persons, whether healthy or unwell.[10] If this eventuates, the use of troponin in ACS will need to be redefined.

As indicated above, troponin concentration may be increased for reasons other than the acute coronary syndrome. With improvements in both cTnT and cTnI assays as described above, it is very apparent that a troponin concentration should be considered only in the clinical context of that particular patient. Detectable troponin does not by itself equate to the acute coronary syndrome.

◗ Cardiac troponins in patients with renal failure

In Australians undergoing chronic dialysis in 2008, there were 15 deaths per 100 patients and the most common cause of death in these patients was cardiac death—predominantly myocardial infarction and cardiac arrest.[11]

It is reported that a large proportion of asymptomatic dialysis patients have detectable cTnT in their blood and that effectively all the cardiac deaths come from this group.[12] While some of these patients may also have detectable cTnI in their blood, the proportion is much lower. Investigation of cardiac risk in renal haemodialysis patients appears to be one area where cTnT is more informative than cTnI.

While it is known that cardiac disease in dialysis populations is heterogeneous, it has been shown that in the one population of dialysis patients NT-proBNP predicts early death and TnT predicts later death; testing presumably identifies subpopulations with cardiac failure and hypertrophy/ischaemia, respectively.[13]

◗ Problems with assays for cardiac troponin I

Cardiac troponin I is prone to modification in the circulation. It may be phosphorylated and oxidised and can exist as a complex with either cTnT or cardiac troponin C. This has some clinical relevance because the different antibodies used in commercial assays may recognise these different molecular forms to varying extents. A major problem with cTnI assays is that the different assays are calibrated with different standards. The same blood sample may give quite different apparent concentrations in different assays. Progress is being made in standardising cardiac troponin I assays and these differences between assays are being reduced but it is unlikely that they will be totally resolved.

○ B-type natriuretic peptide (BNP)

Commercial assays for BNP and its precursor NT-proBNP are both available. These two forms are often referred to interchangeably as 'BNP'.

The cardiac natriuretic peptide family of neuro-endocrine hormones has a complex physiological role in modulating blood volume and pressure. This involves natriuresis and diuresis as well as antagonism to the renin-angiotensin system. These peptides are also antimitotic and may modulate cardiac hypertrophy.[14] In the presence of left ventricular dysfunction with worsening cardiac failure, the concentration of plasma BNP increases in proportion to the New York Heart Association (NYHA) classification of severity. However, there are a number of other pathophysiological states in which BNP may be elevated, such as hypertension and cardiac hypertrophy, pulmonary hypertension, and renal disease.

While the most appropriate use of this marker remains to be defined, a systematic review has shown that BNP is a strong prognostic indicator of relative risk of death or cardiovascular events for both asymptomatic individuals and patients with heart failure at all stages of disease.[15]

A proposed use for this marker has been to reduce hospitalisation and length of stay in persons presenting to the emergency department with shortness of breath.[16] Recent work suggests that using BNP has little effect on health outcomes or use of health services.[17]

As with cTnI, several different assays for BNP or its associated peptides (e.g. NT-proBNP) have been used in the published studies. As these assays are not yet standardised, numerical values from one assay cannot be compared quantitatively with those from another.

○ C-reactive protein (CRP)

CRP is an acute phase reactant produced by the liver in response to cytokine release during inflammation. It has long been used in clinical practice to follow systemic inflammation, especially bacterial infection. More recently, epidemiological evidence has shown that basal levels of CRP in the absence of apparent inflammatory disease (so-called high sensitivity or hs-CRP) may predict future myocardial or cerebrovascular events.[18]

The value of hs-CRP appears to relate to activity in the atherosclerotic plaque. Among the cellular elements of the atherosclerotic plaque are inflammatory cells that, by releasing interleukin-6, cause secretion of CRP into the circulation. There are a number of biological and analytical problems in using CRP measurements to predict the likelihood of future cardiovascular events. Biological variability in basal CRP concentration is considerable—even mild, subclinical infections can cause significant increases in CRP concentration that are unrelated to cardiovascular disease. The standard deviation for each individual varies from 30% to 63% of the mean value.[19] Thus it might be highly misleading to contemplate using a single measurement to guide possible therapy. A recent large clinical trial found that CRP offered minimal additional benefit over conventional risk markers for cardiac disease.[20]

There are outstanding laboratory problems with use of hs-CRP: not all assays produce identical results and no laboratory has the resources to determine its own reference ranges (the transportability of results between assays is obviously of great importance in defining the concentrations that relate to the different quartiles of basal CRP concentration). At the present time it appears undesirable to use hs-CRP in individual risk stratification.

In patients with coronary artery disease:
- the presence of any cardiac troponin indicates a worse prognosis.
- CK-MB is no longer the preferred marker in the diagnosis of myocardial infarction.
- high sensitivity C-reactive protein and B-type natriuretic peptide are not currently recommended for routine clinical use.

○ References

1. Thygesen K., Alpert J.S., White H.D. et al. Universal definition of myocardial infarction. *J Am Coll Cardiol* 2007; 50:2173–95.
2. Bonaca M.P. and Morrow D.A. Defining a role for novel biomarkers in acute coronary syndromes. *Clin Chem* 2008; 54: 1424–31.
3. Sanger A.K. and Jaffe A.S. Requiem for a heavyweight. The demise of creatine kinase-MB. *Circulation* 2008; 118: 2200–6.
4. Ammann P., Pfisterer M., Fehr T. and Rickli H. Raised cardiac troponins. *BMJ* 2004; 328: 1028–9.
5. Gunnewiek J M. and van der Hoeven J.G. Cardiac troponin elevations among critically ill patients. *Curr Op in Crit Care* 2004; 10: 342–6.
6. Morrow D.A. Evidence-based decision limits for cardiac troponin: low-level elevation and prognosis. *Am Heart J* 2004; 148: 739–42.
7. Hamm C.W and Braunwald E. A classification of unstable angina revisited. *Circulation* 2000; 102: 118–22.

8. Venge P., Johnston N., Lindahl B., James S. Normal plasma levels of Troponin I measured by the high-sensitivity Troponin I Access prototype assay and the impact on the diagnosis of myocardial ischaemia. *J Am Coll Cardiol* 2009; 54: 1165–72.

9. Mingels A., Jacobs L., Michielsen E. et al. Reference population and marathon runner sera assessed by highly sensitive cardiac troponin T and commercial cardiac troponin T and I assays. *Clin Chem* 2009; 55: 101–8.

10. Bergmann O., Bhardwaj R.D., Bernard S. et al. Evidence for cardiomyocyte renewal in humans. *Science* 2009; 324: 98–102.

11. McDonald S., Excell L. and Livingston B. Chapter 3, Deaths. *Thirty-second Annual Report, Australia And New Zealand Dialysis And Transplant Registry, 2009.* www.anzdata.org.au/anzdata/AnzdataReport/32ndReport/Ch03.pdf (accessed 23 April, 2010).

12. Dierkes J., Domrose U., Westphal S., Ambrosch A., Bosselman H-P., Neumann H. and Luley C. Cardiac troponin T predicts mortality in patients with end-stage renal disease. *Circulation* 2000; 102: 1964–9.

13. McGill D., Talaulikar G., Potter J. et al. Over time, high-sensitivity TnT replaces NT-proBNP as the most powerful predictor of death in patients with dialysis-dependent chronic renal failure. *Clin Chim Acta* 2010;doi:10.1016/j.cca.2010.03.004.

14. Chen H.H. and Burnett J.C. Jr. The natriuretic peptides in heart failure: diagnostic and therapeutic potentials. *Proc Assoc Am Physician* 1999; 111: 406–16.

15. Doust J.A., Pietrzak L., Dobson A. and Glasziou P.P. How well does B-type natriuretic peptide predict death and cardiac events in patients with heart failure: systematic review. *BMJ* 2005; 330: 625–7.

16. Mueller C., Scholer A., Laule-Kilian K. et al. Use of B-type natriuretic peptide in the evaluation and management of acute dyspnoea. *NEJM* 2004; 350: 647–54.

17. Schneider H-G., Lam L., Lokuge A. et al. B-type natriuretic peptide testing, clinical outcomes and health services use in emergency department patients with dyspnoea. *Ann Intern Med* 2009; 150: 365–71.

18. Ridker P.M. High-sensitivity C-reactive protein: potential adjunct for global risk assessment in the primary prevention of cardiovascular disease. *Circulation* 2001; 103: 1813–18.

19. Campbell B., Badrick T., Flatman R. and Kanowski D. Limited clinical utility of high-sensitivity plasma C-reactive protein assays. *Ann Clin Biochem* 2002; 39: 85–8.

20. Melander O., Newtone-Cheh C., Almgren P. et al. Novel and conventional biomarkers for prediction of incident cardiovascular events in the community. *JAMA* 2009; 302: 49–57.

20 B-type natriuretic peptide: a new diagnostic tool for congestive heart failure

B. Ewald

Synopsis

B-type natriuretic peptide (BNP) and the related NTproBNP are released
from the ventricle of patients with heart failure. High concentrations
help to distinguish heart failure (HF) from other causes of dyspnoea.
The test detects heart failure with either diastolic or systolic ventricular
dysfunction but is also elevated in left ventricular hypertrophy. Trials in
general practice show it to be of most use in excluding heart failure
in patients with concurrent respiratory disease.

◯ Introduction

The diagnosis of heart failure rests on three elements: suitable signs and
symptoms, objective evidence of ventricular dysfunction and response to
treatment. While the diagnosis is generally clear when the patient has obvious
clinical or radiological pulmonary oedema, it can be difficult to make when
the condition is less advanced or the patient has comorbidities such as lung
disease. Symptoms can be scored using the Framingham criteria. However,
one recent study compared the Framingham criteria against diagnoses made
by two cardiologists with access to echocardiographic results for 1586 acutely
dyspnoeic patients presenting to emergency wards and found concordance
in only 73% of patients.[1] Improved ways of detecting heart failure would
therefore be of great clinical benefit.

It is now recognised that only half the patients with clinical heart failure
have left ventricular systolic dysfunction (LVSD) as measured by a reduced
ejection fraction. Many have good systolic contraction but impaired diastolic
relaxation, so a diagnostic test for heart failure must detect the condition both
with and without reduced ejection fraction.

Objective evidence of ventricular dysfunction is currently obtained from
echocardiography, nuclear medicine or catheter studies. Catheter studies
and nuclear medicine are invasive, expensive and not widely available.
Echocardiography is more widely available but requires waiting for and

travelling to an appointment, which can be difficult for frail, aged or rural patients. Confirmation of HF by a simple blood test would therefore be a very attractive alternative.

○ Physiology

Four neurohormonal systems are activated by ventricular dysfunction. These are the sympathetic nervous system, the renin-angiotensin-aldosterone system, the endothelin pathway and the natriuretic peptides. All these systems maintain systemic tissue perfusion and the first three also maintain blood pressure, which is advantageous in the short term but deleterious to the heart in the long term.

The natriuretic peptides produce diuresis, natriuresis and vasodilatation. These effects reduce the load on the heart and work in opposition to the renin-aldosterone system and the sympathetic nervous system. Although natriuretic peptides are increased in heart failure their effects are overwhelmed by the activated renin-angiotensin-aldosterone system and sympathetic nervous system. B natriuretic peptide (BNP) was originally called 'brain natriuretic peptide' as it was found in the brains of pigs. It is produced by the ventricle in response to increased end diastolic pressure or volume.

○ B-type natriuretic peptide (BNP)

When stimulated by stress or stretch, ventricular myocytes produce the 108 amino acid peptide ProBNP. Before excretion this peptide is cleaved to produce an inactive 76 amino acid N-terminal fragment (NTproBNP) and the C-terminal 32 amino acid with hormonal activity (BNP). The plasma half-life of BNP in vivo is 18–22 minutes while that of NTproBNP is 60–120 minutes.

Available assays measure either NTproBNP or BNP. There are currently several assays available that do not give directly comparable results. Individual laboratory reference ranges should therefore be used. BNP results in pg/mL can be converted to pmol/L by multiplying by 0.289, and NTproBNP results in pg/mL can be converted to pmol/L by multiplying by 0.118.

When BNP rises in response to ventricular stretch it tends to go very high, which gives it good discriminatory power in separating ventricular causes from other causes of dyspnoea. In one series of patients presenting to an emergency department with shortness of breath, those without heart failure had a mean BNP concentration of 38 pg/mL while those with heart failure averaged 1 076 pg/mL.[2] There are several commercial kits for measuring BNP and NTproBNP on laboratory autoanalysers and one kit for bedside measurement (although at approximately $60 per test it is about double the cost of the laboratory-based test). Due to its longer half-life NTproBNP is more strongly affected by age and renal impairment than BNP and it is proposed that a different cut point should be used for those over 75 years of age. In head-to-head tests there is generally a small advantage of BNP over NTproBNP in diagnostic accuracy.

In normal populations the level of BNP is higher in women than men and increases with age. It is also higher in patients with renal impairment, lower in the obese and shows a transient peak in the week after myocardial infarction.

◯ Test validity

A systematic review found 21 published studies examining the diagnostic validity of BNP to detect clinical (systolic or diastolic) HF in symptomatic hospital patients or outpatients.[3] Meta-analysis showed that diagnostic performance was quite good with a sensitivity and specificity of around 85%. There was no difference in test performance between inpatient and outpatient settings; however, diagnostic accuracy decreased with age, so the test is of less use in the very elderly. While a new test has to have adequate sensitivity and specificity, to be useful it also has to provide information beyond that available from existing tests. This was nicely demonstrated in a randomised controlled trial of the contribution of natriuretic peptide results to the diagnosis of heart failure by GPs in New Zealand, which showed that NTproBNP made a significant contribution to diagnostic accuracy beyond signs, symptoms, other blood tests and chest X-rays. The main value was the exclusion of HF in those who did not have it.[4] Similar work has been done in emergency departments where randomised trials in dyspnoeic patients showed that the availability of BNP or NTproBNP led to shortened ED visits, fewer readmissions over the subsequent 60 days and cost savings.[5,6]

◯ False positives

BNP is generally higher in women and increases with age, ventricular hypertrophy and renal failure. It can also be elevated in cor pulmonale and in pulmonary embolism. Patients with background HF but an alternate cause of acute dyspnoea will also have high BNP levels.[7]

◯ Cut points

The cut points used in research have varied widely and the values from the various analytic methods are not equal. Laboratories will provide cut points that match their analytic method, which should preferably be age and sex specific.

○ Availability

BNP and NTproBNP are increasingly available at hospital laboratories, and since November 2007 have attracted funding under the Medical Benefits Schedule (MBS) for use in dyspnoeic patients in hospital emergency departments. For patients in general practice, most pathology labs can either do the test or send it on to a reference lab, but there is a patient charge of about $50. The 2007 Medical Services Advisory Committee review of BNP in non-hospital settings concluded that it was a valuable test but recommended against funding it as the potential cost was 4–11 million dollars annually and the patient benefit was not yet quantified. This is despite patient benefit from outpatient echocardiography never having been quantified but still attracting MBS funding of $81.4 million in 2008–9. While it is relatively simple to generate evidence about short duration visits to emergency departments it is unlikely there will ever be evidence about the contribution of a valuable diagnostic test in the outpatient setting where its chief use is in ruling out a diagnosis.

○ Other uses

BNP has been investigated as a screening test for early detection of HF in the elderly and as a management tool in treating HF according to a BNP target. Neither of these is of sufficient value that it can be currently recommended.

○ Summary

BNP and NTproBNP are useful tests for the work up of a patient who is short of breath. The greatest value is to rule out HF in patients with comorbidities, particularly respiratory disease. An elevated BNP needs further investigation, usually with echocardiography to distinguish the various possible causes. The lack of MBS funding is a barrier to efficient diagnosis for patients who cannot afford to pay for the test.

References

1. Maisel A., Krishnaswarmy P. and Nowak R. Rapid measurement of B-type natriuretic peptides in the emergency diagnosis of heart failure. *NEJM* 2002; 347: 161–7.
2. Dao K., Kazanegra H., Amirnovin L., Clopton A. and Hlavin M. Utility of B-type natriuretic peptide in the diagnosis of congestive heart failure in an urgent care setting. *J Am Coll Cardiol* 2001; 37: 379–85.
3. Ewald B., Ewald D., Thakkinstian A., Attia J. et al. Meta-analysis of B type natriuretic peptide and N-terminal pro B natriuretic peptide in

the diagnosis of clinical heart failure and population screening for left ventricular systolic dysfunction. *Intern Med J* 2008; 38: 101–13.

4. Wright S.P, Doughty R.N, Pearl A., Gamble G.D, Whalley G.A., Walsh H.J. et al. Plasma amino-terminal pro-brain natriuretic peptide and accuracy of heart-failure diagnosis in primary care 1: A randomized, controlled trial. *J Am Coll Cardiol* 2003; 42): 1793–800.

5. Moe G.W., Howlett J. et al. N-Terminal Pro-B-Type natriuretic peptide testing improves the management of patients with suspected acute heart failure: primary results of the Canadian prospective randomized multicenter IMPROVE-CHF study. *Circulation* 2007; 115(24): 3103–10.

6. Schears R.M., Olson L.J. et al. Information value of serum BNP in the emergency department for prediction of congestive heart failure diagnosis at discharge. *Ann Emerg Med* 2008; 51(4): 531.

7. Chung T., Sindone A. et al. Influence of history of heart failure on diagnostic performance and utility of B-type natriuretic peptide testing for acute dyspnea in the emergency department. *Am Heart J* 2006: 152(5): 949–55.

R.H. Mortimer

Synopsis

Thyroid disorders can be difficult to detect clinically, but thyroid function tests can assist in making a diagnosis. Measuring thyroid stimulating hormone (TSH) is the first step. If it is abnormal, free thyroxine should be measured. A raised concentration of TSH with a low concentration of free thyroxine suggests hypothyroidism. A low concentration of TSH with a high concentration of free thyroxine suggests hyperthyroidism. Measuring thyroid autoantibodies may help establish the cause of the dysfunction. Different assays can give different results and tests of thyroid function may be affected by drugs and intercurrent illness.

○ Introduction

The thyroid gland secretes thyroxine (T_4) and triiodothyronine (T_3). These hormones are essential for normal growth, development and metabolic function.

Altered thyroid function is common. For example, the prevalence of hypothyroidism may be up to nearly 10% of the general population.[1] As thyroid disorders may not present with classical clinical signs, it is essential to have accurate assays of thyroid function to assist in the diagnosis.

○ Thyroid physiology

The thyroid gland actively transports diet-derived iodide from the blood by means of a cell membrane iodide pump called the sodium-iodide symporter. Iodide then combines with tyrosines in thyroglobulin, mediated by thyroperoxidase, to form T_4 (four iodine atoms) or T_3 (three iodine atoms). The uptake of iodide and the release of T_4 and T_3 are enhanced by TSH, which is secreted by the pituitary gland.

About 90% of thyroid hormone released is T_4 and 10% is the more biologically active T_3. In some hyperthyroid states the ratio of T_3 to T_4 is higher. Both hormones are co-secreted with thyroglobulin and circulate in blood bound to thyroid hormone binding proteins (thyroxine binding globulin, transthyretin and albumin). A very small unbound ('free') fraction is available for uptake by cells. Much of the T_3 in the blood is generated by the liver, after enzymatic removal of an iodine atom from T_4.

TSH secretion is mainly regulated by circulating T_4 (which is deiodinated to T_3 in the pituitary) and to a lesser extent by circulating T_3. There is a classical negative feedback loop between T_4 and TSH. This is log-linear (log TSH is inversely proportional to free T_4), which means that small changes in free T_4 cause large inverse changes in TSH concentrations. Additionally, TSH secretion is regulated by the hypothalamic hormones thyrotrophin releasing hormone (stimulating) and somatostatin (inhibiting) (Fig. 21.1).

Figure 21.1 Pituitary-thyroid physiology

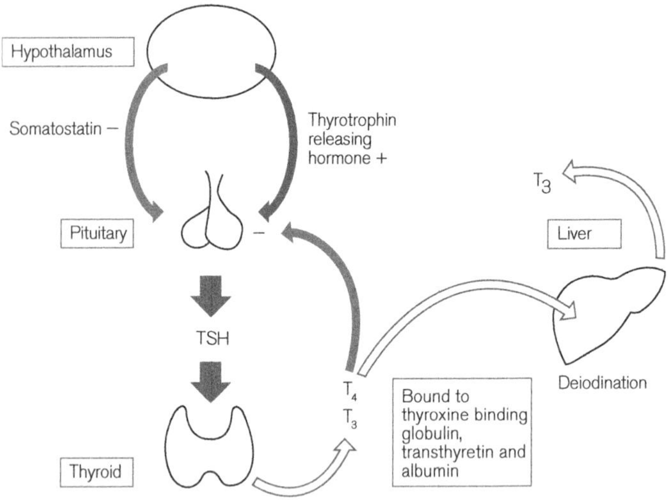

○ Blood tests relevant to thyroid disease

TSH is the hormone which is usually tested. It is the only test funded by the Medicare Benefits Scheme to screen for thyroid disease when there is no history of thyroid problems.

Thyroid stimulating hormone

TSH is a sensitive marker of thyroid function because it is influenced by small changes in free T_4 concentrations. A low TSH usually indicates hyperthyroidism whereas raised TSH usually means hypothyroidism. Over the years the lowest concentration of TSH that can be detected by assays has progressively fallen, allowing better separation of normal and hyperthyroid states.

Thyroid hormone assays

Only very small fractions of thyroid hormones are not bound to protein. These free thyroid hormones are the physiologically important thyroid hormones in blood. Modern immunoassays that estimate free hormone concentrations are widely available.

Altered serum albumin concentrations, abnormal binding proteins, free fatty acids and drugs such as heparin, frusemide and phenytoin may interfere with these assays. Most laboratories now use chemiluminescent methods that are more (but not completely) resistant to such interference. When results do not fit into a recognised pattern the laboratory should be consulted to identify such interferences.

Thyroid-related autoantibodies

If a person has altered thyroid function, testing for thyroid antibodies helps to determine if they have an autoimmune condition.

Thyroperoxidase autoantibodies

Thyroperoxidase antibodies are also known as thyroid microsomal antibodies. They are present in autoimmune thyroid disease, but there is debate about whether low levels are always pathological. Unfortunately, there are significant differences between laboratories when the same sera are studied, and lower detection limits are variable. Assay sensitivities and reference ranges can therefore vary quite widely.

Thyroperoxidase antibodies can cause hypothyroidism in at least two ways. First, they can block thyroperoxidase, thereby inhibiting T_4 and T_3 synthesis; second, they can act through antibody-dependent cell cytotoxicity and thyroid inflammation. Low concentrations may not be associated with evidence of thyroid dysfunction, but the incidence of raised TSH increases as antibody levels rise. The prevalence of positive antibody levels and mild hypothyroidism increases with age.

The concentration of thyroperoxidase antibodies may fluctuate in patients with autoimmune thyroid disease. This has no clinical significance and repeated measurements are not recommended. Maternal thyroperoxidase antibodies cross the placenta, but their effects on fetal thyroid function are unclear.

Thyroglobulin autoantibodies

Thyroglobulin autoantibodies are also markers of autoimmune thyroid disease, but are less common than thyroperoxidase antibodies. Thyroglobulin autoantibodies do not inhibit thyroperoxidase or mediate antibody-dependent cell cytotoxicity and are therefore markers rather than mediators of autoimmune thyroid disease. There are considerable variations in sensitivity and reference ranges between assays. Other autoimmune diseases can also increase the concentration of thyroglobulin autoantibodies.

TSH receptor autoantibodies

TSH receptor autoantibodies may stimulate or less commonly block the TSH receptor. Stimulating antibodies cause Graves' disease and probably also cause the associated ophthalmopathy. Blocking antibodies can cause hypothyroidism. The assay of TSH receptor autoantibodies done in clinical laboratories cannot distinguish between stimulating or blocking antibodies. This is not usually relevant as clinical hyperthyroidism would suggest that the dominant antibody is stimulatory.

Measuring TSH receptor autoantibodies can be useful if the cause of hyperthyroidism is not apparent. However, initial hopes that remission of Graves' could be predicted by falling autoantibody levels have not been supported by most studies.

Measurements of TSH receptor autoantibodies do have an important role in managing pregnant women with Graves' disease. High concentrations of maternal TSH receptor autoantibodies can predict fetal and neonatal hyperthyroidism. It is important to recognise that TSH receptor autoantibodies do not always fall after successful treatment, so pregnant women with a previous history of Graves' disease should be screened for TSH receptor autoantibodies.

Thyroglobulin

Thyroglobulin, a large glycoprotein, represents about 80% of the wet weight of the thyroid and is co-secreted with thyroid hormone. Concentrations are high in patients with raised TSH concentrations or nodular goitres, but it is not clinically useful to measure thyroglobulin in these situations.

Most papillary and follicular carcinomas synthesise and secrete thyroglobulin but raised thyroglobulin levels are not a reliable indicator or screening test for thyroid malignancy. Thyroglobulin concentration becomes a useful marker of remaining or recurrent cancer in patients who have had a total thyroidectomy and remnant ablation with radioiodine for papillary and follicular carcinoma.

Unfortunately, up to 20% of patients with differentiated thyroid cancer have thyroglobulin autoantibodies that interfere with the thyroglobulin assay, leading to underestimation of thyroglobulin concentration. Thyroglobulin autoantibodies should therefore be measured, with a sensitive assay, on all thyroglobulin samples.

Reference ranges

As most commercial assays do not physically measure the analyte, results given are always an approximation of actual levels. Each assay, even for the same analyte, will therefore give slightly different results because of intrinsic variations in the reagents used and the effects of interfering illnesses and substances. Free T_3 levels are the most variable between assay methods.

Reference ranges are altered by ethnicity, age and iodine intake. In Australia these factors are probably not clinically significant. Different ranges also apply in pregnancy, neonates and very young children.

Reference ranges are defined as those into which 95% of a normal population fall. (Accordingly 2.5% of normals will have higher and 2.5% will have lower results than the reference range.) Each assay must therefore be interpreted in terms of its own reference range. The practical implications of this are that blood test results from different laboratories may not be directly comparable and their interpretation requires examination of the reference ranges.

Reference ranges change in pregnancy. In early pregnancy chorionic gonadotrophin is secreted by the placenta in large amounts. This is structurally similar to TSH (but is not measured by the TSH assay) and stimulates the maternal thyroid. This leads to increased maternal thyroid hormone secretion and a reduced maternal TSH. Occasionally women develop mild hyperthyroidism in the first trimester, especially if they have hyperemesis.

Detecting and confirming thyroid dysfunction

The inverse log-linear relationship between free T_4 and TSH means that TSH concentrations are sensitive indicators of thyroid dysfunction. A raised TSH suggests hypothyroidism while a low TSH suggests hyperthyroidism.[2] There are other causes of low TSH concentrations, notably hypothalamic-pituitary disease, but this is very uncommon in the general population. The finding of an abnormal TSH should lead to measurement of free T_4 levels.

Interpreting thyroid function tests may be particularly difficult if the patient is systemically ill. Starvation or severe illness can be associated with dysregulation of TSH secretion and reduced deiodination of T_4 to T_3 (the 'sick euthyroid syndrome'). Low TSH and T_3 levels are typical and can cause diagnostic confusion.

Very occasionally a raised TSH with a normal free T_4 relates to interference in the TSH assay. Very rarely, thyroid hormone resistance or a pituitary TSH-secreting adenoma is associated with a mildly raised TSH in the presence of a raised free T_4.

Treatment with amiodarone is often associated with abnormal thyroid function tests. The most common finding is a raised TSH caused by inhibition of pituitary T_4 to T_3 conversion but true hypothyroidism and hyperthyroidism can occur. Diagnosis and management may be complex and require expert advice.

◐ Hyperthyroidism

A low TSH and raised free T_4 indicate hyperthyroidism and should lead to consideration of causation and treatment. The majority of younger patients will have Graves' disease but older patients are more likely to have nodular thyroid disease.

Transitory hyperthyroidism can be seen in patients with viral thyroiditis. Most have had a recent upper respiratory tract infection and present with neck tenderness and pain, which may be referred to the ear.

Some patients have a low TSH but normal free T_4. Measurement of free T_3 can then be helpful as some patients will have T_3 toxicosis caused by overproduction of T_3. If T_3 is not raised a repeat measurement of T_4 and TSH is warranted. This may show normal values but a persistently low TSH with a normal free T_4 suggests autonomous thyroid function and a diagnosis of 'subclinical hyperthyroidism', which is usually associated with a nodular goitre (or, unusually, hypothalamic-pituitary disease). Subclinical hyperthyroidism in the elderly is associated with an increased risk of atrial fibrillation, stroke and osteoporosis.

◐ Hypothyroidism

A raised TSH and a low free T_4 indicate primary hypothyroidism, almost always due to autoimmune thyroid disease but sometimes due to previous surgery or radioiodine administration. The incidence of raised TSH and thyroid antibody levels and hypothyroidism increases with age and is significantly more common in women.

It is not uncommon to find a raised TSH but normal free T_4. In most cases this suggests autoimmune thyroid disease. This subclinical hypothyroidism is more likely to progress to overt hypothyroidism when higher levels of TSH and thyroid autoantibodies are present.

Asymptomatic patients with a raised TSH and normal free T_4 require regular monitoring, especially if they are elderly or have high levels of anti-thyroperoxidase autoantibodies. Every six months is probably sufficient.

There is considerable debate about the normal upper limit of the TSH reference range. The high background prevalence of autoimmune thyroid disease as well as the age, iodine status, smoking prevalence and ethnicity of the 'normal' population has raised the 'normal' upper limit. In people without these factors the upper limit is probably 2.5 mIU/L. While mildly raised TSH levels rarely require treatment, a concentration above 4.0 mIU/L and the presence of thyroid antibodies is predictive of eventual hypothyroidism and indicates that these patients need to be followed up.[3]

Common results of thyroid function tests are summarised in Table 21.1.

Table 21.1 Common results of thyroid function tests

TSH	Free T$_4$	Free T$_3$	TPO and Tg autoantibodies	Comment
↔	↔	↔	↔	Normal
↑	↓	↓	↑	Primary hypothyroidism (Hashimoto's)
↑	↔	↔	↑	Subclinical hypothyroidism (Hashimoto's)
↓	↑	↑	↑	Hyperthyroidism (consider Graves', measure TSH receptor autoantibodies)
↓	↔	↔	↔	Subclinical hyperthyroidism (consider nodular thyroid disease)
↔↓	↓	↓	↔	Consider pituitary disease
↓	↔	↑	variable	T$_3$ toxicosis

↔ normal, ↑ raised, ↓ reduced; T$_3$ triiodothyronine; T$_4$ thyroxine; Tg thyroglobulin; TPO thyroperoxidase; TSH thyroid stimulating hormone

○ Adjusting thyroxine treatment

Replacement thyroxine in hypothyroid patients should be adjusted to maintain TSH at about 2 mIU/L. It takes about six weeks for a change in thyroxine dose to achieve stable concentrations of free T$_4$. Changes to the dose of thyroxine and tests of thyroid function should not be done more frequently, unless clinically indicated. It is not uncommon for patients who are less than optimally compliant with recommended thyroxine treatment to take several tablets before a doctor's visit. This may be associated with a raised TSH but normal free T$_4$.

Many patients with a history of differentiated thyroid cancer are advised to take suppressive doses of thyroxine. Guidelines suggest that with persistent disease TSH should be kept below 0.1 mIU/L.[4] Patients who presented with high-risk disease, but who are clinically free of disease, are advised to maintain TSH between 0.1 and 0.5 mIU/L for 5 to 10 years. Advice from commercial pathology laboratories that thyroxine doses be reduced in these patients should be resisted.

�‍ Adjusting treatment for hyperthyroidism

TSH may remain suppressed for weeks or even months after a patient starts antithyroid medications. It is useful to monitor free T_4 and free T_3 every 6 to 12 weeks to judge the adequacy of treatment. A rise in TSH indicates overtreatment. Patients with severe hyperthyroidism may need more frequent monitoring.

◍ Summary

Thyroid dysfunction is common in the general population and TSH measurements provide a sensitive method for detection. An abnormal TSH requires further investigation, including at least measurement of free T_4. Interpretation of the results of thyroid function tests is facilitated by an understanding of thyroid hormone physiology, especially the normal inverse relationship between free T_4 and TSH concentrations. Variations in assay performance mean that it may be helpful to consistently use the same laboratory for an individual patient. An understanding of the effects of severe illness and medications on test results is also important.

References

1. Canaris G.J., Manowitz N.R., Mayor G. and Ridgway E.C. The Colorado thyroid disease prevalence study. *Arch Intern Med* 2000; 160: 526–34.
2. Ladenson P.W., Singer P.A., Ain K.B., Bagchi N., Bigos S.T., Levy E.G. et al. American Thyroid Association guidelines for detection of thyroid dysfunction. *Arch Intern Med* 2000; 160: 1573–5.
3. Walsh J.P., Bremner A.P., Feddema P. et al. Thyrotropin and thyroid antibodies as predictors of hypothyroidism: a 13-year, longitudinal study of a community-based cohort using current immunoassay techniques. *J Clin Endocrinol Metab* 2010; 95: 1095–104.
4. Cooper D.S., Doherty G.M., Haugen B.R., Kloos R.T., Lee S.L., Mandel S.J. et al. Revised American Thyroid Association management guidelines for patients with thyroid nodules and differentiated thyroid cancer. *Thyroid* 2009; 19 :1167–214.

22 Evaluating adrenocortical function in adults

J.T. Ho and D.J. Torpy

Synopsis

Adrenocortical disease encompasses overproduction of cortisol, aldosterone or (less frequently) adrenal sex steroids from generally benign tumours/hyperplastic processes or rarely from high mortality malignant adrenal cancer. The diagnosis of early Cushing's syndrome due to cortisol overproduction, or of primary aldosteronism, requires clinical suspicion or a judicious screening strategy along with appropriate biochemical testing. Primary or secondary adrenal insufficiency (apart from that following prolonged corticosteroid therapy) is uncommon, but delayed diagnosis leads to unnecessary morbidity. Widespread use of abdominal imaging has led to increased recognition of the high frequency of benign adrenal tumours in adults—around 15% of these produce excess steroid hormones and early diagnosis may prevent later frank hypersecretory syndromes. Consensus guidelines exist for screening for primary aldosteronism and for endocrine dysfunction in incidentally discovered adrenal tumours. The optimal clinical criteria for screening for Cushing's syndrome in at-risk groups or among individuals without a recognisable clinical syndrome remain controversial. The following brief summary outlines the essential strategies to achieve early diagnosis of adrenocortical disease. The problem of congenital adrenal hyperplasia is beyond the scope of this article.

○ Introduction

The adrenal cortex consists of three functionally separate layers. The outer *zona glomerulosa* produces aldosterone under the stimulatory control of the renin-angiotensin system and potassium. Aldosterone increases sodium reabsorption and potassium excretion in the kidney, gut and sweat glands. The *zona fasciculata* produces cortisol under the control of pituitary adrenocorticotropic hormone (ACTH). ACTH is principally regulated by hypothalamic corticotrophin-releasing hormone (CRH) and responds to diurnal rhythm, stress and negative feedback from circulating cortisol. Cortisol regulates metabolism and during stress restrains and redirects the immune system and accentuates cardiovascular responses. The inner *zona reticularis* produces the adrenal androgens dehydroepiandrosterone (DHEA) and androstenedione. These androgens are elevated in states of increased ACTH release but are regulated independently in fetal life and in early puberty (adrenarche) through incompletely understood mechanisms. The adrenal medulla is part of the sympathetic nervous system and produces noradrenaline and adrenaline. Adrenaline synthesis is facilitated by cortisol from the neighbouring adrenal cortex.

Adrenal testing is based on hormone measurement driven by clinical evaluation. Imaging of the adrenal and pituitary is confounded on the one hand by the frequent presence of non-functioning tumours and on the other hand by hyperfunctional states where the cells do not form tumours that can be resolved by CT scan of the adrenal or MRI of the pituitary. Adrenal testing procedures follow principles common to other endocrine systems. These principles include the use of basal hormone levels for screening, measurements of trophic hormones to diagnose the site of endocrine lesion (e.g. ACTH levels to separate an adrenal from a pituitary lesion in hypercortisolism) and suppression or stimulation tests to diagnose definitively the site and cause of hormone excess or deficiency, respectively.

◯ Testing for hypercortisolism (Cushing's syndrome)

Cushing's disease is defined as excessive ACTH secretion by the pituitary with secondary adrenal hyperactivity. Cushing's syndrome includes conditions of glucocorticoid excess either from exogenous steroid intake, primary adrenal gland hypersecretion or ectopic ACTH secretion from extrapituitary neuroendocrine tumours. The features of Cushing's syndrome are familiar as they are seen with exogenous glucocorticoids which are widely used for their anti-inflammatory efficacy. However, early endogenous Cushing's syndrome is notoriously difficult to diagnose because weight gain, hypertension, diabetes mellitus and mood change are frequent in patients with metabolic syndrome or polycystic ovary syndrome. Later, catabolic features—such as osteoporotic fractures, muscle weakness and skin fragility—may lead to clinical diagnosis but early diagnosis will avoid disability and reduce mortality risk.

There are two major confounders inherent to cortisol testing for Cushing's syndrome. One is that there is a broad reference range for cortisol production, and some Cushing's patients have cortisol production rates within this range. Moreover, this cortisol production may be intermittent or cyclic. Second, some individuals may have transient hypercortisolism and features consistent with early Cushing's but without the progressive catabolic effects of Cushing's. These individuals have 'pseudo-Cushing's', in some cases associated with alcohol abuse or depression. Pseudo-Cushing's may be a consequence of a disordered stress system with a multifactorial basis, perhaps representing the tip of the iceberg in stress-induced disease. No single test is infallible in Cushing's syndrome and values close to literature cut-offs must be regarded with suspicion.[1]

○ Screening tests for Cushing's syndrome

Most cases can be readily diagnosed with a 24-h urine free cortisol (UFC). However, as many as 15% of new Cushing's cases operated on in larger centres have a normal UFC. The overnight 1-mg dexamethasone suppression test (DST) also has a substantial false positive and false negative rates with their relative proportions dependent on the cortisol cut-offs used. The DST appears to have particularly high sensitivity in the diagnosis of early or subclinical Cushing's following the detection of an adrenal incidentaloma. Midnight salivary cortisol levels have been shown to have good validity in research settings and our own experience would bear this out. However, a locally validated assay with high sensitivity for the very low cortisol levels in saliva is essential. Furthermore, indiscriminate use of salivary cortisol testing is likely to lead to excessive numbers of false positives and unnecessary follow-up testing among those with low pretest probability of Cushing's.

24-hour urine free cortisol (UFC)
The UFC provides an integrated assessment of cortisol secretion, thereby avoiding the pitfalls of blood measures including circadian rhythm, pulsatile cortisol release and altered levels of corticosteroid binding globulin. If the laboratory uses a radioimmunoassay (RIA) the result largely reflects cortisol metabolites due to the relatively non-specific antibodies used. High performance liquid chromatography (HPLC) UFC are more specific and results are typically around one-third of those using RIA methods. However, current diagnostic schemata have mostly been developed using immunoassays. In addition, high urine volumes (above 4 L per day) may elevate cortisol excretion. Cortisol excretion rates vary diurnally but urine creatinine excretion does not. Hence, it is not possible to correct an incomplete or over-collection with the 24-h urine creatinine. The creatinine is useful in determining if the urine collection timing was likely to be adequate (e.g. a low 24-h urine creatinine in a large person may suggest under-collection). In addition, in sequential measurements the 24-h urine creatinine should not vary by more than 10%.

False negatives may be seen in patients with early or mild Cushing's syndrome or in those with cyclic hypercortisolism; the latter occurs in 10% or more of Cushing's, depending on how it is defined. Patients with factitious Cushing's syndrome due to exogenous glucocorticoid may have low urine cortisol levels, depending on the assay reactivity of the steroid taken, but pointers to early diagnosis include low ACTH and adrenal atrophy on CT scan. False positive UFCs can be seen in patients with chronic alcoholism, depression, idiopathic pseudo-Cushing's or serious illness.

Late night salivary cortisol

Salivary cortisol levels reflect plasma free cortisol. Only 5–6% of plasma cortisol is free, the remaining portion is bound to corticosteroid binding globulin or albumin. It is this free fraction of cortisol that is closely regulated and biologically active. In Cushing's syndrome cortisol levels are often normal in the morning but elevated at midnight, a time when cortisol secretion is at a diurnal nadir. To measure cortisol at the diurnal nadir, home collection of saliva at midnight or late night/bedtime has been shown to provide a convenient, valid test for excessive cortisol secretion. Saliva collection is achieved with a commercial salivette collection tube with a cotton cylinder. A midnight salivary cortisol measurement is a useful test for the diagnosis of Cushing's syndrome but appropriate assay-specific normative values must be used for its interpretation. Currently, using the Roche assay on the E170 immunoassay analyser in Adelaide we have found a cut-off of 13 nmol/L reliably distinguishes Cushing's from non-Cushing's patients but internationally cut-offs have ranged widely.[2]

Midnight plasma cortisol

Cortisol levels peak around the time of waking, decrease rapidly through the morning and reach a nadir around midnight. Most patients with Cushing's syndrome have early morning plasma cortisol concentrations within or slightly above the normal range. In contrast, their midnight plasma cortisol concentrations are almost always high (> 207 nmol/L). A midnight value less than 120 nmol/L virtually excludes Cushing's.

Low-dose dexamethasone suppression testing (DST)

The overnight dexamethasone suppression test is commonly used as a screening test for Cushing's syndrome. Dexamethasone, 1 mg orally, is given at 11 pm and plasma cortisol measured at 8–9 am the next day. Recently, it has been shown to have high sensitivity in the evaluation of adrenal incidentaloma, where hypercortisolism is the commonest endocrine lesion. However, there is a lack of data to define the natural history of these early or 'preclinical' Cushing's patients. The DST has been variously validated in the past, often with inappropriate controls such as normal volunteers. The ideal cut-off is generally quoted as between 50–140 nmol/L with lower values increasing the false positive test rate. Further, a small proportion of true

Cushing's disease patients suppress below 50 nmol/L.[3] Low cut-off values (50 nmol/L or less) tend to over diagnose Cushing's and high cut-off values (140 nmol/L or above) tend to miss Cushing's cases. False positive results (non-suppression) can occur in acute illness, depression, anxiety, alcoholism, high oestrogen states and drugs that accelerate dexamethasone metabolism.

○ Testing in ACTH-dependent Cushing's

Patients with ACTH-dependent Cushing's should have a high-dose (8 mg) dexamethasone suppression test, corticotrophin releasing hormone stimulation test and in many cases petrosal sinus sampling. These tests are directed towards distinguishing the source of ACTH (pituitary versus ectopic) and are beyond the scope of this chapter.

○ Testing for primary hypoadrenalism (Addison's) and ACTH deficiency

Although fatigue is a key symptom of hypoadrenalism, most fatigued individuals have normal adrenal function. Clinical factors suggesting a need for adrenal testing include low blood pressure, postural hypotension, weight loss, hyperpigmentation, hyponatraemia and hyperkalaemia. Rarely, hypoglycaemia or hypercalcaemia are seen, usually in association with cardiovascular collapse ('adrenal crisis'), often precipitated by stressors such as sepsis, trauma or surgery.

Most cases of Addison's are due to autoimmune adrenal destruction and sometimes there is a personal or family history of other autoimmune diseases. Autoimmune adrenal dysfunction is slowly progressive. Often, aldosterone deficiency, heralded initially by elevated plasma renin levels, develops before hypocortisolism. Testing for 21-hydroxylase antibodies, where available, may be positive in early autoimmune adrenal disease. In general, testing for adrenal hypofunction is most often done by use of a synthetic ACTH stimulation test (measuring cortisol response), ACTH levels (for differential diagnosis) and plasma aldosterone and plasma renin activities with a serum sodium and potassium. A high morning cortisol level may obviate the need for a Synacthen test and can be taken with the other tests described prior to a Synacthen test[4].

Plasma cortisol

An early morning plasma cortisol level below 200 nmol/L, performed within 1 hour of waking, strongly suggests adrenal insufficiency. Conversely, a plasma cortisol level greater than 500 nmol/L excludes the diagnosis. Intermediate cortisol levels may require investigation with a Synacthen stimulation test. The early morning cortisol level is particularly useful within

6 weeks of acute ACTH deficiency (e.g. after pituitary surgery) when adrenal atrophy may not have yet developed and Synacthen testing will be normal.

Plasma ACTH

Measuring plasma ACTH will help localise the cause of adrenal insufficiency—adrenal (primary or Addison's) or pituitary (secondary) or hypothalamic (tertiary). In primary adrenal insufficiency, plasma ACTH is greatly elevated due to a lack of cortisol negative feedback on the hypothalamic-pituitary unit. In secondary or tertiary adrenal insufficiency, ACTH levels are low or inappropriately normal.

Cosyntropin (Synacthen) ACTH stimulation testing

In most cases of suspected hypoadrenalism, a stimulation test using the 1-24 fragment of the complete 39 amino acid ACTH molecule (cosyntropin, marketed as Tetracosactrin or Synacthen) is needed to definitively diagnose cortisol deficiency. Patients with both primary and secondary adrenal insufficiency have an inadequate cortisol peak response to a Synacthen injection. In Addison's disease, a destructive process has left insufficient residual adrenal tissue to respond to ACTH; in secondary insufficiency, loss of the trophic action of ACTH results in adrenal atrophy.

The traditional Synacthen dose of 250 mcg was based on a miscalculation and is more than 100 times the peak dose–response relationship. A 1 mcg dose produces high physiological ACTH levels as opposed to the pharmacological levels achieved with 250 mcg. However, it appears that the benefits of the lower Synacthen dose are marginal in practice, perhaps producing slightly higher diagnostic accuracy in secondary hypocortisolism. Use of the 250 mcg dose, which is the dose available commercially, is preferred. As adrenal atrophy develops slowly, Synacthen testing for adrenal insufficiency should be delayed at least 6 weeks after pituitary surgery. A normal response to IV Synacthen is a cortisol peak value at either 30 or 60 min of > 500 nmol/L. Older fluorometric assays were less specific and led to low cut-off values of 500 nmol/L. The previously recommended additional criterion of a cortisol increment greater than 200 nmol/L is highly dependent on basal cortisol and hence time of day and rarely contributes to diagnosis, except in cases of cortisol binding globulin deficiency where incremental cortisol levels are normal but peak values are low.

It is important to recognise that cases of missed adrenal insufficiency after normal Synacthen testing are described, the reproducibility of testing is imperfect and the test has not been validated against clinical endpoints but has been validated against the 'gold-standard' of the insulin hypoglycaemia test.

Insulin-induced hypoglycaemia (IIH) test

Insulin-induced hypoglycaemia has been extensively evaluated for testing hypothalamic-pituitary-adrenal function. It has several distinct advantages. The test induces endogenous ACTH and cortisol release through activation of hypothalamic CRH release, acting via higher CNS centres. The IIH leads to growth hormone (GH) release and is the test of choice when GH prescription for adults is contemplated. However, IIH is contraindicated in patients with epilepsy, coronary artery disease or arrhythmia. It should probably be avoided in older patients (over 55) because of the risk of occult coronary disease. IIH must be performed with medical supervision as resuscitation with IV glucose is needed for reduced consciousness or hypoglycaemic complications or after satisfactory hypoglycaemic stress is achieved. The standard insulin dose (0.15 U/kg) may be modified in likely hypoadrenalism (to 0.1 U/kg) or in insulin resistance (to 0.20–0.25 U/kg). Hypoglycaemia begins 30–45 min after insulin and the test may be terminated 10 min after the onset of profuse sweating. Glucose reflectance meters have insufficient accuracy for determining onset of severe hypoglycaemia, yet there are usually delays in getting a formal blood glucose from the laboratory. The test aims to produce blood glucose levels of less than 2.0 mmol/L. A normal cortisol peak exceeds 500 nmol/L. Despite the theoretical advantages, the risks, side effects and need for medical monitoring have led clinicians to favour Synacthen testing. Consequently IIH is rarely used in modern practice, even in specialised endocrine clinics, but may be adopted if GH replacement in adults becomes more popular.

Corticotropin-releasing (CRH) hormone test

The use of CRH to test ACTH and cortisol reserve assesses pituitary and adrenal function directly. Other than minor flushing, CRH (1 mcg/kg IV) rarely produces side effects. Cortisol responses are comparable to those seen with 1 mcg/kg Synacthen testing. The test is not widely used for hypocortisolism as CRH is relatively expensive and available only in Australia via the TGA IPU scheme, and Synacthen testing is generally satisfactory. However, CRH is used for separating Cushing's disease from ectopic Cushing's patients. This relies on the observation that patients with Cushing's disease show an exaggerated response to CRH relative to normal, whereas ectopic Cushing's patients show no ACTH or cortisol response. CRH is also used to stimulate the pituitary during petrosal sinus sampling.

○ Testing for primary aldosteronism

Conn's syndrome—hypertension and hypokalaemia due to an aldosterone-secreting adrenal tumour—was described in 1955. Although Conn predicted that hyperaldosteronism, which has since been also shown to result from bilateral adrenal aldosterone secretory autonomy, would be recognised as a common cause of hypertension, estimates of around 0.1% of hypertensive cases persisted until the 1990s. At this time, widespread use of screening using the plasma aldosterone concentration to plasma renin activity ratio (PAC:PRA), as described by Hiramatsu et al. in 1981, led to increased diagnosis of hyperaldosteronism.[7] Most of these additional cases were normokalaemic. Overall, primary aldosteronism appears to be a more common form of curable hypertension (estimates vary from 1 to 10%) than renovascular hypertension and phaechromocytoma.

Screening for primary aldosteronism appears to be indicated in all hypertensives with spontaneous or thiazide-induced hypokalaemia, all cases without excellent blood pressure control on two antihypertensives and perhaps in all hypertensives, although rigorous health outcome studies do not exist in the community context. Testing the PAC:PRA ratio is also indicated in patients with adrenal incidentaloma[5].

The PAC:PRA ratio

Screening can be performed on a mid-morning sitting blood sample on a normal diet. The initial evaluation should consist of documenting that plasma renin activity is reduced and that plasma aldosterone concentrations are high, resulting in a plasma aldosterone concentration (pmol/L) to plasma renin activity (ng/mL/h) ratio of greater than 30. An elevated PAC:PRA ratio may occur even with low aldosterone levels if the PRA is very low, for example in individuals taking a high salt diet. Hence, an elevated PAC:PRA ratio may not suggest primary aldosteronism if the PAC is less than 400 nmol/L. Serum potassium should be taken simultaneously as a low serum potassium will reduce the PAC and indicate a requirement to fully replace potassium prior to testing. Recently many laboratories have begin measuring renin directly (direct renin concentration, DRC) rather than measuring the ability of a sample to catalyse angiotensin production in vitro. The ALDO:DRC ratio may vary in different laboratories due to use of different units so that the laboratory range should be noted. Either assay appears valid for the diagnosis of primary aldosteronism.

Importantly, if PAC:PRA ratios are measured, knowledge of the pitfalls will prevent invalid testing and unnecessary follow-up tests. The differential diagnosis of hypertension and hypokalaemia includes renovascular disease. Less common causes include Cushing's syndrome, licorice ingestion, certain forms of congenital adrenal hyperplasia, and rare renin-secreting tumours. Antihypertensive drugs can interfere with the PAC:PRA ratio. Diuretics and aldosterone receptor blockers, such as spironolactone, need to be stopped for 6 weeks prior to testing. Beta-blockers suppress the PRA but they can be stopped 24–48 h prior to testing. The effects of angiotensin converting enzyme (ACE) inhibitors and angiotensin receptor blockers (ARBs) are generally minor but in a patient treated with an ACE inhibitor or ARB, a detectable PRA level or a low PAC:PRA ratio does not exclude the diagnosis of primary aldosteronism. Dihydropyridine calcium antagonists, such as nifedipine and amlodipine, can reduce the PAC in patients with an aldosterone-secreting adenoma. Renal impairment may elevate the PAC:PRA ratio by two mechanisms: increased potassium elevates the PAC and salt and water retention suppresses the PRA.

Confirming primary hyperaldosteronism and its subtype

Confirmatory testing is directed towards demonstrating aldosterone secretory autonomy, using measurements of plasma or urine aldosterone under salt-loading conditions. The final step is to determine if one or both adrenals are the source of aldosterone; this generally requires adrenal vein sampling.

◐ Adrenal incidentaloma

An unanticipated adrenal mass (incidentaloma) is found in approximately 4% of upper abdominal CT scans. Clinical, imaging and biochemical evaluation is necessary to exclude malignancy and hormone excess[6].

◐ Evaluation for malignancy

The a priori risk of adrenocortical cancer (ACC) is very low, considering that adrenal tumours are present in 3% of individuals over 50 years and ACC has an incidence of 1 per million per year. CT imaging characteristics that assist with excluding malignancy include CT density (less than 10 Hounsfield units is likely to be benign) and size (tumours less than 4 cm in diameter are likely benign). A follow-up CT scan at 6–12 months is indicated and, if the lesion is stable, imaging can be discontinued. Adrenal metastases are common, are not always bilateral and need to be considered in all those with past malignancy or those at high risk. Chemical shift magnetic resonance imaging (MRI), in some hands, has differentiated metastasis from benign adenoma with an accuracy of 100%. Needle aspiration should never be performed in cases of likely adrenocortical carcinoma due to the risk of seeding but may be necessary in cases of suspected metastases where management would be altered by the biopsy.

Evaluation for hormonal function

Up to 15% of adrenal incidentalomas are functional from the in vivo biochemical standpoint, with cortisol secretion the commonest abnormality, followed by aldosterone secretion. Many resected tumours are phaeochromocytomas but most are clinically silent and non-secretory.

Clinically significant sex steroid secretion is rare. Screening tests include the 1-mg overnight DST; if the cortisol is > 140 nmol/L then consider work up for early Cushing's. The use of the 1mg DST as a necessary criterion for diagnosing subtle or subclinical Cushing's, with low cortisol cut-offs and the attendant false positive rates, may have led to the conclusion that subclinical Cushing's is common[7]. Catecholamine excess can be screened for with plasma metanephrines or 24-h urine free catecholamines. If the patient is hypertensive, a PAC:PRA ratio and serum potassium should be obtained to help exclude primary aldosteronism. Importantly, hormone over-production may develop and it is prudent to evaluate these patients clinically and biochemically annually for 4 years.

◐ Summary

Disorders of adrenocortical function are uncommon and the symptoms often non-specific. However, application of a small number of biochemical screening tests can separate those patients who do not have a disorder of adrenal function from those that require specialised assessment and more complex dynamic testing procedures.

References

1. Newell-Price J. Bertagna X., Grossman A.B. and Nieman L.K. Cushing's syndrome. *Lancet* 2006; 367: 1605–17.
2. Gagliardi L., Chapman I.M., O'Loughlin P. and Torpy D.J. Screening for subclinical Cushing's syndrome in type 2 diabetes mellitus: low false-positive results with nocturnal salivary cortisol. *Horm Metab Res* 2010; 42: 280–4.
3. Montwill J., Igoe D., McKenna D.J. The overnight dexamethasone test is the procedure of choice in screening for Cushing's syndrome. *Steroids* 1994; 59: 296–8.
4. Nieman L.K. Dynamic evaluation of adrenal hypofunction. *J Endocrinol Invest* 2003;26: 74–82.
5. Mulatero P., Dluhy R.G., Giacchetti G., Boscaro M., Veglio F. and Stewart P.M. Diagnosis of primary aldosteronism: from screening to subtype differentiation. *Trends Endocrinol Metab* 2005; 16: 114–9.
6. No authors listed. NIH state-of-the-science statement on management of the clinically inapparent adrenal mass ("incidentaloma"). *NIH Consens State Sci Statements* 2002; 19: 1–25.
7. Hiramatsu K., Yamada T., Yukimura Y., Komiya I., Ichikawa K., Ishihara M. et al. A screening test to identify aldosterone-producing adenoma by measuring plasma renin activity: results in hypertensive patients. *Arch Intern Med* 1981; 41: 1589–93.

23 The glucose tolerance test

S.K. Gan and D.J. Chisholm

Synopsis

The roles of the fasting plasma glucose (FPG) level and oral glucose tolerance test (OGTT) have evolved over recent years with the use of a lower fasting plasma glucose threshold for the diagnosis of diabetes (≥ 7.0 mmol/L) and the introduction of a category of impaired fasting glucose (IFG) in the classification of glucose tolerance. Thus an OGTT is not required when a diagnosis of diabetes is established by a random plasma glucose ≥ 11.1 mmol/L in a patient with symptoms of hyperglycaemia or by a (replicated) fasting plasma glucose > 7.0 mmol/L, nor usually when a fasting plasma glucose is < 5.5 mmol/L, which indicates a very low likelihood of diabetes.

An OGTT is indicated when the fasting plasma glucose is between 5.5 and 6.9 mmol/L. The 2-h post glucose load reading is then critical in the diagnosis of diabetes (2-h plasma glucose ≥ 11.1 mmol/L) or impaired glucose tolerance (IGT; 2-h plasma glucose 7.8 to 11.0 mmol/L).

◯ Introduction

The use of the fasting plasma glucose level and the OGTT in the diagnosis and classification of glucose intolerance and diabetes mellitus has recently undergone revision. In particular a lower fasting glucose threshold has been used for the diagnosis of diabetes mellitus by both the American Diabetes Association (ADA) and the World Health Organization (WHO) to enhance the diagnostic sensitivity of the fasting glucose level and on the basis that a fasting plasma glucose of 7.0 mmol/L corresponds in population studies to a 2-h OGTT level of 11 mmol/L. In fact the ADA suggested the OGTT should be discarded in favour of using the FPG alone but this was not accepted when epidemiologic data showed that a substantial proportion of people with an FPG < 7.0 mmol/L had a 2-h OGTT plasma glucose diagnostic of diabetes and that the 2-h OGTT plasma glucose correlates better with adverse cardiovascular events than the FPG. The ADA has most recently also adopted a threshold glycated haemoglobin (HbA1c) of ≥ 6.5% as an alternative criterion for diagnosis of diabetes, although the WHO and other international bodies are still considering this recommendation.

The four categories of glucose tolerance are currently defined as:

- normal
- impaired fasting glucose (IFG) (prediabetes)
- impaired glucose tolerance (IGT) (prediabetes)
- diabetes mellitus.

The term 'prediabetes' has recently been adopted internationally to describe the presence of IFG and IGT.

A diagnosis of IGT or IFG does not indicate a necessary progression to diabetes—in fact 2 to 12% of subjects with IGT each year develop diabetes mellitus and many revert to a normal glucose tolerance test. Age, obesity and the degree of glucose intolerance are major risk factors for progression to diabetes. Significantly, the categories of IFG and IGT are associated with other manifestations of metabolic syndrome and an increased risk of cardiovascular disease. The risk of subsequent cardiovascular events seems more strongly associated with IGT than IFG.

◐ Technical aspects

Subjects should receive a relatively high carbohydrate diet (at least 150 g) for 3 days before the test. On the morning of the test 75 g glucose (or 1.75 g/kg up to 75 g in children) is given following an overnight fast. Blood samples are taken while fasting and 2 hours after the glucose load.

Care must be taken to distinguish between glucose levels performed on plasma or blood (plasma levels are approximately 13% higher than whole blood levels) and capillary or venous samples (capillary is higher in the non-fasting state). Venous samples are normally taken during an OGTT. It should be noted that glucose preservatives (e.g. fluoride oxalate) reduce but do not totally prevent glycolysis during sample transport/holding, which can lead to underestimation of the true glucose concentrations.

◐ Physiological aspects

Although it is the best we have, the OGTT is a relatively imprecise test, as biological variation in the response to glucose ingestion is added to any assay error. Undue carbohydrate restriction on the days prior to the test can lead to an impairment of glucose tolerance. If the test has been performed during severe stress or intercurrent illness, mild elevations of blood glucose levels should not be diagnosed as diabetes until the test is repeated under more normal circumstances.

A 'flat' glucose tolerance curve (low peak level) has sometimes been regarded as indicative of malabsorption. However, a flat curve is a fairly common finding in fit, normal people with very efficient glucose disposal.

Some individuals can have an impaired fasting plasma glucose (≥ 6.1 but < 7.0) but a 2-h post glucose load level in the diabetic range. A diabetic OGTT response, however, is rare if the fasting venous plasma glucose is < 5.5 mmol/L. An abnormal fasting plasma glucose with a normal 2-h OGTT level may also occur and some of these variabilities appear to reflect gender variation or different population backgrounds (e.g. IFG is more common in males).

Is the result abnormal?

The current diagnostic criteria as set out in the Australian National Evidence Based Guidelines For Type 2 Diabetes are shown in Table 23.1.

Table 23.1 Values for diagnosis of diabetes mellitus and other categories of hyperglycaemia

	Glucose concentration (mmol/L) in plasma (*whole blood*)	
	Venous	**Capillary**
Diabetes mellitus		
Fasting	≥ 7.0 (≥ 6.1)	≥ 7.0 (≥ 6.1)
or random level	≥ 11.1 (≥ 10.0)	≥ 12.2 (≥ 11.1)
Impaired glucose tolerance (IGT)		
Fasting	< 7.0 (< 6.1)	< 7.0 (< 6.1)
and 2 h post-glucose load	≥ 7.8 (≥ 6.7)	≥ 8.9 (≥ 7.8)
	and < 11.1 (< 10.0)	*and* < 12.2 (< 11.1)
Impaired fasting glucose (IFG)*		
Fasting	$\geq 6.1^*$ (≥ 5.6) and < 7.0 (< 6.1)	≥ 6.1 (≥ 5.6) and < 7.0 (< 6.1)
and 2 h post-glucose load (if measured)	< 7.8 (< 6.7)	< 8.9 (< 7.8)
Normal		
Fasting	$< 6.1^*$ (< 5.6)	< 6.1 (< 5.6)
and 2 h post-glucose load (if measured)	< 7.8 (< 6.7)	< 8.9 (< 7.8)

*Note that the American Diabetes Association has recently recommended that the lower diagnostic plasma glucose level for IFG should be ≥ 5.6 mmol/L but this recommendation has not been adopted by WHO or Australian expert groups at this time.

It should be stressed that the OGTT is often not necessary in the diagnosis of diabetes mellitus. Either a fasting venous plasma glucose above 7.0 mmol/L (blood glucose > 6.1 mmol/L) or a repeated random plasma glucose above 11.1 mmol/L (blood glucose > 10 mmol/L) establishes a definite diagnosis of diabetes mellitus. Nearly all subjects who have symptomatic hyperglycaemia will easily exceed these cut-off points and even asymptomatic patients with glycosuria will generally have fasting or random glucose levels in the diagnostic range if they do have diabetes.

If a diagnosis of diabetes is suspected and the fasting venous plasma glucose is between 5.5 and 7.0 mmol/L or random plasma glucose is less than 11.1 mmol/L, an OGTT is appropriate. The same rules apply when conditions with known tendency to insulin resistance are under investigation, such as polycystic ovary syndrome or acanthosis nigricans.

Unfortunately an OGTT is often requested inappropriately, especially in the following four situations:

1. a newly presenting patient with symptoms of hyperglycaemia or substantial glycosuria (this includes nearly all children with type 1 diabetes). Correct procedure here is to determine a fasting or random plasma glucose level, which will nearly always establish the diagnosis. The performance of an OGTT is unnecessary and will delay appropriate therapy.

2. to determine the type of therapy or the response to therapy in diabetes. An OGTT should not be used here.

3. at times of severe physical or emotional stress or intercurrent illness or in patients on medications (e.g. corticosteroids) that may elevate blood glucose levels. An OGTT should not be used here. If diabetes mellitus is present in these situations a fasting or random blood glucose level will be elevated.

4. in the diagnosis of hypoglycaemia. If fasting hypoglycaemia is suspected, a fasting plasma glucose is the appropriate test (if necessary, with a prolonged fast). If 'reactive' hypoglycaemia is suspected a plasma glucose level at a time the person is symptomatic should be obtained.

○ Testing for gestational diabetes

This represents a special situation where glucose tolerance can be assessed by using either a standard fasting 75 g OGTT (at any time during gestation if gestational diabetes is suspected and repeated at 26–28 weeks if a test earlier in gestation is normal) or a screening test measuring plasma glucose 1 hour after a 50 g or 75 g oral glucose load, performed in the morning, non-fasting, usually at 26–28 weeks gestation. In guidelines published by the Australasian Diabetes in Pregnancy Society (ADIPS) the criteria for diagnosis of gestational diabetes using the 75 g OGTT are a fasting venous plasma glucose

> 5.5 mmol/L and/or a 2-h post load reading > 8.0 mmol/L. If the screening test of a 1-h post 50 g or 75 g glucose load is used, venous plasma glucose readings of > 7.8 mmol/L and > 8.0 mmol/L respectively would need to be followed by a fasting 75 g OGTT to confirm diagnosis of gestational diabetes.

Screening is recommended in all pregnant women and especially those with risk factors (e.g. age > 30, obesity, family history of diabetes, past history of gestational diabetes or high-risk ethnic groups). Maternal follow-up testing with a fasting 75 g OGTT is recommended at 6–8 weeks postpartum and, if normal, at 1–2 yearly intervals during child-bearing years.

◷ What to do about a diagnosis of impaired glucose tolerance or impaired fasting glucose

There is no uniform opinion about the clinical approach to this situation but we recommend the following guidelines:

1. If there is a definite family history of non-insulin dependent diabetes, advise the patient to follow an appropriate diabetic diet and maintain a good level of physical activity but do not label the patient with the diagnosis of 'diabetes' or 'early diabetes' (which may prejudice insurance, superannuation, etc). Warn them of the symptoms of hyperglycaemia and check a fasting glucose level at 12-month intervals.

2. If the glycaemic abnormality persists after at least 6 months of lifestyle modification, use of pharmacotherapy, particularly metformin, may be considered although this would be outside approved indications.

3. If there is not a definite family history of diabetes, warn the person that there is an approximate 2–12% risk of developing diabetes each year, with greater risk associated with obesity and more marked glucose intolerance. Offer the suggestion of reducing this risk by restricting free sugar and fat intake plus regular exercise; aim for weight reduction if obese. Warn them of the symptoms of hyperglycaemia and check a fasting glucose level at 12-monthly intervals.

4. If the person is pregnant, a diabetic diet should be followed and blood glucose levels monitored. It should be noted that epidemiological data suggest that even slight hyperglycaemia represents a risk to the fetus during pregnancy. Thus the patient should be treated as having diabetes for the duration of the pregnancy.

The above advice should be tempered according to the age of the subject. A diagnosis of IGT or IFG at age 75 would be of much less consequence than the same diagnosis at age 40. As impaired glucose tolerance has been associated with an increase in cardiovascular risk, it is sensible to assess other cardiovascular risk factors in this situation and advise the patient accordingly.

◗ What to do about a diagnosis of diabetes mellitus

1. Decide if the diagnosis is likely to be type 1 or type 2 diabetes. Pointers to type 1 diabetes include age less than 30, presence of ketones in the urine, normal or reduced body weight and either (a) absence of family history of diabetes or (b) history of type 1 diabetes. If in doubt, measurement of anti-GAD antibodies can be performed as an indicator of type 1 diabetes.
2. In type 1 diabetes, commence insulin therapy immediately.
3. If the diagnosis is type 2 diabetes, the prescription is diet and exercise ± biguanide (or sulphonylurea) tablets. Insulin is occasionally necessary soon after diagnosis and often becomes necessary after about 10 years. There are also a number of other antidiabetic medications available, usually used as add-on therapy, and these are discussed in recent guidelines by Diabetes Australia and the National Health and Medical Research Council of Australia (see reference below.)

◗ Additional tests

Insulin levels are not usually required for therapeutic decision making. A fasting or postprandial C-peptide level may sometimes be useful in a patient on insulin therapy to indicate whether they have endogenous insulin production, which can have some value in deciding the most appropriate insulin regimen.

As diabetes represents a cardiovascular risk factor it is appropriate to check cholesterol, HDL cholesterol and triglycerides on a regular basis (the latter two may be improved to some extent by good diabetes control and a diabetic diet) and a urine microalbumin level is an indicator of early diabetic nephropathy.

◗ Summary

Epidemiological evidence indicates that a fasting venous plasma glucose of 7.0 mmol/L is a more sensitive (but still reasonably precise) threshold for the diagnosis of diabetes than the previous level of 7.8 mmol/L. In many clinical settings measuring fasting or random glucose will suffice for confirming the diagnosis of diabetes but the OGTT continues to have an important role in the clinical diagnosis of diabetes mellitus when fasting or random glucose levels are non-diagnostic.

Further reading

Alberti K.G.M M. and Zimmet P.Z. Definition, diagnosis and classification of diabetes mellitus and its complications. Part 1: diagnosis and classification of diabetes mellitus. Provisional Report of a WHO Consultation. *Diabet Med* 1998; 15: 539–53.

American Diabetes Association. Diagnosis and classification of diabetes mellitus. American Diabetes Association Position Statement. *Diabetes Care* 2005; 28 (S1): S37–42.

Australian Centre for Diabetes Strategies. *National Evidence Based Guidelines For Type 2 Diabetes.* Available at http://www.diabetes.net.au

Colagiuri S., Davies D., Girgis S. and, Colagiuri R. *National Evidence Based Guideline For Case Detection And Diagnosis of Type 2 Diabetes.* Canberra: Diabetes Australia and the NRMRC, Canberra 2009. Available at http://www.nhmrc.gov.au/guidelines/health_guidelines.htm

Colman P.G., Thomas D.W., Zimmet P.Z. et al. New classification and criteria for the diagnosis of diabetes mellitus. Position Statement from the Australian Diabetes Society, New Zealand Society for the Study of Diabetes, Royal College of Pathologists of Australasia and Australasian Association of Clinical Biochemists. *MJA* 1999; 170: 375–8.

Hoffman L., Nolan C., Wilson J.D. et al. Gestational diabetes mellitus—management guidelines. The Australian Diabetes in Pregnancy Society. *MJA* 1998; 169: 93–7.

Shaw J.E. and Chisholm D.J. Epidemiology and prevention of type 2 diabetes and the metabolic syndrome. *MJA* 2003; 79: 379–83.

Twigg S.M., Kamp M.C., Davis T.M., Neylon E.K. and Flack J.R. Prediabetes: a position statement from the Australian Diabetes Society and Australian Diabetes Educators Association. *MJA* 2007;186: 461–5.

QUICK FLICK 23

24 Diabetes monitoring: use of glycated haemoglobin and glycated protein assays

G. Jones and D.J. Chisholm

Synopsis

The measurement of glycated haemoglobin or haemoglobin A1c (HbA1c) is the test of choice for monitoring mean glycaemic control in diabetic patients. There has been considerable progress towards standardisation of HbA1c assays to allow comparison of results between different laboratories and different measurement technologies. There remains, however, further work in order to fully characterise the fraction of glycated haemoglobin which best reflects recent average blood glucose levels and to ensure high quality testing and standardisation in all laboratories.

○ Introduction

The phenomenon of glycation (or glycosylation) of proteins to form neoglycoproteins has long been recognised in the area of food technology as a cause of the 'browning reaction'. In recent years there has been increasing understanding of the phenomenon of in vivo glycation of proteins, leading to the development of assays which are indicators of mean glycaemic control in patients with diabetes.[1,2] There has also been intensive study of the possibility that the phenomenon of protein glycation is a significant contributor to long-term diabetic complications—either by causing changes in structural proteins such as collagen or by altering function of other proteins such as receptors, enzymes or the apolipoproteins of circulating lipids.

Measurement of circulating neoglycoproteins has now been accepted as a marker of the exposure of circulating proteins to glucose and also of the risk of diabetic complications.[3] Assays of glycated haemoglobin and glycated albumin (fructosamine) are available and each assay reflects the lifespan of that protein in the circulation; for example, HbA1c indicates glycaemic control over 3 months (the life of the red cell) and fructosamine reflects control over 6 weeks (the life of serum albumin in the circulation).

In both cases results are weighted toward recent glycaemic control, as recent changes have affected all the protein present at the time of measurement.[1]

○ Biochemistry of protein glycation

When proteins are exposed to glucose, the carbonyl group of glucose may attach to the α-amino groups of the N-terminal amino acids of the proteins or less rapidly to the ε-amino groups of lysine. This attachment results in the formation of a Schiff base (aldimine) in a reversible reaction. An Amadori rearrangement then results in the non-reversible formation of a ketoamine after which cyclisation generates a glycated protein (Fig. 24.1).

Glycated proteins are quite stable and are not enzymatically degraded in mammals. Exposure of proteins to high concentrations of glucose over a relatively long period of time may result in the formation of advanced glycosylation end products (AGE) or 'browning'.

Glycation of proteins occurs continuously in all individuals and is dependent on the time of exposure and the glucose levels present. In non-diabetic humans at physiological blood glucose levels, approximately 1% of serum albumin is normally glycated as is about 5% of haemoglobin.

Figure 24.1 Glycation of proteins

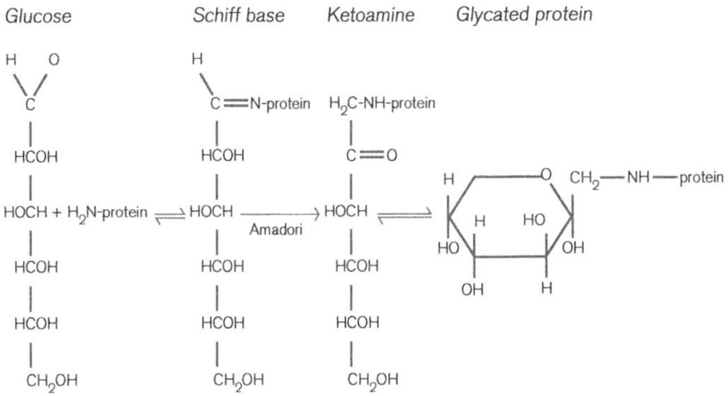

○ Methodology

HbA1c

Several methods are routinely used to measure glycated haemoglobin. These include ion-exchange chromatography, affinity chromatography and various immunoassay systems, but each glycated haemoglobin method measures a different glycated component of haemoglobin.[1,2] Boronate affinity methods separate 'total glycated haemoglobin' according to structural characteristics of the glycated component. Immunoassay methods also rely on structural differences in haemoglobin species but they measure only the glycation of the NH_2 terminus of the β-chain (HbA1c specifically). Ion exchange and electrophoretic methods separate HbA1c from other Hb species according to molecular charge. Because of these methodological differences, glycated haemoglobin results from different laboratories may vary.[1,2]

The International Federation of Clinical Chemistry set up an international working group (IFCC WG) in 1994 to progress international agreement in regards to HbA1c measurements. Consequent work has led to the definition of HbA1c, the preparation of pure HbAO and HbA1c, the development of reference methods and the preparation of secondary reference calibrators and controls. The IFCC WG has defined HbA1c as β-N valine glycated Hb (β-N-(1-deoxy)-fructosyl Hb). This represents the major glycation site of the HbA1c molecule. Batches of purified HbAO (> 99.5% pure) and purified HbA1c (> 98.5% pure) were prepared by several preparation chromatography steps (CE/AC/CE) from human blood. The batches have been consistent and stable and have been used to generate standards for the reference methods.[4]

Two reference methods have been developed based on proteolytic cleavage of HbA1c by endoproteinase Glu-C to form hexapeptides that are then analysed by HPLC-mass spectrometry or HPLC-capillary electrophoresis. Both methods have been accepted by all member national societies of the IFCC as reference methods for HbA1c. Both methods yield identical percentage HbA1c values in all samples and mixtures analysed.[5] Secondary reference materials (SRM) have been prepared with values assigned by the IFCC network laboratories.

It is important to align the method used in the Diabetes Control and Complications Trial (DCCT), which showed a correlation between levels of HbA1c and microvascular outcomes in type 1 diabetic patients) with the new reference methods and this has been done.[6] The original DCCT method was an in-house HPLC method which is not commercially available; however, a US group, the National Glycohemoglobin Standardisation Program (NSGP), has certified methods and laboratories against this method and is now also using the newer secondary reference materials. Most of the commonly used methods in Australia today are referenced against these standards. While there is agreement in regards to the reference methods and the reference materials, the values reported by the new reference methods are lower than the DCCT values for HbA1c due to less background correction. A vigorous discussion is currently ongoing about whether to (1) change the values for HbA1c, which would require widespread re-education of practitioners and patients, (2) adjust the new reference methods to the old DCCT values to allow clinicians to remain with their known values or (3) change to a new parameter such as mean glucose equivalent.[7] This matter is still under discussion in 2010.

Assay precision is a further important matter. Most immunoassay systems struggle to reach the recommended within-laboratory precision of a coefficient of variation (CV) of less than 3%. The importance of the assay precision can be seen with the example of an assay with CV of 5%. A result from such an assay of 9.0% HbA1c indicates 95% confidence interval for the result of between 8.1% and 9.9%. Obviously this represents a wide range of possibilities for the state of glycaemic control and also makes detecting significant changes in results difficult. Some variant haemoglobins continue to give grossly different values in some systems.

Despite referencing of methods back to the DCCT trial, a sample may still give significantly different results when measured in different laboratories. However, due to common reference materials that have been supplied to the different manufacturers this difference should become less. Nevertheless it is still preferable to monitor patients with results from a single laboratory and if differences are seen on changing laboratories, these should be discussed with the laboratories concerned before assuming that a true change in the patient's glycaemic control has occurred.

○ Glycated serum proteins

With the rise in understanding and acceptance of HbA1c testing there has been a reduction in the use of other glycated proteins such as fructosamine. The fructosamine assay is largely a measure of glycated albumin and therefore reflects the average blood glucose over the previous 2 to 3 weeks, reflecting the half-life of albumin in the circulation. In general this test is now used in circumstances where HbA1c is inappropriate either due to a desire to investigate shorter time intervals or because there is interference with HbA1c measurement. It is also potentially useful in late pregnancy when short term changes in glucose level may occur.

○ Clinical use of glycated protein assays

The particular use of HbA1c (or fructosamine) assay is to provide an index of medium- to long-term control of the diabetes (Table 24.1). This contrasts with the use of self blood glucose monitoring to indicate hour-to-hour or day-to-day changes in control, which may be used to adjust therapy on a daily basis, for example in the type 1 patient who may alter insulin doses or carbohydrate intake in response to such things as changes in physical activity.

Table 24.1 Correlation between HbA1c level and mean plasma glucose levels (from DCCT data)

HbA1c (%)	Mean plasma glucose (mmol/L)
6	7.5
7	9.5
8	11.5
9	13.5
10	15.5
11	17.5
12	19.5

HbA1c measurements have a particular value in diabetic patients who are unwilling or unable to do regular fingerprick blood glucose measurements or in situations where there may be doubt as to the validity of the measurements, such as a faulty monitoring device. Patients attending a physician or clinic may be affected by stress or altered lifestyle routine on that day and have higher than usual blood glucose measurements ('white coat hyperglycaemia')—a satisfactory HbA1c level on these occasions is very reassuring.

Although HbA1c levels correspond to the initiation and progression of diabetic complications (especially microvascular disease) physicians need to be realistic in setting target goals. Even with the intense supervision and aggressive therapy in the DCCT few patients with type 1 diabetes achieved a normal HbA1c and the mean of the intensively treated group was approximately 7.0%—about 15% above the upper limit of normal. Even at this level of control there was a three-fold increase in hypoglycaemic reactions and a similar proportionate increase in severe hypoglycaemic reactions. Most diabetologists would feel happy if type 1 diabetic patients could achieve HbA1c levels around the 7 to 7.5% range. In patients with hypoglycaemia unawareness and problems with severe hypoglycaemic reactions the target HbA1c may need to be a little higher. Newer monitoring systems under development may help to alleviate this problem by allowing better identification of asymptomatic hypoglycaemia.

In type 2 diabetic patients, who are less susceptible to hypoglycaemia, and especially in those on low levels of medication, it is desirable and often possible to achieve HbA1c levels in the 6 to 7% range. However, the United Kingdom Prospective Diabetes Study clearly demonstrated the difficulty in maintaining this control over the long term with presently available therapies and indicated the need to aggressively add further medication when a satisfactory HbA1c level is not achieved.[7]

There is some evidence for individual biological variation in the degree of haemoglobin glycosylation for a given level of glycaemia and it has been suggested from analysis of DCCT data that 'high glycosylators' are more susceptible to microvascular complications.[8] However, the measure of mean blood glucose used in this analysis was a seven-point BG profile done one day every 3 months, which may not have been representative of the true mean blood glucose level. Consequently, the degree of variation in 'glycosylating ability' and its importance as a determinant of diabetic complications require further investigation.

HbA1c levels are closely correlated with the development or progression of microvascular disease and neuropathy but the relationship with cardiovascular events and mortality is less impressive, and a number of studies indicate that attention to blood pressure and lipid control has great importance with regard to cardiovascular outcome.

In the chronic stable situation the performance of a glycated haemoglobin or fructosamine assay at 3 to 6 month intervals would be considered reasonable by most physicians expert in diabetes management.

Glycated haemoglobin and fructosamine have not been considered suitable for the diagnosis or exclusion of the diagnosis of diabetes mellitus or impaired glucose tolerance, but this is an area of intense current discussion and there is increasing evidence that a HbA1c level above 6.5% is a reliable diagnostic value. However, as an index of metabolic control in individual patients these assays have great importance in research studies assessing the relationship of glycaemic control to progression of complications or other outcome measures; they may also be used as an important parameter for auditing outcome for clinic populations.

○ Sources of error in interpreting HbA1c results

One source of error in HbA1c estimation is the presence of unusual haemoglobin, which may or may not produce an aberrant result depending on the method used. Another important source of variation is increased red cell turnover, where the red cell has had a shorter duration of exposure to blood glucose: an example would be a haemolytic anaemia where the HbA1c level may be considerably lower than would be expected from the level of glycaemia. High intakes of vitamin C or E have also been reported to falsely lower results, possibly by inhibiting glycation of haemoglobin. A variety of other conditions or medications may interfere depending on the method, including hypertriglyceridaemia, hyperbilirubinaemia, uraemia, chronic alcoholism, chronic salicylate ingestion and opiate addiction.[1]

References

1. Goldstein D.E., Little R.R., Lorenz R.A., Malone JI, Nathan D., Peterson C.M. et al. Tests of glycaemia in diabetes. *Diabetes Care* 2004; 27: 1761–73.
2. Sacks D.B., Bruns D.E., Goldstein D.E., Maclaren N.K., McDonald J.M. and Parrott M. Guidelines and recommendations for laboratory analysis in the diagnosis and management of diabetes mellitus. *Diabetes Care* 2003; 25: 750–86.
3. The Diabetes Control and Complications Trial Research Group. The effect of intensive treatment of diabetes on the development and progression of long-term complications in insulin-dependent diabetes mellitus. *NEJM* 1993; 329: 977–86.
4. Finke A., Kobold U., Hoelzel W., Weykamp C., Jeppsson J-O. and Miedema K. Preparation of a candidate reference material for the international standardisation of HbA1c determinations. *Clin Chem Lab Med* 1998; 36: 299–308.
5. Jeppsson J-O., Kobold U., Barr J., Finke A., Hoelzel W., Hoshino T. et al. Approved IFCC reference method for the measurement of HbA1c in human blood. *Clin Chem Lab Med* 2002; 40: 78–89.
6. Hoelzel W., Weykamp C., Jeppsson J-O., Miedema K., Barr J.R., Goodall I. et al. IFCC reference system for measurement of haemoglobin A1c in human blood and the National Standardisation Schemes in the United States, Japan and Sweden. A method comparison study. *Clin Chem* 2004; 50: 166–74.
7. Turner R.C., Cull C.A., Frighi V. and Holman R.R. Glycemic control with diet, sulfonylurea, metformin, or insulin in patients with type 2 diabetes mellitus: progressive requirement for multiple therapies (UKPDS 49). UK Prospective Diabetes Study (UKPDS) Group. *JAMA* 1999; 281: 2005–12.
8. McCarter R., Hempe J.M., Gomez R. and Chalew S.A. Biological variation in HbA1c predicts risk of retinopathy and nephropathy in type 1 diabetes. *Diabetes Care* 2004; 27: 1259–64.

Synopsis

Hormone testing is helpful in the investigation of infertility but excessive testing is rarely valuable. The history of infertility and examination of both partners usually enables a simple approach to testing. Tests of ovulation rely on measuring serum progesterone 7 days before an expected period. Measurement of serum testosterone is sufficient to exclude ovarian or adrenal tumours as a cause of hyperandrogenism while prolactin and thyroid stimulating hormone may be valuable in women with irregular periods. Semen analysis is essential in the infertile male.

○ Introduction

The general practitioner is usually the first person to see the 10–15% of couples who are concerned about their fertility. At some time in their lives approximately half of these couples will seek medical advice. A third of these people will need to be referred to a specialist or assisted reproductive technology unit. In a third of infertility cases there is a female factor, in another third a male factor and in the remaining third there will be a combination of both or no detected cause. The investigation depends upon the couple's history, their ages and the findings on examination (Fig. 25.1). Patients who present with less than 12 months of infertility should have minimal testing unless a clear cause is found from clinical assessment. Selection of tests after this will depend on the potential cause of infertility indicated by the history and examination.

○ Female infertility

A detailed history of the menstrual cycle often provides a clue to problems such as anovulation or ovarian failure. A general examination should be carried out in addition to a pelvic examination to look for problems such as hypothyroidism or hirsutism.

Figure 25.1 Investigation and management of the infertile couple in general practice

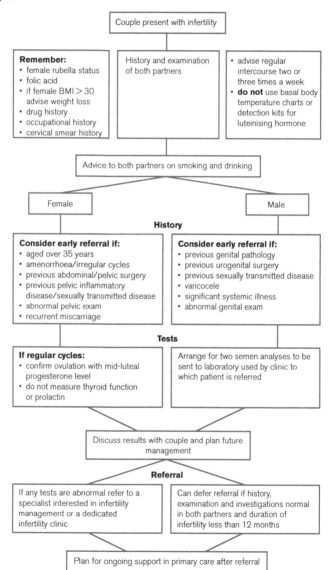

Issues to consider when measuring female hormones

The concentrations of most hormones fluctuate during the menstrual cycle and in the case of luteinising hormone (LH) and follicle stimulating hormone (FSH) there is also a minute-by-minute pulsatile variation. Most hormones should be measured in the first 7 days of the cycle when there is little fluctuation in their concentrations but the pulsatile release of hormones such as LH may lead to quite variable results between specimens. The measurement of hormones such as prolactin can be significantly affected by stress and medication. Progesterone and 17-hydroxyprogesterone vary substantially between the follicular and luteal phases of the cycle. In perimenopause the concentrations of FSH can fluctuate markedly as the ovarian sensitivity to gonadotrophins varies.

Tests for detection of ovulation

The most appropriate test for detecting ovulation is a serum progesterone concentration. This is performed approximately 7 days before the predicted date of a menstrual period (day 1). The day can be calculated on the basis of a 14-day luteal phase, so if the menstrual cycle is 28 days, test on day 21; test on day 23 of a 30 day cycle and day 25 of a 32 day cycle.

A progesterone concentration above 20–25 nmol/L confirms ovulation occurred in that cycle. Lower values mean either anovulation or inappropriate timing of the blood test. A low concentration can be checked by taking two measurements of progesterone a week apart in the next cycle or alternatively recalculating the day of testing.

Urinary dipsticks for LH are also widely used for ovulation detection but are expensive, open to problems of interpretation and are only of value when periods are regular. Blood or urinary LH tests are of no value in general practice.

Tests for hirsutism

The commonest cause of hair growth in women with abnormal periods is polycystic ovary syndrome. The most appropriate test for hyperandrogenaemia is a serum total testosterone. This will normally be below 2 nmol/L but reference ranges can vary from laboratory to laboratory and also during the menstrual cycle. Values of testosterone above 10 nmol/L are suggestive of a testosterone-producing tumour of the ovary or adrenal. As testosterone is bound to sex hormone binding globulin, an estimate of free androgen can be obtained by calculating the ratio of testosterone to sex hormone binding globulin (the free androgen index). Direct measurement of free testosterone is technically flawed and a useless test.

Tests for other androgens, such as androstenedione and dehydroepiandrosterone, are of little value in general practice. The commonly used LH:FSH ratio is also of little value although a raised LH with a normal FSH is helpful in the diagnosis of polycystic ovary syndrome. Measuring 17-hydroxyprogesterone is occasionally helpful where late onset congenital adrenal hyperplasia (an inherited condition affecting one of the enzymes in the adrenal gland) is suspected.

Many women with polycystic ovary syndrome will develop diabetes. When the syndrome is diagnosed in an overweight patient, diabetes mellitus and hypertriglyceridaemia should be excluded.

Tests for early menopause

The only test of any value where the diagnosis is uncertain is serum FSH. The concentration may be raised above 20–30 IU/L but this test should be repeated on several occasions as the condition of ovarian failure fluctuates remarkably. There is no place for measuring oestradiol or LH in this situation.

Tests for early pregnancy

Human chorionic gonadotrophin is the best test for early pregnancy. Values over 25 U/L in the blood or urine are usually diagnostic of pregnancy. Concentrations below this are reported as equivocal or negative. If the result is equivocal it can be repeated 2 days later and should have at least doubled in value. While modern laboratory assays for human chorionic gonadotrophin are reliable, urinary home pregnancy tests are often less satisfactory. There is usually a 1:1 relationship between concentrations of human chorionic gonadotrophin in blood and urine. However, blood testing is more reliable and is positive 1–2 days earlier.

Tests for menstrual irregularity

Where abnormal periods are present, measuring serum prolactin is of value. Prolactin concentrations are increased by stress, hypothyroidism, dopamine-depleting drugs and microadenoma of the pituitary as well as by pregnancy and lactation. When periods are irregular, measuring thyroid stimulating hormone is important to exclude primary hypothyroidism. Routine measurement of FSH, LH and oestradiol for infertility is of little value except in early menopause. Chromosome analysis is needed in cases of primary amenorrhoea.

○ Male infertility

After a history and examination, semen analysis is the essential test.

Semen analysis

Infertility in a couple requires analysis of a sample of semen. A semen specimen should be produced, after 3 days abstinence from ejaculation, into a clean wide-topped jar and delivered to the laboratory within 20 minutes. Previous illness and some drugs (e.g. anabolic steroids, testosterone) can seriously affect the amount and motility of the sperm.

Analysis required

The volume, concentration, motility and morphology of the seminal specimen are measured. Sperm numbers should be above 20×10^6 per mL, motility should be at least 50% and morphology should be above 20% normal. Morphology is poorly assessed by most laboratories other than those routinely dealing with infertility but it predicts the chances of fertility. Single, double or triple defects necessitate the measurement of a second specimen in a specialist laboratory and probable referral to a specialist.

Other tests

In patients with azoospermia, small testes and a high FSH, chromosome analysis may be required to exclude conditions such as Klinefelter's syndrome (XXY). Other disorders of semen analysis may require the measurement of FSH and LH to show whether the defect is in the testis (high result) or in the hypothalamus or pituitary (low result). Serum testosterone is normally well above 10 nmol/L and low values may necessitate testosterone replacement or injection of human chorionic gonadotrophin depending on the cause and desire for fertility. Occasionally microadenomas of the pituitary can present with high prolactin values and male infertility. Sperm antibody testing is important.

○ Summary

Infertility is a condition initially best dealt with by the general practitioner. After history and examination, selective testing of hormones is helpful for making the diagnosis and for decisions regarding referral. Inappropriate hormone testing is expensive and a waste of resources.

26 Biochemical tests in pregnancy

H.A. Tran

Synopsis

Pregnancy is a normal physiological phenomenon with many biochemical changes ranging from alterations in electrolyte concentrations to more complex changes in cortisol and calcium metabolism. The results of biochemical tests during pregnancy may therefore differ from the usual reference ranges so they may be mistakenly interpreted as abnormal. This can lead to unnecessary and potentially dangerous therapeutic actions. If there is doubt about a result, contact the laboratory to ask if the result reflects the physiological changes that occur during pregnancy. Further investigation and treatment can be recommended if appropriate.

○ Introduction

Pregnancy is associated with normal physiological changes that assist the nurturing and survival of the fetus. Biochemical parameters reflect these adaptive changes and are clearly distinct from the non-pregnant state. The woman's renal function, carbohydrate and protein metabolism and, particularly, hormonal pattern are affected. It is critical to appreciate both normal and abnormal changes as laboratory results can influence the management of both mother and child.

○ Renal function

During pregnancy the serum sodium is about 3–5 mmol/L lower than non-pregnancy because of an increase in intravascular volume and resetting of the osmostat. Cardiac output and renal blood flow are also increased. This leads to an increased glomerular filtration rate (GFR) with resultant decrease in concentrations of serum urea, creatinine and uric acid (Table 26.1).

Table 26.1 Normal reference ranges and their interpretation during pregnancy*

Analytes	Normal (non-pregnant)	Pregnancy	Abnormalities and possible interpretations
Haemoglobin (g/L)	115–165	110–150	
White cell count (× 10⁹ per L)	4.0–11.0	Unchanged	Abnormal results need to be considered in conjunction with the patient's clinical state
Platelets (× 10⁹ per mL)	150–450	Unchanged	
Sodium (mmol/L)	135–145	132–140	
Potassium (mmol/L)	3.5–5.5	3.2–4.6	
Urea (mmol/L)	2.5–6.8	1.0–3.8	↑ in dehydration, hyperemesis gravidarum, late stage pre-eclampsia, renal impairment
Creatinine (mmol/L)	60–100	40–80	↑ in renal impairment, late stage pre-eclampsia
Fasting glucose (mmol/L)	3.0–5.4	3.0–5.0	↑ in gestational diabetes mellitus (refer to reference 2 for diagnostic criteria)
Total calcium (mmol/L)	2.2–2.6	2.0–2.4	↑ in primary hyperparathyroidism, hyperemesis gravidarum
Ionised calcium (mmol/L)	1.16–1.30	1.16–1.30	
Magnesium (mmol/L)	0.6–1.0	0.6–0.8	↓ in vomiting, hyperemesis gravidarum
Albumin (g/L)	33–41	24–31	↓ in malnutrition, recurrent vomiting, hyperemesis gravidarum
Bilirubin (micromol/L)	3–22	3–14	↑ in intrahepatic cholestasis of pregnancy, HELLP, late stage pre-eclampsia, acute fatty liver, viral hepatitides
Alanine aminotransferase (U/L)	1–40	1–30	↑ in intrahepatic cholestasis of pregnancy, HELLP, late stage pre-eclampsia, acute fatty liver, viral hepatitides

QUICK FLICK 26

continues

Table 26.1 Normal reference ranges and their interpretation during pregnancy*
continued

Analytes	Normal (non-pregnant)	Pregnancy	Abnormalities and possible interpretations
Aspartate aminotransferase (U/L)	1–30	1–21	↑ in intrahepatic cholestasis of pregnancy, HELLP, late stage pre-eclampsia, acute fatty liver, viral hepatitides
Alkaline phosphatase (U/L)	25–100	125–250	↑ in metabolic bone disorders but placental serum alkaline phosphatase needs to be excluded

*Adapted from reference 7
↑ increased concentration; ↓ decreased concentration; HELLP haemolysis-elevated liver enzymes-low platelets
Note: Each laboratory, where practicable, should develop its own reference ranges for pregnant women. Care should be exercised in comparing results from different laboratories due to differences in assay methodologies.

In most cases renal function during pregnancy can be adequately assessed by the serum urea and creatinine. If required the GFR can be estimated using the Cockcroft-Gault or Method of Disease Renal Diet formulae[1] (current laboratory policy is to supply the eGFR) but it is necessary to take into account the pregnant state specifically. The GFR can also be calculated using urinary volume and urinary and serum creatinine. Radioactive studies of urinary excretion are clearly not appropriate. The validation of cystatin-C as an accurate marker of GFR during pregnancy is promising although it is not yet common in clinical practice.[2] Serum bicarbonate falls by about 4 mmol/L to compensate for the respiratory alkalosis, a result of the high progesterone level which in turn stimulates respiratory drive.[3]

The renal tubular threshold is also lowered in pregnancy. This results in an increased excretion of uric acid, amino acids and glucose. Urinary testing for glycosuria can therefore be misleading. Similarly urinary testing to assess metabolic changes should not be used during pregnancy and is best delayed until well into the postpartum period. The best practical uses of urine testing during pregnancy are to diagnose pregnancy itself, to detect asymptomatic bacteriuria and to warn of imminent pre-eclampsia where there is significant proteinuria.[4]

◗ Liver function tests

All markers of liver function are generally reduced or low during pregnancy due to the expansion of extracellular fluid. Hence serum albumin, transaminases (AST and ALT) and total bilirubin are low compared with the non-pregnant state. The only exception is serum alkaline phosphatase (ALP) which is elevated due to ALP of placental origin.

Causes of abnormal liver function tests specific to pregnancy include intrahepatic cholestasis of pregnancy, pre-eclampsia, haemolysis-elevated liver enzymes-low platelets (HELLP) and, rarely, acute fatty liver of pregnancy (Table 26.1). All of these can cause significant fetal and maternal morbidity and mortality. Newly acquired hepatitides during pregnancy and adverse drug reactions should also be considered when assessing abnormal liver function tests.

○ Calcium metabolism

During pregnancy, serum total calcium, phosphate and magnesium tend to be low due to the expanded intravascular space. Concentrations of calcium are also affected by the reduced albumin concentration. However, the results all remain within the reference range. If there is any doubt regarding the calcium result, measure the ionised calcium concentration, as it remains unchanged during normal pregnancy despite changes in vascular volume and binding proteins. The concentration of serum parathyroid hormone tends to be 50% lower in pregnancy despite the increased urinary excretion of calcium as a result of the increased GFR.[5] Although primary hyperparathyroidism is rare, it remains the commonest cause of hypercalcaemia during pregnancy. However, differentiating it biochemically from familial hypocalciuric hypercalcaemia (which has non-surgical management) is difficult and evaluation at a specialist endocrinology clinic is recommended.

○ Carbohydrate metabolism and gestational diabetes mellitus

The concentration of fasting glucose is reduced during pregnancy because of increased substrate utilisation (Table 26.1). With the increasing incidence of obesity there will be an increased prevalence of gestational diabetes and type 2 diabetes developing or detected during pregnancy. It is therefore prudent to be familiar with the diagnostic criteria.[6] It is essential to screen for gestational diabetes at 26–28 weeks of gestation so that the correct interpretation can be made. The test is positive if the plasma glucose concentration is 7.8 mmol/L or more than 1 hour after a 50 g glucose load, and a full 75 g oral glucose tolerance test is then necessary.[6] Recently, the American Diabetes Association recommended the latter be performed on all women without known diabetes antecedent pregnancy.[7]

◐ Hormonal changes

Pregnancy causes a remarkable number of hormonal changes that continue to evolve throughout the gestational period. This makes the interpretation of biochemical and hormonal results a challenging task. The changes are a continuation of the luteal phase of the menstrual cycle. Once pregnancy has occurred concentrations of progesterone and oestrogen continue to rise, suppressing the secretion of luteinising hormone and follicle stimulating hormone. However, these changes are non-specific and should not be used to confirm pregnancy.

To confirm pregnancy serum human chorionic gonadotrophin (HCG) is the test of choice. The concentration of HCG is likely to be elevated by trophoblastic activity as early as day 8 after implantation. Concentrations peak at approximately 10 weeks and then decline to plateau out at a lower level.

◐ Thyroid function

Thyroid function tests are not uncommonly ordered during pregnancy and interpreting the results is challenging. Physiologically the concentration of thyroid stimulating hormone (TSH) normally decreases during the first trimester of pregnancy during which there is maximal cross-stimulation of the TSH receptor by HCG. In different series the lower limit of 'normal' pregnancy has been reported to be between 0.02 and 0.1 mU/L and the upper limit between 2.15 and 3.4 mU/L; this may reflect different genetic make up and dietary intake of iodine.[14,15] The TSH concentration returns to its pre-pregnancy level in the second trimester and then rises slightly in the third. However, most of the changes still occur within the normal non-pregnant reference range. Serum free thyroxine concentration decreases slightly but significantly and this is most marked in the third trimester.[8] The assays for free thyroid hormones during pregnancy remain problematic generally.[9] Total concentrations, which include both free and protein-bound fractions, are significantly elevated due to increased circulating binding globulins.[8] Clinical indicators are usually confusing due to symptoms of pregnancy that can mimic thyrotoxicosis, such as nausea, vomiting, heat intolerance, fatigue, anxiety and palpitations. The presence of a goitre, especially in patients with a borderline iodine deficiency, can further confound the diagnosis.

Graves' disease is the commonest cause of true thyrotoxicosis in pregnancy. Where there is prolonged and intractable nausea and vomiting, Graves' disease should be distinguished from hyperemesis gravidarum of pregnancy and transient hyperthyroxinaemia of pregnancy. It is important that they are distinguished from Graves' disease as the prognoses and management are distinctly different (Table 26.2). Hyperemesis gravidarum and transient hyperthyroxinaemia of pregnancy are often self-limiting and can be treated expectantly with general support and/or beta-blockade.[10] Graves' disease needs to be optimally controlled in order to optimise both fetal and maternal outcome.[8]

In patients with a previous history of Graves' or Hashimoto's disease, consideration should be given to checking whether antibodies are still present, because they can cross the placenta and affect the fetus.

Table 26.2 Distinguishing hyperemesis gravidarum and thyrotoxicosis during pregnancy

	Reference range in pregnancy	Graves' disease	Hyperemesis gravidarum
Thyroid stimulating hormone (mU/L)[14]		< 0.05	< 0.05
First trimester	0.1–3.4 (but see text)		
Second trimester	0.37–3.8		
Third trimester	0.4–4.0		
Free tetra-iodothyronine (pmol/L)*	10.0–25.0	+++	+ to ++
Free tri-iodothyronine (pmol/L)*	3.5–6.0	+ to +++	+ to +++
Human chorionic gonadotrophin	Normal* for gestational age	Normal* for gestational age	+++ for gestational age
Thyroid stimulating immunoglobulin	Absent	Present	Absent
Thyroid–myeloperoxidase antibodies	Absent or present in low titre	Absent	Absent or low

+ increase
*Reference ranges often vary between laboratories

QUICK FLICK
26

○ Haematology

In pregnancy there is a gradual increase in circulating blood volume of up to 1.5 L by the third trimester. As there is a relatively smaller increase in red cell mass, there is a decrease in haematocrit and haemoglobin concentrations. Platelet concentrations remain essentially stable throughout (Table 26.1).[11] While white cell count can be as high as $15–16 \times 10^9$/L, the majority do not exceed the non-pregnancy reference range.[12] Erythrocyte sedimentation rate also rises significantly, peaking between 50 and 70 mm/h depending on gestational age.[13] Thus, where this range is exceeded, it is important that active inflammation or infection is thoroughly excluded.

○ Summary

Pregnancy leads to many changes to laboratory tests which can be misinterpreted as abnormal. In general most of the analytes have lower concentrations than in the non-pregnant state due to increased intravascular volume while the free active fractions, such as ionised calcium, remain unchanged. It is uncommon for a particular analyte to become elevated and this is a useful pointer to recognising abnormal laboratory results during pregnancy. When there are clinically discrepant results, it is prudent to seek further advice from the laboratory.

References

1. Levey A.S., Coresh J., Balk E., Kausz A.T., Levin A., Steffes M.W. et al. National Kidney Foundation practice guidelines for chronic kidney disease: evaluation, classification, and stratification. *Ann Intern Med* 2003; 139: 137–47.

2. Larsson A., Palm M., Hansson L.O. and Axelsson O. Cystatin C and modification of diet in renal disease (MDRD) estimated glomerular filtration rates differ during normal pregnancy. *Acta Obstet Gyn Scand* 2010; 54: Mar 25 [Epub ahead of print].

3. McAuliffe F., Kametas N., Krampl E., Ernsting J. and Nicolaides K. Blood gases in pregnancy at sea level and at high altitude. *Brit J Obstet Gynaecol*, 2001; 108: 980–5.

4. Lowe S.A., Brown M.A., Dekker G.A., Gatt S., McLintock C.K., McMahon P.L. et al. Guidelines for the management of hypertensive disorders of pregnancy 2008. *Aust NZ J Obstet Gynaecol* 2009; 49: 242–6.

5. Seely E.W., Brown E.M., DeMaggio D.M., Weldon D.K. and Graves S.W. A prospective study of calciotropic hormones in pregnancy and post

partum: reciprocal changes in serum intact parathyroid hormone and 1,25-dihydroxyvitamin D. *Am J Obstet Gynecol* 1997; 176: 214–7.

6. Hoffman L., Nolan C., Wilson J. D., Oats N. J. J. and Simmons D. Gestational diabetes mellitus—management guidelines. The Australasian Diabetes in Pregnancy Society. *MJA* 1998; 169: 93–7.

7. International association of diabetes and pregnancy study groups consensus panel. International association of diabetes and pregnancy study groups recommendations on the diagnosis and classification of hyperglycemia in pregnancy. *Diabetes Care* 2010; 33: 676–82.

8. Glinoer D. The regulation of thyroid function in pregnancy: pathways of endocrine adaptation from physiology to pathology. *Endocr Rev* 1997; 18: 404–33.

9. Demers L.M. and Spencer C.A. Laboratory medicine practice guidelines. Laboratory support for the diagnosis and monitoring of thyroid disease. Free thyroxine and free triiodothyronine estimate tests. *Thyroid* 2003; 13: 21–32.

10. Hershman J.M. Physiological and pathological aspects of the effect of human chorionic gonadotropin on the thyroid. *Best Pract Res Cl En* 2004; 18: 249–65.

11. Hytten F. Blood volume changes in normal pregnancy. *Clin Haematol* 1985; 14: 601–12.

12. Hiss R.G. Evaluation of the anaemic patient. In: Laros R.K, Jr., ed. *Blood Disorders In Pregnancy.* Phildelphia; Lea & Febiger, 1986. p.9.

13. Van den Broe N.R. and Letsky E.A. Pregnancy and the erythrocyte sedimentation rate. *Brit J Obstet Gynaecol*, 2001; 108: 1164–67.

14. Larsson A., Palm M., Hansson L-O. and Axelsson O. Reference values for clinical chemistry tests during normal pregnancy. *Brit J Obstet Gynaecol* 2008; 115: 874–81.

15. Gilbert R.M., Hadlow N.C., Walsh J.P. et al. Assessment of thyroid function during pregnancy: first trimester (weeks 9–13) reference intervals derived from Western Australian women. *MJA* 2008; 189: 250–3.

QUICK FLICK 26

27 Biochemical tests for abnormalities in pregnancy

H.A. Tran

Synopsis

Pregnancy induces major physiological, hormonal and biochemical changes to achieve optimal outcomes for the baby and mother. When the pregnancy deviates from its normal course, there are many biochemical markers that can be used to assess these abnormalities. As biochemical assessments are only one part of obstetric care, results should be interpreted in conjunction with clinical and medical imaging data. Imaging is especially important and can be used to assess many placental and fetal abnormalities. Ultrasonography continues to improve and be refined in the early detection of fetal structural defects. It has equalled, if not superseded, biochemical testing in many aspects of obstetric care.

○ Introduction

Biochemical markers are used to assess maternal, placental and fetal health. They help to diagnose and monitor maternal conditions such as gestational diabetes and pre-eclampsia, trophoblastic disease and fetal chromosomal abnormalities such as Down syndrome (Table 27.1). These biochemical and hormonal tests constitute only one aspect of obstetric care. They should be used together with clinical findings and imaging, particularly ultrasonography.

Table 27.1 Biochemical tests for common maternal, placental and fetal conditions

	Condition	Test
Maternal	Gestational diabetes	Glucose screening tests at 24–28 weeks: 50 g challenge test OR 2-h 75 g oral glucose tolerance test

	Condition	Test
	Pre-eclampsia*	1. Urinary protein (by dipstick testing or formal quantitation)
		2. Serum uric acid
		3. Renal function tests
		4. Full blood count (for Hb concentration and platelet count)
Placental	Trophoblastic disease* (hydatidiform mole or choriocarcinoma)	1. HCG
		2. Free β-HCG
		3. Urinary HCG when indicated
Fetal	Down syndrome*	Maternal serum alpha-fetoprotein, HCG, pregnancy-associated plasma protein-A and transnuchal ultrasound at 11–13 weeks gestation
		Maternal serum alpha-fetoprotein, HCG, pregnancy-associated plasma protein-A and serum unconjugated oestriol in various combinations at 15–18 weeks gestation
	Neural tube defects	Maternal serum alpha-fetoprotein OR amniotic fluid alpha fetoprotein (less common)

*Potential use of fetal DNA in maternal circulation
HCG human chorionic gonadotrophin

○ Biochemical assessment of maternal health

Common problems in pregnancy include gestational diabetes and pre-eclampsia.

Diabetes

The prevalence of gestational diabetes mellitus ranges from 1 to 14% depending on the populations studied.[1] In Australia the prevalence ranges from 5.5 to 8.8%.[2] Screening for gestational diabetes mellitus in Australia is strongly advocated at 26–28 weeks of gestation. This enables early intervention which results in significant improvements in both fetal and maternal outcomes.[3]

Occasionally, the serum glucose is unexpectedly found to be in the diabetic range in the first trimester. By definition, this is gestational diabetes mellitus but testing does not distinguish between diabetes preceding or occurring at the same time as pregnancy. The diagnosis can be confirmed by further tests of fasting glucose concentration or a 75 g oral glucose tolerance test. These patients should be reassessed in the postpartum period for evidence of diabetes. The woman's glycated haemoglobin (HbA1c) should be maintained in the normal range or as near normal as possible to ensure optimal fetal outcome but hypoglycaemia must be strenuously avoided.

Pre-eclampsia

Pre-eclampsia occurs typically in the third trimester and affects 4–8% of pregnancies.[4] It consists of a triad of pregnancy-associated hypertension (that is, there is no pre-existing hypertension), marked proteinuria (greater than 300 mg daily) and pathological oedema. It is thus critical that urinary dipstick testing for protein, which can be fully quantitated if required, is performed at each antenatal visit together with blood pressure measurement and careful examination for oedema. Other findings include rises in serum uric acid (which can antedate the onset of hypertension), urea and creatinine. Low haemoglobin and platelet concentrations are informative if the patient is suspected to have the severe form of pre-eclampsia: haemolysis-elevated liver enzymes-low platelets (HELLP). In the absence of pre-existing pathology, these biochemical parameters should return to normal after delivery.

◗ Biochemical assessment of placental health

Ultrasonography has added another dimension to first trimester obstetric care to such an extent that many traditional biochemical tests have been rendered redundant. Maternal serum human placental lactogen and serum or urinary oestriol concentrations, which were previously used extensively in the assessment of placental function, are rarely used nowadays.

Human chorionic gonadotrophin (HCG)

As pregnancy progresses, the patient's hormonal profile continues to evolve with steadily rising concentrations of progesterone and oestrogen. These continue to rise well into the first trimester while concentrations of luteinising hormone and follicle stimulating hormone are low or suppressed. To maintain progesterone production from the corpus luteum in order to keep the pregnancy viable in its early stage, the placenta starts to secrete HCG. The serum HCG concentration is therefore the test of choice for confirming pregnancy.

Physiologically, serum HCG arising from trophoblastic activity is elevated as early as the eighth day after implantation. Concentrations double every 2–3 days and peak at approximately 10 weeks. They then decline and plateau at a lower concentration until parturition (Fig. 27.1).

In addition to confirming pregnancy, serum HCG can be used as a marker to assess various abnormalities in the first trimester. A failure to rise at the appropriate rate suggests the impending loss of the pregnancy from spontaneous miscarriage or an unviable/ectopic pregnancy. A markedly elevated serum HCG suggests the presence of multiple pregnancies,

Figure 27.1 Human chorionic gonadotrophin (HCG) and thyroid stimulating hormone (TSH) concentrations

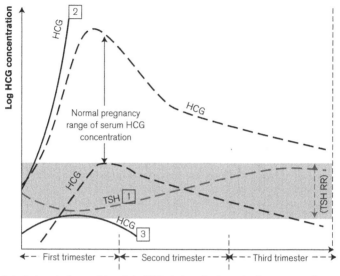

Note the broad reference intervals for HCG which peaks during the first trimester of pregnancy.

1. Represents the normal response of serum thyroid stimulating hormone (TSH) during pregnancy. The reference range (RR) for TSH is in the shaded area. Note the drop in TSH concentration in the first trimester corresponding with the peak HCG concentration. This is due to negative feedback on TSH secretion resulting from the stimulating effect of HCG on TSH receptors.

2. The high baseline HCG concentration with markedly shortened doubling time suggests multiple pregnancy or a trophoblastic tumour. .

3. Failure of HCG to rise or double with time. This suggests the presence of an unviable or ectopic pregnancy or threatened miscarriage.

especially with assisted fertilisation, or the presence of gestational trophoblastic disease including chorionic carcinoma and hydatidiform mole. A hydatidiform mole typically appears as a 'snow storm' on ultrasound. Confirmatory biochemical tests should include the *free* β-HCG concentration because this form of HCG is secreted in disproportionately high amounts.[5]

HCG can be used to assess the effectiveness of therapy and monitor for recurrence following surgery for gestational trophoblastic disease. A rapid decline or the disappearance of serum HCG is to be expected after successful surgery. False positive results at low HCG concentrations have been reported and have led to unnecessary surgery.[6] It is therefore important that, when the HCG concentration is contrary to the clinical assessment, parallel *urinary* HCG concentrations should be analysed. (If the serum concentration of HCG is low but detectable in a clinically cured patient, the absence of urinary HCG raises the suspicion of a false positive serum result. If HCG is also present in the urine a residual tumour is more likely.) In these complex situations, ongoing communication with the laboratory is critical to the care and outcome for patients.

In the second trimester an elevated serum HCG concentration has been associated with a two- to three-fold increased risk of fetal growth retardation.[7]

◐ Biochemical assessment of fetal health

The major aim of fetal assessment is to ensure satisfactory growth in utero. There are many factors that can cause fetal growth retardation. These range from poor maternal nutritional state to placental insufficiency and fetal abnormality. As with placental function, medical imaging is increasingly used to detect fetal abnormalities, thus reducing the utility of biochemical markers.

Alpha-fetoprotein
Alpha-fetoprotein is a fetal protein arising from the yolk sac and fetal liver. It can be detected in increasing concentrations in maternal serum until 32 weeks of normal gestation.

Neural tube defects
In neural tube defects such as spina bifida and anencephaly, the concentration of alpha-fetoprotein in the maternal serum is unusually high in the first trimester because cerebrospinal fluid leaks into the amniotic fluid.[8] Other causes of elevated alpha-fetoprotein, such as incorrect gestational date and multiple pregnancy, need to be excluded. As a marker of neural tube defects maternal serum-alpha fetoprotein should be ideally measured between 15 and 18 weeks of gestation. Any suspicion of a neural tube defect can be further assessed with ultrasound, usually at 18–20 weeks. This scan also assesses for other fetal morphological abnormalities and placental placement.

Down syndrome
Down syndrome is one of the common causes of fetal growth retardation. It is the result of either partial or total trisomy of chromosome 21 and is a major obstetric concern, particularly in older women. Important biochemical markers include alpha-fetoprotein, HCG, unconjugated oestriol, pregnancy-associated plasma protein-A, serum inhibin-A and free β-HCG. These markers are used in various combinations and together with ultrasound to

increase the detection rate of Down syndrome. It cannot be overemphasised that the gestational age must be correct in order for screening parameters to be accurate.

Between 11 and 13 weeks (that is late *first* trimester), serum pregnancy-associated plasma protein-A, free β-HCG and ultrasound assessment of nuchal thickness (the physiological space between the back of the neck and the overlying skin of the fetus) are most commonly used tests when assessing the risk of Down syndrome. Due to the changing concentrations of these markers in the normal pregnant population, the results are mathematically corrected for easy comparison. The nuchal thickness is increased in Down syndrome and approximately 70% of cases will be detected by ultrasound in experienced centres. In combination with biochemical markers, the detection rate increases to 85–90%.[9,10] Abnormal results can be followed up with direct karyotyping using chorionic villous sampling but this carries a 0.5–1.0% risk of pregnancy loss in the first trimester.

In the *second* trimester, screening for Down syndrome traditionally employs the triple test of maternal serum HCG, serum unconjugated oestriol and alpha-fetoprotein at 15–18 weeks of gestation. Some laboratories also measure serum pregnancy-associated plasma protein-A. The combination of these markers and maternal age delivers a 60–65% detection rate but this includes the 5% of women who have a false positive result. Transnuchal thickness in the mid to late second trimester does not correlate well with Down syndrome and does not add to the value of biochemical markers.[11]

The results of Down syndrome screening in the first and second trimester are expressed as the proportion of affected pregnancies, for example, 1 in 488 chance of having Down syndrome. This is accomplished using a risk-assessment program that incorporates nuchal thickness (only in the first trimester), biochemistry results and maternal age.

Other approaches

Another biochemical method of assessing fetal health is the analysis of amniotic fluid. Measuring bilirubin concentration in amniotic fluid is critical for assessing fetal intravascular haemolysis in the presence of Rhesus incompatibility. The lecithin-to-sphingomyelin ratio in amniotic fluid can be used to assess fetal lung maturity in preterm labour but is rarely used these days due to the widespread availability of synthetic surfactant.

Recently there has been a resurgence of interest in using maternal growth hormone and insulin-like growth factor levels during the first and second trimester of pregnancy as predictors of fetal outcome, but these are yet to be of routine clinical use.[12]

Fetal DNA

A major advance in molecular biology has been the possible detection and isolation of fetal DNA in the maternal circulation.[13] This exciting discovery has opened up new horizons in the non-invasive assessment of fetal-maternal health. High concentrations of fetal DNA in the maternal circulation have been found in Down syndrome, pre-eclampsia, invasive placenta and preterm labour. This technique has also allowed for the prenatal non-invasive diagnosis of rhesus D genotype, myotonic dystrophy and achondroplasia.[14]

◗ Summary

Biochemical markers are important in the assessment of maternal, placental and fetal health. They remain critical in supporting and diagnosing many associated conditions despite the increasing quality and use of ultrasonography. As normal values continue to change with gestational age, these markers should be measured at the correct gestational age to enable accurate interpretation.

References

1. Diagnosis and classification of diabetes mellitus. American Diabetes Association Position Statement. *Diabetes Care* 2005; 28: S37–42.
2. Hoffman L., Nolan C., Wilson J.D., Oats J.J. and Simmons D. Gestational diabetes mellitus—management guidelines. The Australasian Diabetes in Pregnancy Society. *MJA* 1998; 169: 93–7.
3. Crowther C.A., Hiller J.E., Moss J.R., Mc Phee A.J., Jeffries W.S. and Robinson JS. Effect of treatment of gestational diabetes mellitus on pregnancy outcomes. *NEJM* 2005; 352: 2477–86.
4. Lyell D.J., Lambert-Messerlian G.M. and Giudice L.C. Prenatal screening, epidemiology, diagnosis, and management of preeclampsia. *Clin Lab Med* 2003; 23: 413–42.
5. Cole L.A. Immunoassay of human chorionic gonadotropin, its free subunits, and metabolites. *Clin Chem* 1997; 43: 2233–43.
6. Rotmensch S. and Cole L.A. False diagnosis and needless therapy of presumed malignant disease in women with false-positive human chorionic gonadotropin concentrations. *Lancet* 2000; 355: 712–5.
7. Onderoglu L.S. and Kabukcu A. Elevated second trimester human chorionic gonadotropin level associated with adverse pregnancy outcome. *Int J Gynaecol Obstet* 1997; 56: 245–9.
8. Mitchell L.E., Adzick N.S., Melchionne J., Pasquariello P.S., Sutton L.N., Whitehead A.S. Spina bifida. *Lancet* 2004; 364: 1885–95.
9. Roizen N.J. and Patterson D. Down's syndrome. *Lancet* 2003; 361: 1281–9.

10. Nicolaides K.H. Nuchal translucency and other first-trimester sonographic markers of chromosomal abnormalities. *Am J Obstet Gynecol* 2004; 191: 45–67.

11. Cuckle H. Integrating antenatal Down's syndrome screening. *Curr Opin Obstet Gynecol* 2001; 13: 175–81.

12. Reis F., D'Antona D. and Petraglia F. Predictive value of hormone measurements in maternal and fetal complications of pregnancy. *Endocr Rev* 2002; 23: 230–57.

13. Lo YD, Corbetta N, Chamberlain PF, Rai V, Sargent IL, Redman CW, et al. Presence of fetal DNA in maternal plasma and serum. *Lancet* 1997; 350: 485–7.

14. Simpson J.L. and Bischoff F. Cell-free fetal DNA in maternal blood: evolving clinical applications. *JAMA* 2004; 291: 1135–7.

Further reading

Human Genetic Society of Australasia (HGSA) and the Royal Australian and New Zealand College of Obstetricians and Gynaecologists. *Prenatal Screening Tests for Trisomy 21 (Down Syndrome), Trisomy 18 (Edwards Syndrome) and Neural Tube Defects.* 2007. Available from www.ranzcog.edu.au/publications/statements/C-obs4.pdf [cited Mar 8, 2006].

28 Interpreting paediatric biochemistry results

P. Verras and R. Greaves

Synopsis

When interpreting biochemical test results in paediatric patients, consider a number of issues that are associated with and specific to childhood. These include the age of the patient, which may vary from approximately 16 weeks prematurity to more than 18 years, and their body weight, which may range from approximately 500 grams to more than 100 kg. Body size is also a factor in certain situations and is of special concern in the current epidemic of childhood obesity. Children are not miniature adults; however, as they age their biochemistry becomes more like that of adults. Added to these patient factors are the effects of the collection process on the blood sample, the method used to analyse the sample, the source of the reference range quoted with the result and the interpretation placed on the result by laboratory staff.

Introduction

Historically the biochemical testing of children, especially very young children, tended to be the province of dedicated 'paediatric' laboratories located in specialist paediatric hospitals. This was usually because small samples of blood were not sufficient for the methods and equipment used in general pathology laboratories at the time. Nowadays almost all of the testing equipment can be adapted to process low-volume samples, although it must be recognised that some of these instruments are more adaptable than others. Most laboratories can now competently analyse small samples without much effect on workflow and consequent productivity but this does not guarantee that the information provided is adequate for the needs of the referring clinician. The results must be interpreted with a knowledge of the factors that affect children's biochemistry.

○ Age-dependent factors

Age-related variation is the single most important factor impacting on the interpretation of paediatric results (Table 28.1). To make matters difficult, chronological age is not a completely reliable guide for interpretation of results, as developmental processes are not uniformly linked to the age of the patient. It is often more useful to consider results in terms of the four stages of childhood development:

- neonate—the first 4 weeks of life
- infant—4 weeks to 2 years
- child—2 years to puberty
- adolescent—puberty to adulthood.

Most laboratories report results with reference intervals that are applied to finite age ranges by computer data systems, sometimes causing large and sudden changes in what is considered to be 'normal' when a patient ages by only a few hours. Prematurity, age of onset of adrenarche, puberty and body mass index (BMI) are additional important factors that are not fully taken into account but can impact significantly on the interpretation of selected biochemical results.

Table 28.1 Examples of common analytes where age-related reference ranges need to be considered for the correct interpretation of paediatric results

Analyte	Reference intervals
Albumin	Lower in children, rising from lowest levels in the neonate and infant to adult levels in adolescence
Alkaline phosphatase	Higher in neonates and until post-puberty. Spikes occur during puberty in association with rapid bone growth.
Bilirubin	Higher in neonates due to immature metabolic pathways
Calcium	Lower values are seen in neonates, especially in prematurity. The upper reference limit is higher in paediatric patients. Adult ranges apply at about 1 year.
Cortisol	No diurnal variation in neonates
Creatinine	Lower due to lower muscle mass in children. Adult ranges apply in late adolescence.
Drug concentrations relative to dose	Concentrations may be higher in neonates due to immature metabolic pathways and lower during childhood due to increased metabolic rates. Reference ranges are usually as for adults.

continues

Table 28.1 Examples of common analytes where age-related reference ranges need to be considered for the correct interpretation of paediatric results *continued*

Analyte	Reference intervals
Free triiodothyronine	Higher in paediatric patients. Adult ranges apply from late adolescence.
Follicle stimulating hormone	Change to adult levels at puberty
Glucose	Lower in neonates, especially in prematurity. Adult ranges apply at one month.
Insulin-like growth factor	Continuous change throughout life
Luteinising hormone	Change to adult levels at puberty
Magnesium	Lower in neonates, especially in prematurity. Adult levels apply by about 1 year.
Oestradiol	Change to adult levels at puberty
Steroid hormones	Change with age. Assay interference is possible in premature neonates. Special pre-assay preparation of the sample is required to remove interferences for immunoassay-based analyses. Some centres now offer mass spectrometry based measurement, which does not suffer from these interferences.
Testosterone	Change to adult levels at puberty
Thyroid stimulating hormone	Slightly higher in neonates. Adult levels apply at 1 month.
Urea	Higher in neonates, falling to adult levels during infancy
Urine catecholamines	Vary with age until adulthood

◗ Prematurity

Despite advances in perinatal care, preterm birth remains a significant problem affecting as many as 7% of all pregnancies.[1] There are more than 16 000 preterm deliveries per year in Australia.[2] Immature and developing organ systems contribute to considerable differences in the concentrations of hormones, proteins, enzymes, metabolites and therapeutic drugs in comparison with adults. It is important to attempt to correct for gestational age especially in the first 6 months of life. However, most laboratory information systems do not provide such a correction and often this relevant information is not included in the request for the test.

○ Puberty

Biochemically, puberty is characterised by the secretion of gonadal hormones. In females puberty can start as early as 8 years and is usually completed by the age of 16 years, whereas in boys it generally commences around 10 to 12 years of age and is generally completed by 18 years of age. Reference ranges for biochemical tests are based on chronological age and not on Tanner staging, so results should always be interpreted carefully in this group. There are marked changes in the concentrations of gonadotrophins and steroid hormones during puberty.

○ Pre-analytical factors

The lack of availability of suitably skilled staff for collecting samples from children may affect the quality of the samples received for testing. Collection problems are encountered mainly in neonates and infants because collecting capillary blood requires some skill and experience to obtain samples that are likely to yield accurate results for all analytes. Excessive squeezing of a capillary collection site may result in haemolysis, leading to elevation of intracellular analytes such as potassium, magnesium, phosphate and lactate dehydrogenase. Dilution of the sample with tissue fluid can have varying effects on other test results. The consequential small blood sample volume is also more susceptible to the deleterious effects of light, heat, contamination and evaporation than larger-volume venous collections. A frequently encountered problem in small samples is the loss of carbon dioxide into the remaining air space in the tube, leading to falsely low bicarbonate values. The use of inappropriately large specimen containers, especially EDTA and fluoride-oxalate tubes, will exacerbate this and other problems. These factors occasionally generate aberrant results, which can only be clarified by repeat collection and analysis.

Collection of timed urine specimens is also often difficult in neonates and infants and an unusually low timed urine volume must always be viewed with suspicion. Urine output starts at around 100–300 mL per day in infants (3–10 days), increasing with age to adult volumes after puberty.[3]

○ Analytical factors

For the paediatric biochemist, hormone assays tend to provide the largest challenge in attempting an appropriate balance between cost, turnaround time and method quality. This is particularly true for full-term and premature babies and for assays that attempt to cater for both the male and female populations. Reference ranges provided by different laboratories may vary considerably.

◐ Assay interference

Fetal adrenal steroids persist until at least 40 weeks post-conception, that is, until at least the equivalent of term, despite early delivery. Interference by fetal steroids is not routinely assessed or accounted for by some assay manufacturers, as the premature neonate may not be their main consideration when developing the assay. The potential presence of fetal adrenal steroids should be taken into account when performing and interpreting steroid hormone assays in children less than 6 months of age. These steroids may interfere with the routine steroid assays available in most laboratories.[4] It is possible to mitigate these problems by adapting assay methods but not all laboratories appear to apply these procedures. Even then different methods may vary widely in their analytical specificity, complicating interpretation even further. A recent alternative, through advances in technology, is to refer samples to specialised laboratories employing mass spectrometry based techniques that do not suffer from such interferences. As a general rule of thumb, when in doubt, hormone assays should be repeated at an age equivalent to or greater than that of a full-term pregnancy, or alternatively the tests may be referred to a specialist paediatric laboratory.

◐ Assay imprecision

In some instances the choice of assay may be applicable for one section of the population but may be less than ideal for another section of the population such as children. This was illustrated by a study examining the reliability of results of testosterone assays in females, who have testosterone concentrations comparable to those seen in childhood. The ten assays examined were the most common assays used in clinical biochemistry laboratories but they were found to have poor sensitivity and precision for low concentrations of testosterone.[5]

◐ Assay bias (accuracy)

Bias is a major issue for any laboratory test and will determine the relevance of quoted reference ranges. Routine tests such as electrolytes and lipids may be closely comparable between different laboratories. However, many others tests—including steroids, peptide hormones, therapeutic drugs and tumour markers—will show potentially misleading variation if performed by different laboratories, which may use different kits with different antibody content and specificity.

○ Interpretation of the results

Providing appropriate reference ranges is crucial to the interpretation of any test result, regardless of the patient group involved. The determination of accurate reference intervals is a considerable burden to any laboratory, which is increased by the variations in analyte concentrations frequently encountered in young children.

It is therefore possible that a laboratory which does not have access to a large paediatric patient base may not have the resources to determine paediatric reference intervals applicable to its own specific methods and analytical systems. In these circumstances the laboratory may have to depend upon data supplied by the manufacturer of their testing materials or perhaps determined by other laboratories. Consequently, the ranges accompanying results may not always be entirely appropriate. Clinicians are well advised to enquire about the source of the reference range(s) when faced with diagnostic uncertainty. Published guidance on paediatric ranges at different ages is available.[6]

Examples of variations which occur in childhood are:

- In the perinatal period, the reference ranges for glucose, calcium and magnesium are lower while that of bilirubin is higher than those of other age groups. In addition, when measuring total calcium concentration it is essential to correct for albumin in newborns or preferably measure their ionised calcium.
- In the term neonate, bilirubin and drug metabolism pathways are immature, and significant changes in concentrations may occur as these pathways mature during the first few weeks following birth. Urea is higher but falls to adult levels during infancy. These effects are more pronounced in premature neonates.
- From infancy through childhood, serum creatinine and urinary catecholamine excretion are lower, eventually reaching adult levels during adolescence.
- From infancy to adolescence, alkaline phosphatase and insulin-like growth factor-1 change considerably over time.
- Hepatic drug metabolism increases from neonatal levels during childhood, eventually decreasing to adult levels after puberty. Thus even weight-adjusted doses required to achieve a therapeutic plasma level may be different from those for adults.

Caution needs to be exercised in the interpretation of hormone results from premature babies because apparently abnormal hormone levels may not be indicative of an underlying pathological process. Hormone assays that have negligible interference (such as mass spectrometry based assays) and the availability of age-appropriate reference ranges are essential for correct and timely interpretation of biochemical results in this age group. More work needs to be conducted by laboratories and manufacturers to develop appropriate reference ranges for gestational age for these analytes.

The adrenarche and pubertal period present considerable difficulties when assigning reference ranges since a child may reach puberty earlier or later than may be anticipated. Results may occasionally be seen significantly outside the reference intervals without any apparent pathology. It may therefore be prudent for laboratories not to quote reference ranges for this patient group, especially if there is automated assignment of ranges. Clinicians could consider encouraging their pathology provider(s) to apply interpretative comments instead of possibly incorrect reference intervals. Providing adequate clinical information to the laboratory will enhance the value of these comments.

�‍○ Summary

Interpretation of laboratory results from paediatric patients may be made difficult by a number of factors. Where uncertainty remains it may be advisable to refer further testing to a laboratory that receives relatively larger numbers of paediatric samples and which should consequently have more data and greater experience in interpreting the results.

References

1. Riley M., Davey M-A. and King J. *Births In Victoria 2003–2004*. Victorian Perinatal Data Collection Unit. Melbourne: Victorian government Department of Human Services, 2005. http://www.health.vic.gov.au/ perinatal

2. National Health and Medical Research Council. *Care Around Preterm Birth. Clinical Practice Guidelines*. Canberra: Australian Government Publishing Service, 1997.

3. Burtis C.A. and Ashwood E.R. *Tietz Textbook of Clinical Chemistry*. 3rd edn. Philadelphia: WB Saunders Company, 1999. p. 1 838.

4. Greaves R., Kanumakala S., Read A. and Zacharin M. Transient 3 beta HSD deficiency and ambiguous genitalia in premature babies. *J Paediatr Child Health* 2004; 40: 233–6.

5. Taieb J., Mathian B., Millot F., Patricot M-C., Mathieu E. and Queyrel N. Testosterone measured by 10 immunoassays and by isotope-dilution gas chromatography-mass spectrometry in sera from 116 men, women and children. *Clin Chem* 2003; 49: 1381–95.

6. Soldin S.J., Brugnara C. and Wong E.C. *Pediatric Reference Ranges*. 4th edn. Washington DC: AACC Press, 2003.

Synopsis

The two common types of drug screens are rapid tests and specific assays. Rapid tests are for a restricted range of substances (usually just drugs of abuse) and have limited sensitivity and specificity. When there are important medicolegal considerations the results must be confirmed by more specific assays. Specific assays are labour intensive tests that can detect most drugs but take much longer to perform. They are required where the concentration of the drug may lead to specific interventions (such as in certain overdoses). Conversely even the most comprehensive negative screen cannot entirely rule out drug ingestion as some substances are difficult to detect. The knowledge of the laboratory staff should be utilised when ordering and interpreting the tests.

○ Introduction

'Drug screens' are simply tests for a range of drugs or other substances. They have a wide variety of uses and almost any bodily fluid can be screened. Routine use of drug screens does not improve clinical outcomes but selective use may assist patient management and occasionally yield an unexpected diagnosis.

○ Types of drug screens

There are two main types of drug screens. Immunoassays screen for a limited range of selected substances. These assays are relatively quick and some can even be performed at the bedside. They are commonly used to detect drugs of abuse or to test for commonly ingested substances in overdose but they do not quantify the concentration. There may be cross-reactivity with some chemically related substances and the test cannot detect uncommon or unsuspected drugs. Different brands of immunoassays have different problems with sensitivity and specificity. These problems should be outlined in the product information of the assays.

The second form of drug screening involves chromatography with or without mass spectrometry. This can detect and quantify most substances that are present in significant concentrations. Testing is relatively expensive and depends heavily on the skill and experience of the laboratory staff. Unless only specific substances are of interest the turnaround time varies from days to weeks, so these tests are less likely to influence the acute management of a patient. There are some rapid high-throughput methods that combine the advantages of both methods but these are not widely available.

Screening tests most commonly use urine but serum can also be used. In forensic studies, vitreous humour, pleural effusions, hair, bone or nails may be screened. Saliva, breath, sweat and breast milk can also be screened when looking for drugs of abuse.

◯ Indications for screening

Overall, screening is most frequently used in medicolegal situations. These include determining cause of death; detecting performance-enhancing drugs in athletes and drug abuse in the workplace; drug and alcohol rehabilitation programs; suspicion of date rape; or for psychiatric patients. In most cases detecting a drug, in any concentration, gives sufficient information.

In acute poisoning and other toxicological screening the drug concentration may be important so screening the urine may not be the appropriate investigation. Drug screens of the urine do not reveal the amount of drug or the time it was taken because the urinary concentration correlates poorly with serum concentrations. Detecting the presence of a drug does not tell you if it is at a toxic concentration or explain the clinical status of the patient. In these circumstances serum may be a better body fluid to screen. This is particularly so for substances such as paracetamol, salicylates, anticonvulsants, alcohol, ethylene glycol, methanol, lithium and theophylline, as their concentrations determine the treatment. In these situations specific assays are usually more appropriate than a 'drug screen'. Paracetamol is so commonly taken in overdose that a routine specific assay in unconscious patients is generally warranted. However, routine specific assays for other substances are not indicated unless there are signs or biochemical changes that raise suspicion of their ingestion. Quantitative screening for drugs is also important in patients with suspected brain death.

◯ Technical aspects

To optimise the usefulness and the cost effectiveness of drug screens there are several important factors. These include selection of a screening test appropriate to the patient, correct collection of samples, communication with the laboratory and follow-up tests where appropriate.

Selecting an appropriate screen

The most common clinical reason for requesting a drug screen is suspected ingestion of an unknown substance or substances. Examples include suspicions of overdose (e.g. coma, seizures, acidosis), malingering or child abuse (e.g. unexplained hypoglycaemia or ataxia) and illicit drug abuse (e.g. psychosis, mood swings). Where possible the drug screen should relate to the patient's clinical presentation. For example, a patient with severe acidosis may be suspected of taking a number of substances. However, most immunoassay techniques do not detect many of the drugs and poisons that lead to acidosis. They are designed to detect only commonly used drugs of abuse and drugs that lead to coma, such as alcohol, benzodiazepines, opiates, amphetamines, tricyclic antidepressants, LSD, cocaine and marijuana. A 'negative' drug screen of the urine in a patient with acidosis would be largely unhelpful or misleading. Specific screening of the serum for ethylene glycol, methanol and salicylates and chromatography to detect other unusual substances may be quicker and much more useful investigations.

In many cases drug screens are done for legal or quasi-legal purposes and the screen must accurately detect substances relevant to that purpose (e.g. drugs that might impair driving). Testing for other substances is irrelevant.

In contrast relatively few laboratories have the capacity to do rapid (non-quantitative) screening for hundreds of different drugs (what many clinicians believe they are ordering when they request a drug screen). Such screens are the only means of identifying toxicological epidemics due to increased toxicity of a substituted illicit drug such as the more toxic paramethoxyamphetamine being sold as 'ecstasy'. Similarly such screening techniques may be critical in suspected chemical terrorist incidents. However, such intensive (and expensive) screening has no role in routine management as it has been repeatedly shown not to improve outcome in individual patients with suspected drug intoxication or overdose.

Communication with the laboratory

Most laboratories performing drug screens do large numbers of tests for non-clinical reasons. If you anticipate that the drug screen may alter your clinical management it is important to discuss the case with the laboratory. A history of the drugs the patient is known to take will help the laboratory to identify the substances you are not concerned about. Knowing which specific substances are suspected on clinical grounds helps the laboratory to tell you whether or not it can identify such substances, for how long they can be detected after ingestion and whether serum or urine is preferred. The laboratory may also alter the methods used to prepare the sample to maximise the sensitivity of the testing for those substances.

Collection of the sample and follow-up tests (medicolegal cases)

Correct and explicit identification of the patient and sample, prevention of tampering during collection and a secure chain of custody are very important in medicolegal cases. If the result has important medicolegal implications the accuracy of the result should be confirmed by using more specific and accurate methods such as gas or liquid chromatography and mass spectrometry. Depending on the drug involved these tests are done on the same specimen or a different specimen.

◯ False positive results

The most common cause of false positive results in clinical settings is the therapeutic use of barbiturates, benzodiazepines and/or opiates for sedation, anaesthetic induction or analgesia. Many immunoassays do not differentiate between drugs in these classes and may cross-react with related therapeutic substances. For example, codeine (and poppy seeds) may lead to positive opiate reactions and decongestants such as pseudoephedrine and phenylpropanolamine may lead to positive amphetamine reactions. Only discussion with the laboratory and further specific testing can clarify such results.

◯ False negative results

False negatives can relate to the time of sampling (too soon or too late), the body fluid tested or the method used. Immunoassays test for a restricted range of chemically related substances. Even within pharmacological drug classes they may not detect substances that have identical effects but an unrelated chemical structure. For example, most immunoassays for opiates do not detect the structurally unrelated methadone, dextromethorphan or pethidine. Metals (e.g. mercury, arsenic) are not detected by the commonly used drug screens and require specific tests. Some toxic substances (insulin, succinylcholine, potassium) cannot be detected by any method, as any avid reader of crime fiction knows.

◯ Other problems of interpretation

The detection of one substance does not exclude the presence of others that cannot be detected by the same method. Drugs with similar chemical structures but different toxicities may give the same result. For example, within the drugs in the amphetamine class (methamphetamine, MDMA, PMA, fenfluramine and pseudoephedrine) there is a non-overlapping spectrum of peripheral and central nervous system stimulant effects and serotoninergic effects which lead to quite different toxicological syndromes. Failure to appreciate that some positive immunoassay screens for amphetamines could indicate ingestion of any or all of these drugs may lead to inappropriate management.

○ Summary

Drug screens are a useful clinical tool if you are selective in their use, have realistic expectations of their sensitivity and specificity and discuss the clinical setting and suspected drugs with the laboratory staff. Otherwise you may be better off disposing of the urine in the traditional and less expensive manner.

Further reading

Braithwaite R.A., Jarvie D.R., Minty P.S., Simpson D. and Widdop B. Screening for drugs of abuse I: Opiates, amphetamines and cocaine. *Ann Clin Biochem* 1995; 32: 123–53.

Eichhorst J.C., Etter M.L., Rousseaux N. and, Lehotay D.C. Drugs of abuse testing by tandem mass spectrometry: a rapid, simple method to replace immunoassays. *Clin Biochem* 2009; 42(15): 1531–42.

Eskridge K.D. and Guthrie S.K. Clinical issues associated with urine testing of substances of abuse. *Pharmacotherapy* 1997; 17: 497–510.

Fabbri A., Marchesini G., Morselli-Labate A. M., Ruggeri S., Fallani M., Melandri R. et al. Comprehensive drug screening in decision making of patients attending the emergency department for suspected drug overdose. *Emerg Med J* 2003; 20: 25–8.

Flanagan R.J. Developing an analytical toxicology service: principles and guidance. *Toxicol Rev* 2004; 23(4): 251–63.

Fortu J.M., Kim I.K., Cooper A., Condra C., Lorenz D.J. and Pierce M.C. Psychiatric patients in the pediatric emergency department undergoing routine urine toxicology screens for medical clearance: results and use. *Pediatr Emerg Care* 2009; 25(6): 387–92.

Hammett-Stabler C.A., Pesce A.J. and Cannon D.J. Urine drug screening in the medical setting. *Clin Chim Acta* 2002; 315(1–2): 125–35.

Simpson D., Braithwaite R.A., Jarvie D.R., Stewart M.J., Walker S., Watson I.W. et al. Screening for drugs of abuse II: Cannabinoids, lysergic acid diethylamide, buprenorphine, methadone, barbiturates, benzodiazepines and other drugs. *Ann Clin Biochem 1997*; 34: 460–510.

Tenenbein M. Do you really need that emergency drug screen? *Clin Toxicol* 2009; 47(4): 286–91.

Wu A.H., McKay C., Broussard L.A., Hoffman R.S., Kwong T. C., Moyer T.P. et al. National academy of clinical biochemistry laboratory medicine practice guidelines: recommendations for the use of laboratory tests to support poisoned patients who present to the emergency department. *Clin Chem* 2003; 49(3): 357–79.

30 Therapeutic drug monitoring: which drugs, why, when and how to do it*

R.A. Ghiculescu

Synopsis

Therapeutic drug monitoring of concentrations of drugs in body fluids, usually plasma, can be used during treatment and for diagnostic purposes. The selection of drugs for therapeutic drug monitoring is important as the concentrations of many drugs are not clearly related to their effects. For selected drugs therapeutic drug monitoring aims to enhance drug efficacy, reduce toxicity or assist with diagnosis. Despite its apparent advantages, it has inherent limitations. Some large hospitals have services that provide support with drug monitoring and interpretation of results.

○ Introduction

The monitoring of therapeutic drugs involves measuring drug concentrations in plasma, serum or blood. This information is used to individualise dosage so that drug concentrations can be maintained within a target range.[1]

Drug concentration at the site of action cannot be routinely measured but the desired or adverse effects may correlate better with plasma or blood concentrations than they do with dose. For a few drugs, concentration measurements are a valuable surrogate of drug exposure, particularly if there is no simple or sensitive measure of effect.

When there is a large inter-individual variation between dose and effect, for example when there is large pharmacokinetic variation, individualising drug dosage is difficult.[1] This is particularly relevant for drugs with a narrow target range or concentration-dependent pharmacokinetics. Similarly, variations within an individual can occur over time for a range of reasons with some drugs, and therapeutic drug monitoring could then be useful.

Therapeutic drug monitoring involves not only measuring drug concentrations but also the clinical interpretation of the result. This requires

---

* This chapter represents an update of R. A. Ghiculescu's article by P. Pillans. (Editor)

knowledge of the pharmacokinetics, sampling time, drug history and the patient's clinical condition.

◐ **Which drugs?**

When an effect—such as changes in blood pressure, pain or serum cholesterol—is readily measured, the dose of a drug should be adjusted according to the response. Monitoring drug concentration is more useful when drugs are used to prevent an adverse outcome, for example graft rejection or to avoid toxicity, as with aminoglycosides. A drug should satisfy certain criteria to be suitable for therapeutic drug monitoring. Examples include:

* narrow target range
* significant pharmacokinetic variability
* a reasonable relationship between plasma concentrations and clinical effects
* established target concentration range
* availability of a cost-effective drug assay.

The most commonly monitored drugs are probably carbamazepine, valproate and digoxin. However, there is little evidence that monitoring concentrations of anticonvulsants improves clinical outcomes when the drugs are used to treat mood disorders.

Table 30.1 shows some of the drugs that meet these criteria.

Table 30.1 Drugs suitable for therapeutic drug monitoring

Drug	Target range*
Drugs regularly monitored in clinical practice	
Aminoglycosides	See text
Cyclosporine	150–400 mcg/L (whole blood) (120–300 nmol/L) Concentrations differ for various clinical settings
Digoxin	0.8–2 mcg/L (1.0–2.5 nmol/L)
Lithium acute mania maintenance	0.8–1.2 mmol/L 0.4–1.0 mmol/L
Perhexiline	0.15–0.6 mg/L (0.5–2.2 micromol/L)
Phenytoin	10–20 mg/L (40–80 micromol/L)
Sirolimus	5–15 mcg/L (whole blood)
Tacrolimus	5–20 mcg/L (whole blood) (6–25 nmol/L)

Drug	Target range*
Drugs for which monitoring may be useful	
Amiodarone	1–2.5 mg/L (1.5–3.0 micromol/L)
Carbamazepine	5–12 mg/L (17–50 micromol/L)
Clozapine	100–600 mcg/L (300–800 nmol/L)
Flecainide	0.2–0.9 mg/L (0.5–2.5 micromol/L)
Lamotrigine	1.5–3 mg/L (6–12 micromol/L)
Salicylate	150–300 mg/L (1.1–2.2 mmol/L)
Sodium valproate	50–100 mg/L (350–700 micromol/L)
Vancomycin	Trough 10–20 mg/L (14–28 micromol/L)

*Concentrations may vary between laboratories

○ Indications (why do it)

Drug assays are costly, so the reason for monitoring and the additional information to be gained (if any) should be carefully considered. For some drugs, therapeutic drug monitoring helps to increase efficacy (vancomycin), to avoid toxicity (gentamicin) and to assist diagnosis (salicylates). Routine monitoring is not advocated for most drugs. Only clinically meaningful tests should be performed.[1]

The appropriate indications for therapeutic drug monitoring (and examples) include:

- toxicity
  - diagnosing toxicity when the clinical syndrome is undifferentiated (unexplained nausea in a patient taking digoxin)
  - avoiding toxicity (aminoglycosides, cyclosporine)
- dosing
  - after dose adjustment (usually after reaching a steady state)
  - assessment of adequacy of loading dose (after starting phenytoin treatment)
  - dose forecasting to help predict a patient's dose requirements[1] (aminoglycosides)
  - single measurement as a yardstick of adequate control
- monitoring
  - assessing compliance (anticonvulsant concentrations in patients having frequent seizures)
  - diagnosing undertreatment (particularly important for prophylactic drugs such as anticonvulsants and immunosuppressants)

QUICK FLICK 30

– diagnosing failed therapy (therapeutic drug monitoring can help distinguish between ineffective drug treatment, non-compliance and adverse effects that mimic the underlying disease).

The target concentration may depend on the indication. For example, the recommended concentration for digoxin depends on whether it is being used to treat atrial fibrillation or congestive heart failure.[2]

◐ Timing of the plasma sample (when to do it)

Unless therapeutic drug monitoring is being used to forecast a dose or there are concerns about toxicity, samples should be taken at steady state (4–5 half-lives after starting therapy).[1,3]

At steady state, plasma concentration is usually proportional to receptor concentration. Some drugs—such as perhexiline, which has a very long half-life in patients who are 'poor' metabolisers—should be monitored before steady state is achieved to prevent toxicity developing after the first few doses. Another example where early monitoring may be useful is after phenytoin loading, where measurement of the plasma concentration can give a preliminary indication of adequate dosing.

The timing of the collection of the sample is important as the drug concentration changes during the dosing interval. The least variable point in the dosing interval is just before the next dose is due. This pre-dose or trough concentration is what is usually measured. For drugs with long half-lives such as phenobarbitone and amiodarone, samples can be collected at any point in the dosage interval.[1,3]

Correct sample timing should also take into account absorption and distribution. For example, digoxin monitoring should not be performed within 6 hours of a dose because it will still be undergoing distribution and so plasma concentrations will be erroneously high.[1,3]

Occasionally, sampling at the time of specific symptoms may detect toxicity related to peak concentrations of, for example, carbamazepine and lithium.

For once-daily dosing of aminoglycosides, the timing of the blood sample is determined by the method of monitoring. For example, it is collected 6–14 hours post-dose when a nomogram is used, or twice within the dosing interval to calculate the area under the concentration–time curve.[4,5] When aminoglycosides are prescribed in multiple daily doses to treat, for example, enterococcal endocarditis, trough samples are measured to minimise toxicity. Note that vancomycin is a glycopeptide and not an aminoglycoside.

○ Therapeutic drug monitoring request (what to document)

Drug assays may be requested for therapeutic drug monitoring or for clinical toxicology purposes.[5] For therapeutic drug monitoring the information required to allow interpretation of the result should include the time of the sample collection, the time of the last dose, the dosage regimen and the indication for drug monitoring.[1,3]

○ Interpretation

Drug concentrations need to be interpreted in the context of the individual patient without rigid adherence to a target range. For example, if a patient has an anticonvulsant drug concentration just below the target range but is not having seizures, an increase in dose is probably not required. For a few drugs, monitoring drug concentration is a helpful adjunctive measure. Before making dose adjustments, it is important to consider if the sample was taken at the correct time with respect to the last dose, if a steady state has been reached and whether the patient has adhered to the treatment. There are other considerations; for example, the serum potassium should be noted when interpreting digoxin concentrations as toxicity can occur at a therapeutic concentration if there is hypokalaemia.

Most drug assays measure total drug concentration (bound and unbound drug) but only the unbound drug interacts with its receptor to produce a response. The unbound fraction may be affected by factors such as serum albumin concentration, displacement by an interacting drug and renal failure. This is important for drugs like phenytoin. If phenytoin's unbound fraction doubles from 10% to 20%, the target range based on total phenytoin concentration should be halved. If dose adjustments are made according to the usual target range, toxicity may result.

○ Measuring and monitoring

Drug concentrations should be measured within a clinically useful timeframe in laboratories with appropriately trained staff and subject to quality assays.[3] The ideal laboratory turnaround time should be shorter than the dosing interval. However, due to cost, assays are performed in batches, which may lengthen the turnaround time.

Plasma drug concentrations are reported either in mass or molar units. Reporting in mass units with attached conversion formulas may assist with interpretation of results.[3]

Differences exist between laboratories, and validated target ranges should accompany results to assist clinicians with safe and effective prescribing.[3]

Some institutions provide drug monitoring and interpretive services which may help to improve the safety, efficacy and cost effectiveness of clinical services. These therapeutic drug monitoring services also have an educational role by promoting the principles of rational prescribing and quality use of medicines.[3]

Limitations

Apart from the limited number of drugs amenable to therapeutic drug monitoring, there are also inherent limitations, including the scientific accuracy of the drug assays, laboratory variability in reporting, limited accessibility in rural Australia and the validity of suggested target ranges.[1,3]

The target range describes a range of drug concentrations associated with a reasonable probability of efficacy without undue toxicity in the majority of patients. It is not well described for most drugs and is often based on a very limited number of data points.[1,2]

Active metabolites (e.g. carbamazepine-10,11-epoxide) may contribute to the therapeutic response but are not routinely measured.

Summary

The drug concentration is complementary to and not a substitute for clinical judgment so it is important to treat the individual patient and not the laboratory value. Drug concentrations may be used as surrogates for drug effects, so therapeutic drug monitoring may assist with dose individualisation. It can also be used to detect toxicity, so therapeutic drug monitoring can optimise patient management and improve clinical outcomes. Careful selection of drugs to be monitored should occur. Regular monitoring of many drugs is not required in a clinically stable patient.

References

1. Birkett D.J. Therapeutic drug monitoring. *Aust Prescr* 1997; 20: 9–11.
2. Chatterjee K. Congestive heart failure: what should be the initial therapy and why? *Am J Cardiovasc Drugs* 2002; 2: 1–6.
3. Gross A.S. Best practice in therapeutic drug monitoring. *Br J Clin Pharmacol* 1998; 46: 95–9.
4. Begg E.J., Barclay M.L. and Duffull S.B. A suggested approach to once-daily aminoglycoside dosing. *Br J Clin Pharmacol* 1995; 39: 605–9.
5. *eTG complete*. Therapeutic Guidelines Ltd. Nov 2007.

Part 3

Haematology Tests

31 The red cells*

W.R. Pitney

○ Introduction

A full blood count (FBC) is one of the most commonly requested of all laboratory tests. It forms part of all multiphasic screening procedures and is requested almost routinely in any patient with more than a minor illness. An FBC is performed using an automated laboratory instrument that measures the haemoglobin and the number of red cells, leucocytes and platelets and generates a number of indices and an automated leucocyte differential count. The reticulocyte count is automated in larger laboratories.

○ Technical aspects

Automated FBC machines measure haemoglobin (Hb), red cell count (RCC) and mean corpuscular volume (MCV). From these measurements the mean corpuscular haemoglobin (MCH), mean corpuscular haemoglobin concentration (MCHC) and haematocrit or packed cell volume (PCV) are calculated (Table 31.1). The red cell distribution width (RDW) is also measured. The RDW is a mathematical representation of the variability in size of the erythrocyte population. The erythrocytes are categorised by volume as they are counted in automated cell counting equipment. Most laboratories no longer examine blood films if the FBC is normal. All abnormal FBCs will have a morphological comment.

The most important red cell aspects of the blood count report are the haemoglobin value and the comment on the blood film, and these should always be considered together.

* This chapter updated by R.A. Dunstan and M. Seldon.

Table 31.1 Measurements and red cell indices

Measurement	Index	Calculation of index	
Haemoglobin concentration (Hb, g/L)	Mean cell volume (MCV)	$\dfrac{\text{PCV}}{\text{RCC}}$	expressed as femtolitres (fL, 10^{-15} L)
Red cell count (RCC, $\times 10^{12}$/L)	Mean cell haemoglobin (MCH)	$\dfrac{\text{Hb}}{\text{RCC}}$	expressed as picograms (pg, 10^{-12} g)
Haematocrit or packed cell volume (PCV, L/L)	Mean cell haemoglobin concentration (MCHC)	$\dfrac{\text{Hb}}{\text{PCV}}$	expressed as g/L

○ Is the result abnormal?

The abnormality reported may be an increase or a decrease in Hb value, RCC and/or haematocrit outside the reference ranges and there may be morphological changes in the red cells in the blood film. There may also be abnormalities in the red cell indices but these should correlate with the red cell morphology; for example, hypochromia should be associated with a low MCH. Minor degrees of anisocytosis (variation in size) and poikilocytosis (variation in shape) are not significant and are found in normal people. A low Hb value due to leukaemia or other malignant blood disorders will usually be associated with abnormalities in white cells and platelets, and the blood film comment should indicate the diagnosis. It will be assumed in what follows that any abnormalities in the blood film are confined to the red cells.

○ Low haemoglobin, red cells normal

The patient appears to have a normocytic normochromic anaemia and the red cell indices are in the normal range. It is important to remember that the normal range of Hb concentration is less in children and in pregnancy. Women of child-bearing age usually have Hb values about 20 g/L lower than men but this difference becomes less after the menopause. Over the age of 75 years Hb may fall secondary to inactivity. Normochromic normocytic anaemia is often a reflection of a general medical or surgical disorder. The patient should be assessed with regard to the conditions listed in Table 31.2. The blood sedimentation rate or C-reactive protein is commonly elevated in these conditions and provides useful information on disease activity. Following haemorrhage and in some types of haemolytic anaemia the red cells may be of normal size and shape but the film report may comment on polychromasia, which indicates increased release of reticulocytes from the bone marrow, and a reticulocyte count should be performed. Haemolytic anaemia is often associated with blood film comments such as the presence of spherocytosis and autoagglutination. A comment of increased red cell rouleaux suggests the possibility of multiple myeloma. A bone marrow examination is usually necessary if there is no obvious cause for normochromic normocytic anaemia with Hb less than 100g/L.

Table 31.2 Important causes of normochromic, normocytic anaemia

Organ failure	Renal failure
	Hypothyroidism
Chronic inflammation	Rheumatoid arthritis
	Chronic infection
Malignancy	Occult
	Non-occult
	Treatment of malignancy (chemotherapy or radiotherapy)
Acute blood loss	
Bone marrow failure	

◑ Low haemoglobin, red cells hypochromic

Usually all three calculated red cell indices will be reduced. The most common cause is iron deficiency anaemia but the alternative diagnosis of thalassaemia trait should be considered and in such patients further investigation is always warranted. The MCV is usually lower and the red cell count higher in thalassaemia trait than in iron deficiency, and stipple cells and target cells may be prominent features of the blood film report. Haemoglobin electrophoretic studies and serum iron studies will usually establish the correct diagnosis. Clinical judgment *is* required to determine whether a patient with iron deficiency warrants further investigation. Menorrhagia and repeated pregnancies are common causes in women of child-bearing age. A site of occult blood loss must always be suspected when iron deficiency is diagnosed in men or in postmenopausal women. Carcinoma of the caecum presents classically as iron deficiency anaemia. A rare cause of hypochromic normocytic anaemia in the elderly is sideroblastic anaemia; bone marrow examination is necessary for diagnosis.

◑ Low haemoglobin, red cells macrocytic

The MCV and MCH will be elevated but the MCHC should be normal. Macrocytosis occurs in liver disease (when the macrocytic cells are usually round and may show a target-cell appearance) and in megaloblastic anaemia (when there is usually prominent poikilocytosis, and ovalling of cells). The commonest cause of macrocytosis in Australia is alcohol, with or without liver disease. The usual causes of megaloblastic anaemia are nutritional (folate deficiency) or pernicious anaemia (vitamin B_{12} deficiency). Measurement of serum B_{12} and folate are indicated. If B_{12} and folate deficiencies are excluded then a bone marrow is indicated. Figure 31.1 summarises the investigation of the anaemias.

○ Raised haemoglobin

An elevated Hb value may be a temporary phenomenon due to haemoconcentration, for example dehydration from excessive use of diuretics. Patients with chronic bronchitis and cigarette smokers may have a moderate elevation of Hb. In cigarette smokers this is initially due to the inhalation of carbon monoxide and the formation of carboxyhaemoglobin, which shifts the oxygen dissociation curve of haemoglobin to the left. Cessation of smoking may result in a considerable fall in Hb value over a period of 6–8 weeks. Chronic hypoxaemia from cardiac or lung disease leads to elevated Hb levels, as do some renal conditions with increased erythropoietin secretion such as polycystic kidney disease. A reduced plasma volume with a normal red cell mass (stress polycythaemia or spurious polycythaemia) sometimes occurs in middle-aged males for no apparent reason. True polycythaemia may be primary or secondary. If the white cells and platelets are normal and there is no splenomegaly, the patient should be investigated for causes of secondary polycythaemia. Primary polycythaemia is marked in 95% of cases by having the JAK2 genetic abnormality.

○ Summary

An abnormality in the blood count always warrants careful consideration. It is unlikely to be due to laboratory error as most laboratories now use automated blood cell counters with a high degree of accuracy and with good methods of quality control. If the results do not fit with the clinical picture, a repeat FBC should be performed. It should be remembered, however, that the quoted references ranges for Hb, RCC and haematocrit are too rigid to include all normal people and an occasional result outside the range may not be abnormal. Furthermore, the references ranges quoted by different laboratories show some variation. *Anaemia is a laboratory finding, not a disease entity, and it is imperative that the cause be found before treatment is commenced. The use of haematinics or blood transfusion without proper characterisation of anaemia is not good practice; it makes subsequent investigation more difficult and may even do harm (e.g. folate can accelerate development of subacute combined degeneration in pernicious anaemia and iron therapy can result in iron overload in thalassaemia trait).*

Figure 31.1 The investigation of anaemia

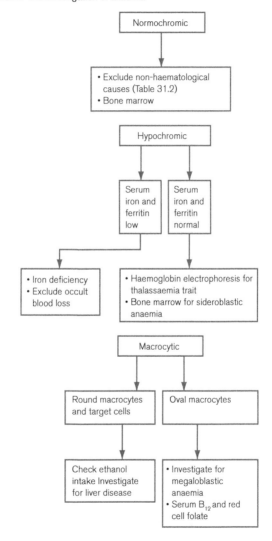

Further reading

Any modern haematology textbook.

32 Interpreting biochemical tests for iron deficiency: diagnostic difficulties imposed by the limitations of individual tests

F. Firkin and B. Rush

Synopsis

Serum biochemical tests that provide indices of iron status play a dominant role in evaluating the cause of microcytic anaemia (a mean red cell volume [MCV] less than 78–80 fL) and assessing the extent to which iron deficiency contributes to anaemia where there are multiple contributory factors. Microcytosis, with or without associated anaemia, is most commonly due to iron deficiency but is also typical in thalassaemia. Microcytosis can also occasionally occur in anaemia secondary to chronic infection, inflammation or malignancy, commonly referred to as anaemia of chronic disease, although the MCV is normal in the majority. Assessment of serum levels of iron, transferrin, ferritin and the percentage saturation with iron of the total iron binding capacity (TIBC) of transferrin constitutes the panel of biochemical tests that is collectively employed as the most common approach to evaluating iron status. It is very important to recognise that any one test performed in isolation, for example the serum iron level, can provide a misleading view of iron status, as the value is frequently skewed by coexisting clinical factors. Coexistence of such modifying factors can usually be recognised by the characteristic difference in the profile of results in the test panel from that typically associated with straightforward iron deficiency. Results of assessment of body iron stores performed in this manner provide such a reliable index of iron status that it is not appropriate to perform endoscopic examinations merely because a patient has anaemia in the absence of haematological or biochemical results that implicate iron deficiency or clinical features suggestive of gastrointestinal disease.

◯ Investigating iron status

The panel of tests that determine levels of serum iron, transferrin (or TIBC), ferritin and the percentage saturation of transferrin with iron represents the appropriate first-line approach for investigating iron deficiency. Determination of only one of these indices can lead to serious misinterpretation of the status of body iron stores.

◯ Pathophysiological aspects

The serum iron/transferrin relationship

The serum (or plasma) iron level falls progressively below the normal range, which is about 10–32 micromol/L for adult males and slightly lower for females (with some inter-laboratory variation in the reference range) in association with a decline in the amount of iron in the body after the reserve stores of iron have become exhausted. The level of transferrin, the major iron transporting protein in the circulation, rises under these circumstances towards or above the upper limit of the normal range. A subnormal level of iron in association with a supranormal level of transferrin is very strong evidence of iron deficiency.

Levels of iron and transferrin in the serum, however, fall rapidly as part of the acute phase response to inflammation despite the presence of normal iron stores. This abnormal state continues as long as the inflammatory process persists and, if sustained, is associated with the development of anaemia usually referred to as 'anaemia of chronic disease'. The low serum iron level in this setting is unfortunately frequently misinterpreted as evidence of iron deficiency, a major diagnostic error that can be avoided by simultaneous examination of the transferrin level, which in this context is subnormal or in the low normal range in contrast to the relatively high or supranormal values seen in uncomplicated iron deficiency. Estimation of the level of serum iron alone is consequently inadvisable in the search for a cause of anaemia (Table 32.1).

Table 32.1 Alteration of serum iron levels by other conditions

False high	False low
Masked by recent iron medication (sometimes unrecognised as a component of vitamin preparations with mineral supplements)	Concurrent inflammatory disorders Postoperative or traumatic wound repair Concurrent infection Concurrent malignancy Hypoproteinaemia

Relation of transferrin level to serum TIBC

The overwhelming majority of iron in serum is bound to the transferrin molecules which serve to transport iron in the circulation. Serum transferrin levels are estimated by immunological assays that indicate a normal range in adults of about 1.9–3.1 g/L, with some variation depending on the method employed. The functional capacity of transferrin can also be expressed in terms of the total amount of iron that it can bind per litre of serum and this value is referred to as the total iron binding capacity (TIBC), with a reference range of about 47–78 micromol/L. Serum TIBC therefore provides an alternative functional expression of the concentration of transferrin in serum. (The conversion factor is that 1 g/L transferrin equates to a TIBC of 25 micromol/L.)

Table 32.2 Alteration of serum transferrin levels by other conditions

False normal	False low
Very uncommon	Concurrent inflammatory disorders
	Postoperative or traumatic wound repair
	Concurrent infection
	Concurrent malignancy
	Hypoproteinaemia

◇ Expressing results as percentage saturation of transferrin

The mean percentage occupation of iron binding sites on transferrin by iron is determined by dividing the serum iron level by the TIBC of the serum, which is now frequently calculated from the level of transferrin determined by antibody-based methods The percent saturation of transferrin in normal adults is about 20–50%. Subnormal values are typical of iron deficiency, but subnormal values are also common in anaemia of chronic disease, where the degree of depression of the serum iron often exceeds the degree of depression of the transferrin level. A subnormal percent saturation of transferrin in isolation is consequently not a specific indicator of iron deficiency.

◇ Diagnostic contribution from assessing serum ferritin

The level of ferritin in serum is normally related to the body's iron stores and provides a valuable indicator of iron deficiency independent of the serum iron level. Subnormal values may be detected when body iron stores are exhausted, even before the serum iron level has unequivocally declined. The quoted normal range is influenced by the particular form of antibody-based assessment that has been employed and by the age and sex of the subject. It is not uncommon for lower values to be quoted for the upper and lower limits of the normal range for menstruating adult women compared with those for adult males. A representative example of the lower limit for adult males is about 15–20 mcg/L, with an upper limit of about 300 mcg/L. The normal range is lower in children.

A subnormal ferritin level is highly specific for iron deficiency but it is essential to recognise that the serum ferritin level increases in a manner independent of its relation to iron stores under some relatively common clinical circumstances, such as inflammatory states and hepatocellular injury, that obscure the normal relation of iron deficiency to the ferritin level. The rise in serum ferritin level in severely iron deficient subjects with a coexisting inflammatory state has been reported to reach the order of 100 mcg/L, occasionally even higher. The extent of this increase in ferritin levels is less than in iron-replete subjects under the same conditions but is nonetheless sufficient to interfere with the capacity of the ferritin level alone to serve as a specific index of iron deficiency under all circumstances.

Table 32.3 Alteration of serum ferritin levels by other conditions

False normal	False low
Concurrent acute and chronic disorders Hepatocellular damage Some malignancies	Very uncommon

○ Evaluating iron status from the overall pattern of iron study test results

Estimations from a single test of either the level of iron, transferrin or ferritin in serum, or the percent saturation of transferrin, are sufficiently commonly affected by coexistent medical conditions to lead to frequent errors in assessing iron status. It is the overall pattern of results that provides a more reliable guide. The subnormal serum iron level in uncomplicated iron deficiency is, for example, associated with a characteristic profile of high normal to elevated transferrin level, a subnormal percent saturation and a subnormal ferritin level. In contrast, the subnormal serum iron level secondary to other disorders, such as infection, is associated with a midrange to low normal transferrin level, often a subnormal percent transferrin saturation and a normal to elevated ferritin level. Such a distinction is dependent on inspecting the overall test result panel and represents an issue of appreciable clinical management importance, as surveys of some series of hospitalised patients have demonstrated that a subnormal serum iron level is more frequently secondary to their current illness than to iron deficiency.

○ Further evaluative steps in inconclusive situations

When the results of the iron study test panel are equivocal and the status of body iron reserves is of major diagnostic importance, it is possible to assess iron reserves by performing a bone marrow aspirate. The marrow particles are stained for iron with the Prussian Blue reaction and examined microscopically. A negative result due to absence of Prussian Blue staining granules is considered to be the gold standard for confirmation of iron deficiency but the procedure is demanding and therefore rarely performed.

An alternative approach is assessment of response to oral iron administration. A rise in the MCV and an increase of > 10 g/L in the haemoglobin level within four to six weeks is evidence that deficiency of iron is contributing to the anaemia. Trials of iron supplements are, however, usually unrewarding in normocytic anaemia where an alternative mechanism is usually responsible for the anaemia.

○ Representative examples of interpretation of abnormal test results

Example A

A 23-year-old man with longstanding microcytic anaemia and low serum iron unresponsive to oral iron supplements:
- Hb 89 g/L, MCV 57 fL (N 80–96)
- Serum iron < 3 micromol/L (N 14–32)
- Serum transferrin 1.5 g/L (N 2.0–3.2)
- Serum ferritin 195 mcg/L (N 40–260)

The pattern of the iron study results and the likely cause of the anaemia are consistent with effects of chronic inflammation. Subsequent determination of the erythrocyte sedimentation rate revealed a very high value of 119 mm/hour. An inflammatory disease was diagnosed and after the underlying disorder responded to specific treatment the haemoglobin level rose to 160 g/L and the MCV to normal.

Example B

The 47-year-old mother of a young teenager who was recently found to have beta-thalassaemia minor was found to have microcytic anaemia on family screening for thalassaemia:
- Hb 65 g/L, MCV 59 fL (N 80–96)

- Serum iron 5.3 micromol/L (N 14–32)
- Serum transferrin 4.6 g/L (N 2.0–3.2)
- Serum ferritin < 5 mcg/L (N 25–155)

This pattern of iron study results is typical of severe iron deficiency and was attributed in this patient to menorrhagia. The haemoglobin level and MCV returned to normal after iron replacement therapy. Subsequent studies revealed no evidence of thalassaemia minor in the mother but did demonstrate beta-thalassaemia minor in the father.

33 Appropriate use of tests for folate and vitamin B$_{12}$ deficiency

J. Metz

Synopsis

A full blood count that shows anaemia and macrocytosis should prompt the practitioner to look for a deficiency of vitamin B$_{12}$ or folate. Tests commonly used for the detection of these vitamin deficiencies are serum folate, red cell folate and serum B$_{12}$ concentrations. Serum folate becomes subnormal in the early stages of negative folate balance before reduction of folate stores. Red cell folate is a direct measure of tissue folate stores. Measurement of both serum and red cell folate yields the maximum information but in practice red cell folate needs to be assayed only when there is macrocytosis and the serum folate is low. Serum B$_{12}$ is a sensitive index of deficiency but a low level does not necessarily indicate deficiency. Following the identification of folate or B$_{12}$ deficiency a cause must be sought.

○ Introduction

Laboratory tests for folate and vitamin B$_{12}$ are essential for the diagnosis of a deficiency of these vitamins and for the investigation of some forms of anaemia. Untreated deficiency of folate or B$_{12}$ may lead to severe anaemia and, in B$_{12}$ deficiency, crippling neurological disease. The clinical indications for testing are broad (Table 33.1). Often the indication for testing is an abnormality found in a full blood examination, such as unexplained anaemia or macrocytosis. Neurological conditions associated with B$_{12}$ deficiency include peripheral neuropathy and subacute combined degeneration of the spinal cord. Deterioration in cognitive ability may also occur. Serum B$_{12}$ should therefore be checked even in the absence of haematological abnormality in patients with some unexplained neurological or neuropsychiatric abnormalities.

Table 33.1 Indications for which testing for folate and B_{12} deficiency might be considered

Unexplained anaemia
Macrocytosis
Suspected malabsorption
Some neurological diseases e.g. peripheral neuropathy
Some psychiatric disorders e.g. unexplained memory loss or dementia
Malnutrition including subjects on restrictive diets e.g. vegetarians
Haematological disease associated with increased cell turnover
Alcohol abuse
Drug therapy e.g. anticonvulsants
Family history of pernicious anaemia
Infertility

○ Investigation of folate and vitamin B_{12} status

Three tests are in common use:
- serum folate
- red cell folate
- serum vitamin B_{12}.

In addition, investigations should always include a full blood examination with assessment of a blood film.

The blood tests must always be taken before specific therapy begins. After such therapy it may be impossible to identify the underlying deficiency.

○ Serum and red cell folate

The usual first test for folate deficiency is assay of serum folate (reference range 7–40 nmol/L). (Reference ranges for serum folate, red cell folate and serum vitamin B_{12} are specific to the methodology used by individual laboratories and may not be identical to the ranges given in this text.) The margin of safety between folate intake and requirement is small so the serum folate concentration may become subnormal after only 3 weeks of negative balance (folate intake less than folate consumption). This is a stage that precedes and may not necessarily progress to body folate depletion with subsequent haematological changes. Subnormal serum folate concentration may imply body deficiency but the serum folate level depends on recent dietary intake and is not strictly a diagnostic test for body folate depletion.

For example, a low serum folate concentration without body depletion occurs with recent alcohol abuse (Table 33.2).

Table 33.2 Problems in interpretation of serum and red cell folate levels in relation to body folate stores

	False normal	False low
Serum folate	Patient given folic acid	Negative dietary folate balance Recent alcohol intake
Red cell folate	Following blood transfusion	Primary B$_{12}$ deficiency

Red cell folate is a direct measure of tissue folate stores. It falls after about 4 months of negative folate balance. Red cell folate will differentiate between negative folate balance and body folate depletion. Low serum with normal red cell folate suggests negative folate balance. Subnormal values for both tests indicate tissue depletion. It is not possible to provide a single reference range for red cell folate as the commercial kits currently in use vary by as much as 100% in their ranges.

A low concentration of red cell folate usually implies significant depletion of folate stores. Subnormal values may also occur in severe vitamin B$_{12}$ deficiency and return to normal following vitamin B$_{12}$ therapy alone. A falsely normal result may occur in a folate-deficient patient who has received a blood transfusion (Table 33.2).

Measurement of serum folate *only* will not differentiate between negative folate balance and tissue folate depletion. Measurement of red cell folate *only* may miss the early stage of negative folate balance. Serum and red cell folate yield complementary data and together the maximum information. However, in practice it is usual to 'screen' with the serum folate assay and to proceed to red cell folate only if the serum folate is subnormal. In a folate-deficient patient recently given folic acid, only red cell folate will detect deficiency.

Serum folate assay is technically easy to perform and is reasonably reproducible but falsely elevated values may occur in folate-deficient patients who have been given folic acid. For technical reasons measurement of red cell folate is not as reliable or reproducible as serum folate and should never be used as the sole test of folate nutrition.

◐ Total serum vitamin B$_{12}$ and the 'active-B$_{12}$' fraction

The B$_{12}$ in serum is carried by two proteins, haptocorrin and transcobalamin. The majority, 70–90%, is bound to haptocorrin and this B$_{12}$ is inert.

Transcobalamin-bound B_{12} is the metabolically active form, which is delivered to developing cells. It was postulated many years ago that measuring transcobalamin-B_{12} ('active-B_{12}') would be a better index of B_{12} status than total B_{12}, but it is only recently that a reliable method for the quantitation of this form of B_{12} has become available.

The most widely used test for B_{12} deficiency is the serum B_{12} assay (reference range 150–600 pmol/L). This is a sensitive index for the detection of B_{12} deficiency but a low concentration does not necessarily indicate tissue deficiency. Conditions where the serum concentrations are low without tissue deficiency include pregnancy, folate deficiency, iron deficiency, simple atrophic gastritis, vegetarian diet, women taking oral contraceptives, low levels of the major B_{12}-carrying protein in plasma (haptocorrin) and certain rare inherited disorders of B_{12} metabolism (Table 33.3). Concentrations below 150 pmol/L are sometimes seen in the elderly or pregnant women who have no neurological or haematological abnormalities, eat a mixed diet and absorb B_{12} normally. Long-term observation indicates that the majority of these people do not develop clinical or haematological features of B_{12} deficiency. The cause of their low B_{12} is likely to be low levels of haptocorrin rather than B_{12} deficiency, but low values should never be regarded as normal for the elderly.

The clinical significance of low or borderline (150–200 pmol/L) serum B_{12} levels in patients with no haematological or neuropsychiatric evidence of B_{12} deficiency is difficult to determine. It Is here that measurement of active-B_{12} (reference range 35–140 pmol/L) is particularly valuable and will identify those patients in whom the low serum total B_{12} is due to reduced haptocorrin. The fall in serum B_{12} in pregnancy is usually due to reduced haptocorrin, and measurement of active-B_{12} should replace that of total B_{12} when deficiency is suspected in pregnant patients.

Table 33.3 Problems in interpretation of serum B_{12} levels in relation to body B_{12} stores

False normal	False low
Patient given B_{12}	Pregnancy
Myeloproliferative disease	Primary folate deficiency
Hepatoma	Iron deficiency
Acute liver disease	Inherited disorders of B_{12} metabolism
Inherited disorders of B_{12} metabolism	Some normal subjects Oral contraceptives Haptocorrin deficiency

○ Blood count and film examination

Changes in the blood count and film are relatively late manifestations of folate or B_{12} deficiency but are often the first clues to the deficiency. Folate and B_{12} deficiency cannot be differentiated, as the haematological changes are identical. The degree of anaemia varies but macrocytosis (raised mean cell volume—MCV) and hypersegmented neutrophils are important features. Many laboratories do not regard macrocytosis as significant until the MCV is greater than 100 fL, but in normal people the MCV should not be more than 95 fL and a mild increase above this size may be the earliest haematological sign of deficiency. If there is associated iron deficiency or thalassaemia, the MCV will often not be raised, despite severe folate or B_{12} deficiency. In addition, while macrocytosis is an important feature of folate or B_{12} deficiency, it occurs in many other conditions such as alcohol abuse, liver disease, hypothyroidism, myelodysplasia and with some drugs including anticonvulsants and oral contraceptives. Macrocytosis may be physiological in pregnancy and the newborn.

○ Bone marrow biopsy

In the past, bone marrow was commonly examined to confirm megaloblastic anaemia when folate or B_{12} deficiency was suspected. Nowadays, with the ready availability of vitamin assays, this expensive and invasive procedure is rarely used for this purpose. It is of most value in differentiating macrocytosis due to myelodysplasia and erythroleukaemia from macrocytosis caused by megaloblastic anaemia.

○ Identifying the deficient vitamin in macrocytic anaemia

In the investigation of patients with macrocytic anaemia it is essential to assay both serum B_{12} and serum and red cell folate in view of the reciprocal changes which may take place in the tests (Table 33.2). As red cell folate may fall moderately in patients with B_{12} deficiency this test alone will not differentiate folate from B_{12} deficiency. Serum folate levels may be elevated, normal or occasionally reduced in B_{12} deficiency. Furthermore serum B_{12} levels may be reduced moderately in patients with folate deficiency. These parallel changes make it difficult to distinguish the combined deficiency of the two vitamins that may occur in malnutrition or with intestinal disorders.

◑ Metabolic assays: serum methylmalonic acid and total homocysteine

The activities of folate and B_{12} in metabolic pathways generate various metabolites, particularly methylmalonic acid (MMA) and homocysteine (Hcy). Assay of these metabolites has been used in the diagnosis of folate and B_{12} deficiency. Serum MMA is raised in B_{12} but not folate deficiency. It is a sensitive but non-specific index of B_{12} deficiency, although the test is not generally available. Serum Hcy is raised in both folate and B_{12} deficiency. Although a sensitive index of deficiency, it has limited specificity because elevations occur in other inherited and acquired disorders, particularly renal impairment, and it is affected also by various lifestyle factors. Measurement of Hcy is of value in that a normal value probably excludes significant folate or B_{12} deficiency, and the assay may help when vitamin measurements are in the indeterminate range or do not correlate with the clinical findings.

◑ Establishing the cause of the deficiency

After folate or B_{12} deficiency has been identified by suitable tests, a cause for the deficiency must be sought. Folate deficiency is commonly the result of undernutrition or malnutrition in association with increased demand (e.g. pregnancy) or excessive alcohol intake. It is important to assess dietary folate intake and to exclude gluten enteropathy (coeliac disease). Dietary fads or reliance on 'junk' foods devoid of green vegetables, an important source of folate, renders members of all socioeconomic groups susceptible to deficiency.[1]

Pernicious anaemia is the most important syndrome of B_{12} deficiency. The diagnosis identifies the need for lifelong B_{12} treatment and the maintenance of a high index of suspicion for complications such as carcinoma of the stomach. In the past, the diagnosis was usually established by assessing B_{12} absorption with and without intrinsic factor in the Schilling test, but this is no longer available. However, valuable information can be obtained from blood tests for intrinsic factor antibodies (IFA), parietal cell antibodies (PCA) and fasting serum gastrin assay. The presence of IFA is virtually diagnostic of pernicious anaemia but it is detected in only about 50% of cases. A false positive IFA result may occur following recent B_{12} injection. PCA and elevated serum gastrin are common but they are not diagnostic. The test for PCA is sensitive to observer subjectivity, and it should be replaced by direct assay for proton pump antibodies. In patients in whom IFA and PCA are not detected and serum gastrin is not elevated, the cause of the B_{12} deficiency is unlikely to be pernicious anaemia. It is controversial as to whether further investigation is warranted before treating these patients.

Reference

1. Stanton R. Dietary sources of essential vitamins. *Aust Prescr* 1992; 15: 80–5.

34 Screening for thalassaemia and haemoglobin variants

D.K. Bowden

Synopsis

The thalassaemias are the commonest single-gene disorders in the world's population and are a common cause of hereditary anaemia. They should be suspected in any individual who has reduced red blood cell indices. A full blood examination and haemoglobin electrophoresis are the tests which should be used first to investigate a suspected carrier of a thalassaemia gene. Iron deficiency can confuse the interpretation of test results, so iron studies are also often required. DNA analysis may be needed to detect the carrier state, particularly in carriers of α-thalassaemia.

○ Introduction

Functioning haemoglobin (Hb) molecules are tetramers made up of two pairs of globin chains, which bind oxygen at the iron porphyrin site attached to each chain. The different types of Hb are characterised by their globin chains, which in adults may be α, β, γ or δ. Normal adult Hb is made up of approximately 97.0% HbA ($\alpha_2\beta_2$), 2.5% minor adult Hb HbA$_2$ ($\alpha_2\delta_2$) and less than 0.8% HbF ($\alpha_2\gamma_2$).

The thalassaemia syndromes are a heterogeneous collection of genetic disorders characterised by a reduced rate of production of one or more of the globin chains of Hb. The α-globin genes are located in the α-cluster on chromosome 16 and are paired ($\alpha\alpha/\alpha\alpha$) whereas the single β-globin gene is found in the β cluster on chromosome 11. The thalassaemia syndromes are usually caused by point mutations or deletions in or close to these globin genes that reduce or abolish expression of the affected gene. The type of thalassaemia is named according to which gene is affected. Hence reduced production of α-chains is called α-thalassaemia and reduced production of β-chains is called β-thalassaemia. The resulting imbalanced globin chain production gives rise to the phenotype of thalassaemia, while the severity depends on which genes are affected and which mutation or combination of mutations is inherited.

A large number of thalassaemia mutations are now known and can all be characterised by DNA analysis. In a carrier these mutations may be silent or may result in the typical haematological phenotype characterised by red blood cell hypochromia and/or microcytosis. The inheritance of a β-thalassaemia mutation from each parent usually causes the severe disease called β-thalassaemia major.

The genetics of α-thalassaemia are more complex as one, two, three or all four genes may be affected. For example, HbH disease—in which HbH is present on Hb electrophoresis—is usually caused by the deletion of three α-globin genes (--/-α) as a result of the inheritance of a single-gene deletion mutation (-α/) from one parent and a two-gene deletion mutation (--/) from the other parent.

Other mutations cause important, clinically significant structural Hb variants such as Hb S, C, D, E, O and Lepore. Certain combinations of these mutations may cause severe disease as outlined in Table 34.1.

Testing in Australia

Australia's population is ethnically diverse and there have always been a significant number of carriers of β-thalassaemia mutations. If both parents are carriers there is a one in four chance in each pregnancy of their having a child with β-thalassaemia major.

Recent immigration to Australia from areas such as South-East Asia, the Indian subcontinent, the Middle East, central and north Africa and southern Europe has introduced large populations of people from areas where the thalassaemias and Hb variants are common. Consequently it has become important in screening programs, particularly antenatal testing, to detect the carrier state for both α- and β-thalassaemia in addition to the Hb variants that, in the homozygous or compound heterozygous form or in combination with β-thalassaemia, may cause severe disease.

The laboratory diagnosis of the thalassaemia carrier state is therefore of increasing importance both for antenatal diagnosis and for clinical management. Thalassaemias are now common in Australia and are a significant public health problem. In recent years in Melbourne approximately 10% of women in their first pregnancy required DNA studies to adequately characterise their carrier state and to provide sufficient information to estimate the risk that their children would have severe disease (Table 34.1).

Table 34.1 Examples of the severe disease risk states identified in recent years in Melbourne's population

β-globin mutations	Homozygous β-thalassaemia
	Hb E/β-thalassaemia
	Hb Lepore/β-thalassaemia
	Sickle cell disease
	HbS/β-thalassaemia
	HbS/HbC disease
	HbS/HbD disease
α-globin mutations	HbH disease (usually mild but occasionally severe, depending on the mutation combination)
	HbH hydrops syndrome (rare)
	Hb Bart's hydrops syndrome

◯ Indications for testing

An accurate diagnosis may be needed to:
- explain a haematological abnormality such as reduced mean cell volume (MCV), mean cell haemoglobin (MCH) or anaemia
- confirm a diagnosis of the severe disorders such as sickle cell anaemia or β-thalassaemia major
- characterise the mutation underlying a thalassaemia carrier state, particularly for α-thalassaemia where the molecular basis can be determined and clarified only by analysis of DNA
- identify silent mutations that may have clinical significance if inherited with a mutation from the other parent, for example silent α- or β-thalassaemia or coexistent α-thalassaemia in a β-thalassaemia or HbE carrier
- provide accurate genetic counselling to individuals and prospective parents
- identify serious disorders in the fetus and hence provide the additional option to couples of termination of pregnancy
- fully characterise a variant haemoglobin.

◯ α-thalassaemia

Each individual normally inherits two pairs of functioning α-globin genes. These are designated as αα/αα. Mutations in this gene cluster causing α-thalassaemia most commonly delete one of the α-globin genes (-α/αα). Point mutations (α^T) within one of the genes may also inactivate the gene. This usually causes a phenotype with a mild carrier state (α^{T}α/αα) equivalent to having a single-gene deletion mutation. Rarely, a point mutation in one globin gene may reduce expression of both genes resulting in a more severe phenotype equivalent to the two-gene deletion carrier. α-thalassaemia mutations are found in most populations but only occur naturally at high frequencies in areas of the world where malaria is or was endemic. The common deletional mutations can have slightly different effects on the patient's red blood cells (Table 34.2).

Table 34.2 Examples of mean values of mean cell volume (MCV) and mean cell haemoglobin (MCH) in adults according to α-thalassaemia genotype*

Genotype	MCV (fL)	MCH (pg)
αα/αα (normal)	89±5	29±2
-α/αα	84±6	27±2
--αα or -α/-α	75±4	23±2

* These figures are a guide only, illustrating typical values. Precise values, which are age- and sex-dependent, are given in the references cited.[1,5]

In South-East Asia up to 10% of the population are carriers of the more severe two-gene deletion mutation (--/αα). These two-gene deletion mutations are also found sporadically in other populations, including from the Mediterranean region.

The mutations of the α-globin genes may be inherited in any combination. The more severe clinical conditions arising from the inheritance of more than one α-thalassaemia mutation include HbH disease (--/-α), Hb Bart's hydrops syndrome (--/--) and the rare HbH hydrops syndrome ($α^Tα/α^Tα$ or --/$α^Tα$). HbH disease varies in severity but is commonly a moderately severe chronic haemolytic anaemia associated with a Hb in the 80–100 g/L range and varying degrees of hypersplenism. The amount of physiologically useless HbH (β4) in patients is usually constant in an affected individual but in different individuals it can vary from 1 to 45% of the total Hb.

○ Hb Bart's hydrops syndrome

This is a serious and significant clinical condition. It not only leads to the death of the baby but may also adversely affect the health of the mother during pregnancy. In unsupervised pregnancies there is up to a 50% maternal mortality with a high incidence of hypertension and haemorrhage.[1] Affected babies usually die at delivery. These at-risk pregnancies should be recognised as early as possible and termination of affected pregnancies is advised on medical grounds.

◖ β-thalassaemia

Each individual inherits from each parent a single β-globin gene located in the β-globin cluster on chromosome 11. The β-thalassaemia carrier state has been known for many decades. There are usually typical hypochromic microcytic red blood cell changes. Hb electrophoresis reveals the diagnostic elevation of the minor adult HbA_2 $(\alpha_2\delta_2)$.

Screening is not always straightforward. Some of the mutations are now known to have a less severe effect on gene expression.[2] Although these mutations are capable of causing severe disease in homozygotes or compound heterozygotes, the indices in carriers may be borderline or normal and the HbA_2 may be minimally elevated or even in the normal range.

In most populations where β-thalassaemia is present there is also a significant incidence of α-thalassaemia. Individuals therefore can inherit both α-thalassaemia and β-thalassaemia carrier states, an interaction which is usually benign and leads to a milder phenotype. The α-thalassaemia carrier state is masked in this setting and ultimately can be excluded only by DNA analysis. In our experience the HbA_2 level usually remains elevated in those who are carriers of both α- and β-thalassaemia.

◖ Structural haemoglobin variants and thalassaemia

Many haemoglobin variants of clinical significance are known. For example, the substitution of one particular amino acid in the β-globin chain produces the HbS associated with the sickling disorders. In Australia we regularly encounter only a small number of variants capable of causing severe disease in the homozygote or in compound heterozygotes. These include Hb E, S, C, D, O and Lepore, which are all readily identified by Hb electrophoresis. It is common for there to be no other haematological change and hence the variants will be overlooked unless Hb electrophoresis is carried out.[3] HbE behaves as a mild β-thalassaemia mutation and is common in South-East Asia where more than 50% of the population in some areas are carriers. Hb Lepore also has a β-thalassaemia phenotype.

Some of these variants in combination with the β-thalassaemia gene may cause severe disease. HbE/β-thalassaemia is common in South-East Asia and varies clinically from a mild condition to the more common severe disease equivalent to β-thalassaemia major. β-thalassaemia combined with HbS results in sickle cell anaemia, although the phenotype may vary considerably from mild to severe disease depending on which combination of mutations is inherited.

○ Laboratory diagnosis

The thalassaemias and structurally abnormal Hbs are common in Australia so accurate laboratory diagnosis is important. Prospective parents expect to be offered options including antenatal diagnosis if there is an identifiable risk of their having a child with severe disease. Hence prepregnancy or testing in early pregnancy is essential. There is also a need to characterise carrier states to provide an explanation of abnormal haematology or to help clarify an otherwise confusing clinical picture, such as the coexistence of α-thalassaemia and iron deficiency anaemia.

Appropriate genetic counselling requires the detection and adequate characterisation of thalassaemia carrier states and the Hb variants. Local policies and practices on screening vary considerably at present.

○ Initial testing

In clinical practice at present I currently recommend that all potential carriers have a full blood examination and Hb electrophoresis. Reduced red blood cell indices (MCV and MCH) are typical of the majority of carriers of β-thalassaemia, Hb Lepore, δβ-thalassaemia and two-gene deletion α-thalassaemia. In δβ-thalassaemia the production of δ chains and β chains is impaired. Significant reticulocytosis is likely to be found in anyone with a significant chronic haemolytic anaemia such as in the HbS disorders and HbH disease. If the indices are reduced, iron studies should be carried out to exclude iron deficiency or to identify it as a coexisting condition.

Electrophoresis is recommended, as the majority of variant Hbs can only be detected by Hb electrophoresis and the indices are often normal in the carrier, such as a carrier of HbS. High-performance liquid chromatography will identify variant Hbs and also quantitate the HbA_2 level. Specialised laboratories may go on to carry out other tests on Hb variants in order to characterise them more fully before deciding whether DNA analysis is required. Most laboratories now provide interpretive reports that give guidance to the requesting practitioner about the significance of the test results.

β-thalassaemia

Nearly all β-thalassaemia carriers have elevated concentrations of HbA_2 and reduced indices. The accurate quantitation of HbA_2 is of particular importance and concern. The upper limit of normal for HbA_2 is 3.5% of the total Hb. Any value above this should be regarded as diagnostic of the β-thalassaemia carrier state irrespective of the indices on the blood test. All but a few individuals, who are further studied by DNA analysis, will have a known mutation.

There are some clinically important β-thalassaemia mutations in which the indices may be normal and/or the HbA_2 may also be normal, minimally elevated or borderline. Other mutations may also confuse the diagnosis of the carrier state. The HbA_2 level may be halved by the coexistence of a δ-gene mutation. These are uncommon but well known in some populations. Iron deficiency may lower a borderline HbA_2 into the normal range.[4]

Some of the less common mutations may have an entirely normal phenotype or normal indices with a mildly elevated HbA_2 level in the 3.5–4.0% range. This is further complicated by the possibility of an individual's having inherited both α- and β-thalassaemia in the carrier states, where there may be an amelioration of haematological abnormality. In these situations the MCV and MCH are variable and may be normal or near normal. In our experience, however, the elevated HbA_2 persists in the presence of coexisting single- or two-gene deletion α-thalassaemia.

α-thalassaemia

The identification of an α-thalassaemia carrier is more complex and relies ultimately on DNA analysis to complete the testing and identify the mutation. Two-gene deletion α-thalassaemia (--/αα) and homozygous single-gene deletion α-thalassaemia (-α/-α) have a similar phenotype and typically show a moderate reduction in the MCV and MCH (Table 34.2).[1] Abnormality is more likely in the MCH rather than the MCV in a carrier of single-gene deletion α-thalassaemia (-α/αα). This has been known for many years; however, there seems to be a reluctance for laboratories to screen using the MCH as the primary critical reference value and some laboratories do not routinely report the MCH.[2,3] Two-gene deletion α-thalassaemia is most common in South-East Asia but also occurs sporadically in other parts of the world. It should always be considered in anyone with suggestive indices, although DNA analysis is required for characterisation.

The majority of individuals with single-gene deletion α-thalassaemia have entirely normal haematology.[1,5] In this situation the carrier state can only be identified by DNA analysis. Consequently, haematologically normal partners of an individual with a two-gene deletion α-thalassaemia require DNA analysis to determine whether or not they are a carrier of a silent single-gene deletion α-thalassaemia mutation and hence whether there is a risk of their having a child with HbH disease (Table 34.3).

Table 34.3 Tests to be performed in the partner of a carrier to determine the risk of having a child with severe disease

Disorder found in one partner	Test to be carried out in other partner to exclude severe disease risk in a child
β-thalassaemia carrier	FBE, Hb electrophoresis (to exclude β-thalassaemia and δβ-thalassaemia carrier state and Hb S, E, O, D, C and Lepore)
Carrier of Hb Lepore, δβ-thalassaemia, Hb S, C, D, E or O	As for β-thalassaemia carrier
Two-gene deletion α-thalassaemia (--/αα)	FBE, Hb electrophoresis, HbH inclusion prep, DNA analysis (to exclude risk of having a child with HbH disease or Bart's hydrops syndrome)
Single-gene deletion α-thalassaemia (-α/αα or -α/-α)	As for two-gene deletion α-thalassaemia (to identify the risk of having a child with HbH disease)

Iron deficiency

Iron deficiency is common in adult women in Australia. In 1997 up to 40% of women attending their first antenatal appointment in Melbourne were iron deficient. This is not a universal figure and is probably disproportionately high for the general population; however, it is a serious potential complicating factor when testing for a thalassaemia carrier state. Both iron deficiency and a thalassaemia carrier state may result in a low MCV and MCH. Erythrocytosis is more likely to be caused by thalassaemia but it is not a diagnostic finding.

In pregnant women with a low MCV and MCH, Hb electrophoresis should be carried out routinely, irrespective of iron status. If possible the father should also be tested. If a non-iron deficient partner has evidence of a thalassaemia carrier state or other haemoglobinopathy then the woman should have full testing including DNA analysis to adequately define the risk of their having a child with severe disease (Table 34.3).

○ Summary

The identification of carriers of thalassaemia and other clinically-significant haemoglobinopathies is a two-stage process. Initially evidence for the carrier state is sought by carrying out a full blood examination and Hb electrophoresis. Iron deficiency can be excluded as a complicating factor by iron studies in individuals who show a haematological abnormality consistent with this diagnosis. In this relatively simple way evidence for all but the silent single-gene deletion α-thalassaemia mutations will usually be obtained. Further studies including DNA analysis can then be carried out for final clarification of the carrier state. It is thus usually possible to identify all but a few mutations and to provide the necessary informative counselling for individuals and couples.

References

1. Higgs D.R. Alpha-thalassaemia. *Ballieres Best Pract Res Clin Haematol* 1993; 6: 117–50.
2. No authors listed. The laboratory diagnosis of haemoglobinopathies. *Br J Haematol* 1998; 101: 783–92.
3. Hendy J.G., Monagle P.T. and Bowden D.K. Antenatal screening and prenatal diagnosis of thalassaemia. *MJA* 1999; 170: 623–4.
4. Wasi P., Disthasongchan P. and Na-Nakorn S. The effect of iron deficiency on the levels of haemoglobins A2 and E. *J Lab Clin Med* 1968; 71: 85–91.
5. Williams T.N., Maitland K., Ganczakowski M., Peto T.E., Clegg J.B., Weatherall D.J. et al. Red blood cell phenotypes in the alpha + thalassaemias from early childhood to maturity. *Br J Haematol* 1996; 95: 266–72.

35 Investigations for thrombotic tendencies

R. Baker

Synopsis

A number of hereditary and acquired thrombophilia factors are associated with the majority of cases of familial or recurrent venous thromboembolism (VTE), including deep vein thrombosis and pulmonary embolism, and some cases of atherothrombosis, namely premature myocardial infarction or ischaemic stroke. They include activated protein C resistance (factor V Leiden), prothrombin gene mutation, natural anticoagulant deficiency (antithrombin III, protein C and protein S), elevated factor VIII levels and antiphospholipid antibodies. Testing for these factors has the potential to identify patients at higher risk of thrombosis who may benefit from prevention and improved treatment strategies. However, these factors are also common in the general population (approximately one in ten people) so a thorough understanding of their significance and clinical management is important. Recent guidelines suggest that indiscriminate routine testing of patients with VTE is not advised and testing should be considered only in selected patients with a strong family history of unprovoked or recurrent venous thrombosis.[1]

○ Introduction

Thrombophilia can be defined as an increased tendency to develop arterial or venous thromboses that are recurrent, familial or present at an unusual site or at a young age. Thrombosis can be catastrophic, leading to death, permanent disability, prolonged periods of hospitalisation or chronic symptoms of lower limb venous insufficiency. The results of appropriate laboratory investigations in selected patients with a strong family history of unprovoked or recurrent VTE can help us develop strategies that will either prevent the occurrence of thrombosis or assist with decisions about effective antithrombotic treatment. Until recently the aetiology of most cases of thrombophilia was largely unknown. This situation has dramatically changed because we now know that over half of patients with thrombophilia and VTE have an abnormality of the natural anticoagulant system.

Clinical assessment is important

Most cases of deep venous thrombosis can be explained by the interaction of plasma coagulation 'thrombophilia' abnormalities and the well-recognised 'clinical' risk factors (such as obesity, major abdominal or orthopaedic surgery, the oral contraceptive pill, pregnancy, malignancy or immobility). The greater the accumulation in the number of either clinical or laboratory risk factors, the more probable is the occurrence of VTE.

Accurate clinical assessment is important to establish the diagnosis, identify family members at risk, prevent recurrence and rule out occult disease. Particular emphasis is made on the site and severity of thrombosis, whether or not it occurred spontaneously or postoperatively and whether the event is associated with a well-identified precipitating factor such as oestrogen therapy or plane travel. A previously undiagnosed malignancy (particularly a mucin-secreting adenocarcinoma) or a myeloproliferative disorder may present with a similar picture of unusual thrombosis. These conditions should be considered before testing for thrombophilia.

Important thrombophilia factors identified

The frequency and the relative risk of first and recurrent venous thrombosis and arterial disease for the thrombophilia factors are found in Table 35.1.[2]

Table 35.1 Frequency and relative risk of venous thrombosis for the thrombophilia factors

	Patients with DVT	General population	Relative risk for first VTE	Relative risk for recurrent VTE	Relative risk for arterial thrombosis
Factor V Leiden	50%	4%	5-fold*	1.4-fold	No association
Prothrombin gene	15%	3%	3-fold	1.4-fold	No association
Antithrombin III, protein C and S deficiency	10%	< 1%	10-fold	2-fold	No association
High factor VIII	36%	17%	5-fold	Up to 5-fold	3-fold
Antiphospholipid antibodies	common	–	10-fold	6-fold	10-fold

*Risk increased to 35-fold in women on the oral contraceptive pill

Activated protein C resistance

Activated protein C (APC) resistance is a hereditary defect of the protein C natural anticoagulant pathway (Fig. 35.1). APC normally acts as a natural anticoagulant. It downregulates the intensity of the clotting cascade by neutralising activated coagulation factor V. This process is inefficient in people with APC resistance. They do not have the crucial APC cleavage site in the factor V molecule because of a point mutation (factor V Leiden).

Activation of the blood coagulation system generates large amounts of thrombin which produces cleavage of fibrinogen to form a stable fibrin clot. Natural anticoagulants downregulate the coagulation cascade. Deficiency of these natural anticoagulants, resistant factor V (factor V Leiden) and increased prothrombin levels impair downregulation. This predisposes the patient to thrombosis.

The heterozygous factor V Leiden mutation is common, occurring in 4% of randomly selected healthy people in Australia.[3] It can be found in up to 50% of patients with recurrent familial venous thrombosis. The mutation

Figure 35.1 Regulation of coagulation activation and thrombophilia abnormalities

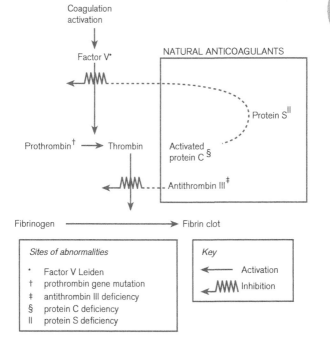

Sites of abnormalities

*	Factor V Leiden
†	prothrombin gene mutation
‡	antithrombin III deficiency
§	protein C deficiency
‖	protein S deficiency

causes a five-fold increased risk of a first venous thrombosis compared to normal. It appears to have a weak and debatable effect on the chance of recurrent VTE. The homozygous form is not infrequent and substantially increases the risk of thrombosis to 100 times normal. The inheritance pattern is autosomal dominant, so there is a one in two chance that other family members may have a similar predisposition to thrombosis.[2] APC resistance is usually detected by a sensitive and specific clotting assay and confirmed by molecular analysis for the factor V Leiden mutation.

Women are especially at risk because oestrogens or pregnancy combined with APC resistance substantially increase the likelihood of thrombosis. The use of a combined oral contraceptive increases the relative risk of thrombosis to 35-fold in those with APC resistance.[4] All oestrogen-containing contraceptive devices should be considered to carry this risk until evidence of their safety has been documented. However, the absolute increased risk for thrombosis is small and is estimated to be 3% over a 10-year period of oral contraceptive use.

In general APC resistance is not associated with ischaemic heart disease or stroke.[3] However, subgroup analysis reveals a 30-fold increased risk of acute myocardial infarction in young women who smoke or who are obese. There are reports of young women who are homozygous for the factor V Leiden presenting with acute myocardial infarction but normal coronary arteries.

Prothrombin gene mutation

A point mutation in the prothrombin molecule (G20210A) causes an increase in its circulating plasma level, predisposing to thrombus formation. The mutation is common in the healthy Australian population (3.3%) and occurs in up to 15% of patients with VTE.[5] It is estimated to increase the thrombotic risk three-fold compared to those without the mutation.[1] The mutation can be detected only by DNA polymerase chain reaction (PCR). The inheritance is autosomal dominant.

Antithrombin III, protein C and S deficiency

Deficiency of antithrombin III, protein C or protein S is rare but is the strongest hereditary risk factors for first and recurrent VTE, with reported incidence rates of up to 4% per year. Over 500 different mutations in these molecules are known, so the relevant family history of VTE can assist in determining the significance of an abnormal laboratory test.

High factor VIII

Elevated factor VIII levels greater than 150% are associated with an increased risk of first and recurrent VTE. The raised levels are independent of an acute phase inflammatory response and often hereditary. The relative risk of venous thrombosis increases to 10-fold when combined with the oral contraceptive use.[2]

Mild to moderate hyperhomocysteinaemia

Although mild to moderate hyperhomocysteinaemia is a graded risk factor for venous and premature arterial thrombosis and vitamin B and folate supplementation effectively lowers the elevated levels, the results of recent large randomised control trials of vitamin B and folate supplementation for the prevention of recurrent VTE or arterial disease have not found benefit or harm.[6] Given these findings, routine testing for mild hyperhomocysteinaemia for thrombophilia is not recommended, although there may still be young people with more severe hyperhomocysteinaemia with arterial or venous thrombosis, who may still benefit from screening and intervention.

Antiphospholipid antibodies

Autoantibodies against phospholipid and other molecules on the platelet surface can be associated with atherothrombosis. The antibody type, class, strength and target antigen(s) are extremely varied, not only among individual patients but also within the same patient at varying times. The three common laboratory methods used to detect these antibodies are the lupus anticoagulant, the anticardiolipin antibody and β2 glycoprotein 1 assays. The lupus anticoagulants are antiphospholipid antibodies detected by clotting methods. β2 glycoprotein 1 and anticardiolipin antibodies are detected by serological methods. Each of these autoantibodies against phospholipids and other coagulation molecules is associated with both arterial and venous thrombosis. Although most of the time both tests are simultaneously abnormal, only one test may be abnormal in one-third of cases despite identical clinical conditions. These antibodies are common in patients with thrombosis. Their detection is important because there may be a substantial increase in the risk of recurrent thrombosis. However, low titres of autoantibodies are frequently found in the normal population, they are of uncertain clinical significance and they may be transient (less than 12 weeks), particularly in response to infection.

Prevention of recurrent thrombosis (especially arterial thrombosis) in patients with persistently high antibody titres may require long-term warfarin therapy. For most cases a target INR of 2–3 is sufficient.[7] Aspirin appears to be less effective in the prevention of recurrent thrombosis than warfarin. Patients with recurrent spontaneous miscarriages may have antiphospholipid antibodies. The combination of low-dose aspirin (100 mg) and standard heparin (5 000 IU twice daily) or low molecular weight heparin substantially reduces fetal loss in any subsequent pregnancy.[8] The detection of antiphospholipid antibodies in patients with thrombosis is frequently the only manifestation of the autoimmune disease known as the primary antiphospholipid antibody syndrome, but antiphospholipid antibodies can also be associated with other autoantibody syndromes such as systemic lupus erythematosus.

▷ Coexisting thrombophilia factors increase thrombosis risk

As thrombophilia factors are relatively frequent, compound heterozygotes (such as factor V Leiden together with the prothrombin gene mutation) are not uncommonly found. This substantially increases the risk of venous thrombosis compared to having only one abnormality.[2] The thrombophilia genes are independently inherited in thrombosis-prone families, so they may be absent or one or other gene may be found or both abnormalities may coexist. This may explain why in some families the thrombosis phenotype is variable. The risk of thrombosis may be further increased by the coexistence of antiphospholipid antibodies or high levels of factor VIII.

▷ Laboratory testing

A diagnosis of thrombophilia in high-risk families should ensure that appropriate counselling for VTE prophylaxis is given in high-risk situations such as after surgery, during periods of immobility (including long plane flights and car trips), during pregnancy and for some time postpartum. Around 80% of VTE cases are caused by a provoking event especially within 3 months of hospitalisation for a medical or surgical illness. Sadly, despite the best efforts only a half of eligible patients receive optimal VTE prophylaxis in hospital. Prevention strategies include measures such as anticoagulant therapy (standard heparin, low molecular weight heparin or oral factor IIa and Xa inhibitors), early mobilisation and increasing lower limb venous blood flow (compression stockings and plantar plexus foot pumps). In affected family members oestrogen-containing contraceptives could be avoided and other choices made, such as progestogen-only implants or barrier methods. The intensity of prophylaxis against venous thrombosis depends on the perceived hazard in each case versus the VTE risk reduction and haemorrhagic threat produced by an intervention. At the very least, diagnosis of a thrombophilia factor should ensure preventive measures are considered in people with previous VTE and even in family members without a history of thrombosis. However there are still families with a strong unprovoked VTE history where no thrombophilia is identified. Caution is still required to prevent VTE in those family members without identified thrombophilia.

○ Whom to test?

Any patient with spontaneous, unusual, recurrent or a strong family history of venous thrombosis or evidence of premature arterial occlusion should be tested. After counselling, it is reasonable to consider testing first-degree relatives for an identified hereditary thrombophilia factor because half the family members will inherit the mutation. Finding the abnormality will provide an opportunity to modify other risk factors and ensure appropriate prophylaxis against venous thrombosis in high-risk situations.

○ Which test and when?

Patients can be tested (Table 35.2) either at the presentation of thrombosis or after finishing anticoagulation. Abnormal results should always be confirmed by repeat testing. This is because the levels of the natural anticoagulant factors may be altered by consumption in the clotting process, blood collection artefacts and standardisation and reproducibility problems inherent in most of the clotting-based laboratory techniques. Testing other family members without thrombosis, to confirm the hereditary nature of the problem, is often helpful for a patient with uncertain results due to acute thrombosis or anticoagulation.

Molecular confirmation of the factor V Leiden mutation is recommended not only to confirm the abnormal clotting result but also to differentiate clearly a homozygote and heterozygote carrier. Protein C and S are vitamin K dependent anticoagulant factors, so deficiency cannot be diagnosed while the patient is on warfarin. However, all the thrombophilia

Table 35.2 Suggested laboratory tests for thrombophilia (consultation with the pathology laboratory is recommended)*

| Full blood examination and erythrocyte sedimentation rate† |
| Factor V Leiden (activated protein C resistance factor) |
| Factor VIII |
| Prothrombin gene mutation |
| Anticardiolipin antibodies |
| Lupus anticoagulant |
| Antithrombin III |
| Protein C, protein S‡ |

*The 85% Medicare rebate is at present approximately $240, including DNA testing for the prothrombin gene mutation. Around 25 mL of blood is required. All tests can be performed when the patient is on heparin.
†Tests for myeloproliferative disorders and occult systemic diseases
‡Should only be done before (or 2 weeks after ceasing) oral anticoagulation

factors can usually be tested while the patient is on therapeutic heparin or low molecular weight heparin.

◐ Summary

Thrombophilia factors are frequently found in the majority of patients with recurrent or familial venous thrombosis. Obtaining a familial history of thrombosis is now analogous to a bleeding history (particularly if the patient has a convincing family history of deep venous thrombosis and is considering surgery or the combined oral contraceptive pill). Laboratory testing can be useful in counselling patients who have a higher risk of thrombosis. This information leads to better informed choices and the development of strategies to prevent thrombosis. However, most patients with these thrombophilia factors will never develop thrombosis in their lifetime and it is important that the testing is integrated into the clinical VTE history. The test result should not be the only guide to the decision process. Long-term anticoagulation could be considered in patients with unprovoked VTE and antiphospholipid antibodies but for the other hereditary factors this recommendation is less certain. The occurrence of thrombosis is explained in people who are at high risk because of the accumulation of an increasing number of either clinical and/or thrombophilia factors.

References

1. Baglin T., Gray E., Greaves M., Hunt B.J., Keeling D., Machin S. et al. Clinical guidelines for testing for heritable thrombophilia. *Br J Haematol* 2010; 149 :209–20.
2. Middeldorp S. and van Hylckama Vlieg A. Does thrombophilia testing help in the clinical management of patients? *Br J Haematol* 2008; 143: 321–5.
3. van Bockxmeer F.M., Baker R.I. and Taylor R.R. Premature ischaemic heart disease and the gene for coagulation factor V. *Nat Med* 1995; 1: 185.
4. van Hylckama Vlieg A., Helmerhorst F.M., Vandenbrouke J.P., Doggen C.J. and Rosendaal F.R. The venous thrombotic risk of oral contraceptives, effects of oestrogen dose and progestogen type: results of the MEGA case-control study. *BMJ* 2009; 339: b2921.
5. Eikelboom J.W., Baker R.I., Parsons R., Taylor R.R. and van Bockxmeer F.M. No association between the 20210 G/A prothrombin gene mutation and premature coronary artery disease. *Thromb Haemostasis* 1998; 80: 878–80.
6. The VITATOPS trial study group. B vitamins in patients with recent transient ischaemic attack or stroke in VITAmins To Prevent Stroke

(VITATOPS) trial: a randomised double blind parallel placebo controlled trial. *Lancet Neurol* 2010; 9: 855–65.

7. Baker R.I. Prevention of recurrent thrombosis in the antiphospholipid antibody syndrome: how long and how high with oral anticoagulant therapy? *MJA* 2004; 180: 436–7.

8. Cohn D.M., Goddijn M., Middeldorp S., Korevaar C., Dawood F. and Farquharson R.G. Recurrent miscarriage and anti-phospholipid antibodies: prognosis of subsequent pregnancy. *J Thromb Haemost* 2010: pub online 5 Aug 2010.

36 Tests of haemostasis: detecting the patient at risk of bleeding

J. McPherson and A. Street

Synopsis

Acquired bleeding disorders are common. They complicate well-defined clinical disorders that can be detected by history and examination. Inherited bleeding disorders are uncommon but can be detected by careful clinical assessment, particularly the personal and family history. Clinical assessment has high sensitivity, although low specificity, for detecting the presence of a bleeding disorder. In contrast the sensitivity and specificity of routine laboratory testing is low. Both false negative and false positive results are common with the basic laboratory 'screening tests'. In a patient without a suggestive history, these tests are inappropriate. In a patient with a suggestive history, they are inadequate.

○ Introduction

Normal haemostasis involves two processes:

- platelet adhesion to areas of vascular injury with the subsequent formation of a platelet thrombus
- activation of coagulation culminating in the formation of a fibrin thrombus.

The earlier 'waterfall' or 'cascade' theory of coagulation described two separate activation pathways: surface or contact-mediated ('intrinsic') activation, and tissue-mediated ('extrinsic') activation. These were seen as involving sequential enzymic reactions. This theory has been replaced by a cellular model of haemostasis, emphasising the close interactions between the contact and tissue-factor activation pathways, with a central role for activated factor VII in initiation of the process.[1] Both models allow for a 'final common pathway' after activation of factor X, leading to thrombin generation and amplification of further thrombin generation through activation by factors VIII and IX leading to fibrin formation.

The two processes of platelet activation and coagulation activation are interactive, although their dominance varies in different sites of the vascular system. Activation of haemostasis is accompanied by activation of the fibrinolytic system, which regulates the size of the clot.

Clinically important abnormalities of these mechanisms are common and a logical and cost-effective approach to the detection of patients at risk of bleeding is required.

◯ Clinical assessment of acquired bleeding disorders

These disorders occur in well-defined clinical settings and the history and physical examination provide a sensitive approach to screening.

The commonest cause of an acquired bleeding disorder is drug therapy:

- aspirin or other non-steroidal anti-inflammatory drugs (NSAIDs) causing platelet dysfunction through inhibition of cyclo-oxygenase. The occurrence and severity of bleeding is variable
- clopidogrel, an inhibitor of ADP-induced platelet aggregation
- cytotoxic drugs causing thrombocytopenia
- oral anticoagulant therapy inhibiting the synthesis of the vitamin K dependent coagulation factors.

Note that some complementary and alternative medications may have aspirin-like activity and contribute to the bleeding risk. Many drugs interact with oral anticoagulants (warfarin) to increase or otherwise alter the bleeding risk. Newer oral antifactor Xa inhibitors are presently registered for thromboprophylaxis for high risk orthopaedic surgery and are likely to have future use in stroke prevention in atrial fibrillation and for the management of venous thromboembolism.

Systemic disease may also be associated with a bleeding tendency:

- Chronic liver disease can result in a variety of haemostatic abnormalities ranging from deficiency of vitamin K dependent coagulation factors through more global coagulation factor deficiencies to low-grade disseminated intravascular coagulation (DIC).
- Biliary obstruction or small bowel malabsorption may cause vitamin K deficiency.
- People with renal failure may have significant platelet dysfunction.
- Patients with severe sepsis, disseminated malignancy, gross trauma or obstetric complications may develop DIC.
- Those with myeloproliferative disorders may have significant abnormalities of platelet function.
- Patients with lymphoproliferative or autoimmune disease may develop autoantibodies to coagulation factors or platelets.

- Paraproteins in patients with plasma cell dyscrasias may interfere with platelet function or fibrin formation.

◒ Clinical assessment of inherited bleeding disorders

These disorders are less common than acquired disorders and the vast majority of patients will have a personal and/or family history of excessive bleeding. The history is a sensitive, though not specific, screen for the presence of an inherited bleeding disorder. It is important to enquire into bleeding during and after surgical or dental procedures; a return to the operating theatre, blood transfusion or need for packing or suture of dental sockets would lead one to suspect an underlying problem.

Menorrhagia, recurrent epistaxis and easy bruising are sensitive indicators, although associated with a high rate of false positives. The perception of menstrual blood loss is variable and often influenced by family norms; the frequency of pad/tampon change may assist in determining its significance. Menorrhagia commencing after pregnancies and childbirth, and uninfluenced by hormone supplements, is unlikely to be due to an inherited haemostatic disorder. Peripartum bleeding is rare in patients with mild von Willebrand disease (the most common inherited haemostatic disorder) and the absence of such a history should not influence the decision as to whether investigation is required.

'Spontaneous' haemarthroses and major muscle bleeds are characteristic of severe haemophilia A (factor VIII deficiency) or severe haemophilia B (factor IX deficiency).

Gastrointestinal bleeding and/or epistaxis as isolated problems are unlikely to be due to an inherited bleeding disorder. However, mucosal surfaces should always be inspected for the characteristic lesions of hereditary haemorrhagic telangiectasia. This condition is underdiagnosed.

If a positive family history is obtained, the pattern of affected individuals may suggest autosomal (e.g. von Willebrand disorder) or X-linked (e.g. haemophilia) inheritance.

Detecting patients with platelet disorders and von Willebrand disorder

The first laboratory test should be the full blood count and blood film. Thrombocytopenia is a common and important cause of bleeding. In addition, thrombocytopenia may coexist with a platelet functional disorder or with von Willebrand disorder. Abnormal platelet morphology may be noted in both acquired and inherited platelet disorders.

Bleeding time (BT)

The BT has been abandoned as a screening test in most laboratories in Australia because it does not reliably detect or exclude abnormalities of haemostasis nor predict the risk of operative or procedural bleeding.[2]

Platelet function studies

There are no 'screening tests' that detect abnormalities of platelet function. Platelet aggregation testing is largely confined to specialist laboratories and remains subject to significant variability in performance and interpretation. This testing cannot be considered as a screen of haemostasis nor can it be used to assess the efficacy of antiplatelet therapies or the clinical phenomenon of 'aspirin resistance' in the absence of standardised definitions, methods and clinical correlation.

Flow cytometry

This technique is best established in diagnosis of well characterised platelet membrane disorders, such as Bernard-Soulier syndrome and Glanzmann's thrombasthenia. It is not useful as a screening test.

Conclusion

The detection of patients with von Willebrand disorder or with an acquired or inherited platelet disorder can only be achieved by careful clinical assessment and supporting specialised laboratory testing. There are no validated or reliable screening tests. Patients with a suggestive history should be investigated by a haematologist. Patients with neither a personal nor family history of bleeding should not be tested.

Detection of patients with a 'coagulation disorder'

While the relevance of in vitro coagulation to in vivo haemostasis is necessarily limited, the simple 'cascade' sequence remains of some value in illustrating how the basic tests of coagulation reflect the levels (activities) of the various coagulation factors (Fig. 36.1). Other tests of coagulation, for example thromboelastography of whole blood under simulated shear conditions or thrombin generation, have not replaced the current basic coagulation tests.

Activated partial thromboplastin time (APTT)

The APTT reflects the activity of coagulation factors in the intrinsic system and the final common pathway of coagulation. It is performed by recalcifying citrated plasma in the presence of a 'surface' activator and a 'partial thromboplastin', with the latter simulating platelet membrane phospholipid.

The APTT may be prolonged by deficiency of a specific coagulation factor (e.g. factor VIII in haemophilia A), a coagulation factor inhibitor, a lupus inhibitor and inhibition of coagulation by heparin. Although the APTT can be

Figure 36.1 Anticoagulant 'targets' of basic tests of haemostasis

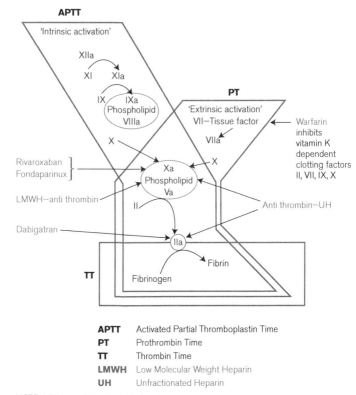

APTT	Activated Partial Thromboplastin Time
PT	Prothrombin Time
TT	Thrombin Time
LMWH	Low Molecular Weight Heparin
UH	Unfractionated Heparin

NOTE: Inhibitors shown in red in figure.

prolonged in patients receiving warfarin or those with vitamin K deficiency or severe liver disease, it is less sensitive to these defects than is the prothrombin time. The APTT is not useful for the assessment of multiple coagulation factor deficiencies, for example after massive transfusion or in DIC, and these situations should be managed in consultation with a haematologist.

Incorrect specimen collection or handling may result in either a false positive (prolonged) or a false negative (shortened) APTT result (Table 36.1).

In practice the main uses of the APTT are:

- monitoring full dose, continuous infusion unfractionated heparin therapy. For the therapeutic interval provided by the laboratory to be meaningful, the heparin sensitivity of the APTT reagent used must have been established by the laboratory. The APTT has no place in the management of patients receiving low molecular weight heparin (LMWH) or heparinoids as the test is insensitive to the amount of factor Xa inhibition incurred by LMWH.

- detecting significant coagulation factor deficiencies in patients with a personal history suggestive of an inherited bleeding disorder or one in appropriate family members. In the absence of such a clinical history, the yield from the APTT is very low. A normal APTT does not exclude a mild but clinically significant coagulation factor deficiency, as most APTT reagents only detect single coagulation factor deficiencies when the level is ≤ 35% of normal. Thus the APTT has little or no value when used as a 'routine' preoperative screening test.[3,4]

- detecting a lupus inhibitor in patients with a history of recurrent fetal loss or recurrent venous and/or arterial thrombosis. Although there are more sensitive screening tests for the lupus inhibitor (e.g. dilute Russell Viper Venom time, dRVVT), in practice many patients are detected because of a prolonged APTT. In spite of sometimes being called the lupus anticoagulant, the causative antiphospholipid antibody or antibodies are associated with a tendency to thrombosis, not bleeding.

- detecting coagulation factor inhibitors (antibodies). Antibodies to factor VIII or, rarely, factor IX may develop in haemophilia but may also occur in patients with autoimmune or lymphoproliferative disorders, in the postpartum period and in previously normal elderly patients. Unexplained bleeding of recent onset with an isolated prolongation of the APTT should arouse suspicion that an inhibitor, usually against factor VIII, may be present.

Table 36.1 Causes of an incorrect APTT

Difficult or slow collection
Delay in mixing blood with the citrate anticoagulant
Addition of an incorrect volume of blood to the citrate
Heparin contamination (e.g. collection in a heparinised syringe or through a heparinised needle)
Prolonged or suboptimal storage of blood before separation of plasma for testing

Prothrombin time (PT and INR)

The PT reflects the activity of the extrinsic system and final common pathway of coagulation (Fig. 36.1). It is measured by recalcifying citrated plasma after the addition of a 'complete' thromboplastin (classically a suspension of human or animal brain or recombinant phospholipids) which simulates tissue factor. Compared with the APTT, the PT is more sensitive to the coagulation defect induced by oral anticoagulant therapy and less sensitive to the effect of heparin.

In practice, the main uses of the PT are:

- monitoring oral anticoagulant therapy. For this purpose the PT is expressed as an international normalised ratio (INR), which provides a result standardised for local reagents and methodology. An INR of 2.0–3.0 is considered to be the appropriate therapeutic interval for the treatment and secondary prophylaxis of venous thromboembolism and primary and secondary prophylaxis against stroke in atrial fibrillation, antiphospholipid antibody syndrome and newer generation prosthetic heart valves. For older prosthetic valves, particularly ball and cage valves, the recommended therapeutic interval is 2.5–3.5.[5] The recommended therapeutic interval varies for specific indications and is not an absolute phenomenon; additionally, oral anticoagulant doses may need to be adjusted for individuals who suffer haemorrhagic or thrombotic events within the specified therapeutic interval.
- assessing patients with hepatocellular disease. The PT is considered to be a sensitive test of liver function. A prolonged PT, particularly in alcoholic liver disease, is often partly due to concomitant dietary vitamin K deficiency.
- detecting vitamin K deficiency, particularly in patients with biliary obstruction, those who abuse alcohol, in small bowel malabsorption and after prolonged fasting or vomiting, especially if associated with broad-spectrum antibiotic therapy.

A prolonged PT may be seen in patients with a lupus inhibitor, although the APTT is generally more sensitive. The PT has only a limited role in the assessment of patients with a history suggestive of an inherited bleeding disorder, as factor VII deficiency is rare. As with the APTT, use of the PT as a 'routine' preoperative screening test has little or no value.[5,6]

Point of care coagulation instruments are available to clinicians and/or patients for testing the INR.[6] The coagulation time is automatically converted to an INR on the result printout. Most detect clot formation in whole blood, rather than plasma, which allows the devices to be used in sites remote from pathology laboratories. There are important issues of operator training, quality control and quality assurance which currently need to be addressed with use of these devices (see Chapter 6).

Thrombin time (TT)

The thrombin time assesses the conversion of fibrinogen to fibrin and is measured by adding thrombin to citrated plasma. The TT only detects abnormalities of fibrinogen and of fibrin formation (Fig. 36.1).

In practice the thrombin time is used by the laboratory, rather than as a requested test, to:

- detect heparin in a specimen with an unexplained prolongation of the APTT. A prolonged TT that corrects with protamine sulfate confirms the presence of heparin in the sample.
- assist in the diagnosis of DIC, in which the TT is prolonged due to the presence of hypofibrinogenaemia and fibrin degradation products (FDP) which interfere with fibrin polymerisation. In DIC, the TT only partially corrects with protamine sulfate.
- detect the rare inherited disorders hypofibrinogenaemia and afibrinogenaemia.
- detect dysfibrinogenaemia (an abnormal fibrinogen molecule with abnormal function). Inherited dysfibrinogenaemia is rare but acquired dysfibrinogenaemia may be seen in patients with hepatocellular carcinoma. A similar functional abnormality may be seen in patients with myeloma, due to the paraprotein interfering with fibrin polymerisation.

◐ Summary

Laboratory testing does not detect the patient at risk of bleeding through 'screening tests'. When the history indicates that a patient is likely to have a bleeding disorder, its nature and severity is defined by specialist laboratory-based testing.

References

1. Hoffman M. and Monroe D.M. A cell based model of hemostasis. *Thromb Haemostasis* 2001; 85: 958–65.
2. Rodgers R.P.C. and Levin J. A critical review of the bleeding time. *Semin Thromb Hemost* 1990; 16: 1–20.
3. Eisenberg J.M., Clarke J.R. and Sussman S.A. Prothrombin and partial thromboplastin times as preoperative screening tests. *Arch Surg* 1982; 117: 48–51.
4. Suchman A.L and Griner P.F. Diagnostic uses of the activated partial thromboplastin time and prothrombin time. *Ann Intern Med* 1986; 104: 810–6.
5. Ansell J., Hirsh J. et al. The pharmacology and management of vitamin K antagonists (The Seventh ACCP Conference on Antithrombotic and Thrombolytic Therapy). *Chest* 2004; 126; 3: S204–33.
6. Tripodi A., Chantarangkul V. and Mannucci P.M. Near-patient testing devices to monitor anticoagulation therapy. *Brit J Haematol* 2001; 113: 847–52A.

37 Abnormal haematology results in children

A.L. Greenway and P. Monagle

Synopsis

Care must be taken when interpreting haematology results in children. They have different physiology from adults so the reference ranges for results differ. The results also vary according to the age of the child. To ensure children are not misdiagnosed or incorrectly investigated it is important to know whether the reporting laboratory has established age-specific reference ranges for children.

Introduction

Pathology tests are an integral part of current medical practice. Accurate and appropriate interpretation of these tests is essential when they are being used for diagnosis or disease monitoring. The critical issues include:

- the choice of the correct test for the clinical situation
- an understanding of the 'normal' or expected results of the test
- an understanding of all of the potential causes of an abnormal result, including spurious causes
- the relative 'weight' that should be given to an abnormal result given the full clinical context.

Children add an additional layer of complexity to each of these issues. For example, issues related to sample collection and the use of capillary blood are particularly relevant causes of spurious results. Perhaps the most misunderstood issue is the concept of 'normal' in different age groups. Countless children are misdiagnosed or over-investigated because of a lack of understanding that they are not just 'little adults' but are physiologically different in many respects. This lack of understanding often extends to the laboratory reporting the results. The clinician may be led astray by reports that would be correct for adult patients but are non-contributory or wrong in children. Nowhere is this more obvious than within haematology. Developmental or age-related changes in haemopoiesis and haemostasis have significant effects on the interpretation of some common pathology tests.

◯ Full blood examination

In the full blood examination the greatest numerical difference between children and adults is seen in the white cell count and differential. The white cell count is significantly higher in children of all ages until mid-adolescence when it approximates adult counts.

Neutrophils

A high neutrophil count is commonly seen, particularly in neonates. The neutrophil count may be up to 14×10^9/L in a normal neonate.[1] These 'normal' differences must be considered, for example in the diagnosis of bacterial infection. Other considerations are the potential response of the child to sepsis (very sick children may have neutropenia) and the effects of concomitant therapies such as steroids in croup or asthma. Features such as neutrophil vacuolation, toxic granulation or left shift with increased band forms are important determinants in the interpretation of neutrophil counts in children.

Lymphocytes

Compared to adults a relative lymphocytosis is common in normal children. Lymphocyte counts up to 11×10^9/L are normal in children under 12 months and elevated counts persist until mid-adolescence.[1] Results that may suggest lymphoproliferative disorders in adult patients are usually either normal or reflect common clinical and subclinical viral infections in children. Less commonly understood is that morphologically normal lymphocytes in young infants often appear atypical or even blast like. Experience with paediatric blood films is required to avoid the unnecessary suggestion of leukaemia in many children or the overdiagnosis of specific viral infections associated with atypical lymphocytes.

Erythrocytes and haemoglobin

Red cell parameters vary significantly between the various age ranges. Relative polycythaemia is normal in the early days of life in both the term and premature newborn. The normal haemoglobin concentration ranges from 135 to 220 g/L in the first weeks of life. This occurs in response to high fetal erythropoietin levels stimulated by the relative hypoxia experienced in utero.

The haemoglobin concentration in normal infants declines after birth to reach the physiological nadir at approximately 8 weeks of age (reference range 90–14.0 g/L). Adverse neonatal events, prematurity and haemolysis (due, for example, to maternal-fetal ABO incompatibility) may impact significantly on the rate and extent of this decline. The causes of the decline include accelerated red cell loss around the time of delivery, reduced survival of neonatal red cells (approximately 90 days vs 120 days) and erythropoietin deficiency as a result of negative feedback from increased oxygenation after the normal neonatal circulation is established. The fall in haemoglobin reactivates erythropoietin production and the normal feedback mechanism that persists for the remainder of life is established.[2]

Red cell size follows a similar pattern to the haemoglobin concentration. Fetal red blood cells are macrocytic relative to adults, with the normal range of mean cell volume (MCV) at birth being 100–120 fL. This drops to 85–110 fL by 1 month and 70–90 fL by 5 months before increasing again from early adolescence to reach normal adult values (80–97 fL) by late adolescence.[2] The initial reduction in MCV occurs as the macrocytic fetal red cells are replaced during the first months of life.

Deviations in red cell size may indicate significant disease in children. Macrocytosis is commonly due to hepatic dysfunction, anticonvulsant therapy, hypothyroidism or B_{12}/folate deficiency and is an early marker of significant bone marrow disorders such as aplastic anaemia. A reduced MCV suggests conditions such as iron deficiency or a thalassaemia syndrome. While iron studies and haemoglobinopathy screening are warranted in adults with an MCV in the high seventies (fL), this result is normal for the majority of children through the years of mid-childhood. In the absence of prematurity or substantial blood loss, microcytosis in the first 6 months of life almost always indicates an α-thalassaemia carrier. Normal fetal iron stores are sufficient during this time, irrespective of diet, and β-thalassaemia carriers do not develop microcytosis until after haemoglobin chain switching (from fetal to adult haemoglobin) is almost complete at around 6 months.

◗ Coagulation studies

Developmental haemostasis can produce significant discrepancies between the reference ranges of coagulation studies, such as the prothrombin time and activated partial thromboplastin time (APTT), depending on age and prematurity.[3] Table 37.1 shows the age-related reference ranges for APTT in our laboratory using a variety of commonly used reagents. The impact of different reagents even when used on the same analyser is obvious.

Most laboratories do not have the resources required to establish age-appropriate reference ranges and until such systems are put in place, over-investigation of normal children whose coagulation results are labelled abnormal will continue. The clinical dilemma is that significant conditions such as von Willebrand's disease may exist in children with a mildly prolonged APTT.

Table 37.1 Normal ranges for activated partial thromboplastin time (APTT) according to age showing reagent/analyser specificity

	APTT results in seconds by age: mean (95th centiles)						
	Day 1	Day 3	1 month– 1 year	1 –5 years	6–10 years	11–16 years	Adults
PTT-A	38.7 (29.8– 54.5)	36.3 (28.4– 69.1)	39.3 (35.1– 46.3)	37.7 (33.6– 43.8)	37.3 (31.8– 43.7)	39.5 (33.9– 46.1)	33.2 (28.6– 38.2)
CK Prest	Not available	Not available	34.4 (31.1– 36.6)	32.3 (29.8– 35.0)	32.9 (30.8– 34.8)	34.1 (29.4– 40.4)	29.1 (25.7– 31.5)
Actin FSL	Not available	Not available	37.4 (33.4– 41.4)	36.7 (31.8– 42.8)	35.4 (30.1– 40.4)	38.1 (32.2– 42.2)	30.8 (27.1– 34.3)
Platelin L	Not available	Not available	36.5 (33.6– 40.4)	37.3 (32.5– 43.8)	35 (31.0– 39.3)	39.4 (32.6– 49.2)	31.3 (27.2– 35.4)

All assays performed on a Stago STA-compact. Minimum 20 samples per age group.

Often the clinical rationale for coagulation testing in children relates to 'abnormal' bruising that may raise questions of non-accidental injury. The interpretation of results then becomes a matter for legal debate as well as clinical management. Simple calculations show that if we used the adult reference range in our laboratory, approximately 30% of all 1–10 year-olds would be labelled abnormal and further investigations would ensue. The direct cost of these further investigations (such as repeat APTT, intrinsic factor assays and von Willebrand's screening) amounts to hundreds of dollars per child.[4] This does not consider the indirect costs such as cancelled surgery, referral for specialist review and missed work (parents) and school to attend hospital appointments.

There is therefore a considerable imperative for all laboratories performing coagulation studies in children to report the results accurately based on age-related reference ranges that are specific to their analyser and reagent systems. The clinician must also be circumspect in the interpretation of all coagulation studies in children. Many of the pitfalls in interpreting coagulation results in children have been recently reviewed.[4]

Abnormalities of coagulation testing have different interpretations in children and adults. For example, a prolonged APTT that fails to correct on mixing studies (mixing studies usually involve a one-to-one mix of patient plasma with normal plasma before APTT testing) is commonly due to a so-called lupus anticoagulant. These non-specific antiphospholipid antibodies can be associated with autoimmune disease in adults and in particular with thrombotic manifestations. While the same is true in children they are far more frequently a transient phenomenon seen after viral illness and in these circumstances are rarely associated with significant pathology.

Summary

Misinterpretation of haematology tests in children is common. Specific issues need to be considered to ensure appropriate interpretation of results. In particular an understanding of 'normal' for different age groups is critical to both full blood examination and coagulation studies. Many laboratories within Australia do not report these parameters appropriately and the clinician must be aware of this to guide subsequent management and investigation.

References

1. Expected hematologic values for term and preterm neonates. In: Christensen R.D., ed. *Hematologic Problems Of The Neonate.* Philadelphia: W.B. Saunders Co, 2000. Ch 7.
2. Smith H. *Diagnosis In Paediatric Haematology.* New York: Churchill Livingstone, 1996. Ch 1, 8.
3. Monagle P., Barnes C., Ignjatovic V., Furmedge J., Newell F., Chan A. et al. Developmental haemostasis: Impact for clinical haemostasis laboratories. *J Thromb Haemost* 2006; 95: 362–72.
4. Monagle P., Ignjatovic V. and Savoia H. Hemostasis in neonates and children: pitfalls and dilemmas. *Blood Rev* 2010; 24: 63–8.

Part 4

Microbiology Tests

38 Hepatitis B: laboratory diagnosis and vaccination

D.S. Bowden and S.A. Locarnini

Synopsis

Automated enzyme immunoassays for hepatitis B surface antigen (HBsAg) have played a major role in the diagnosis of hepatitis B virus (HBV) infection. In conjunction with other hepatitis B serological assays testing it can usually be determined whether a patient has an acute or a chronic HBV infection or past infection and whether vaccination has been successful. Nevertheless interpreting hepatitis B serology is not always straightforward and serology has proved inadequate in determining how new therapeutic agents can be assessed and monitored. Some of these problems can be overcome by new sensitive HBV DNA load assays which use improved signal amplification or real-time PCR. Following a complete course of hepatitis B vaccination, antibodies to hepatitis B surface antigen (anti-HBs) should be checked to confirm seroconversion. Current immunisation protocols ensure adequate anti-HBs coverage in the majority of cases. Revaccination generally converts non-responders/hypo-responders if sufficient courses are used.

◯ Introduction

Hepatitis B is the most common form of viral hepatitis and constitutes a global public health problem with more than 400 million people chronically infected. Of these chronic carriers, about 25% will develop serious liver disease including cirrhosis and hepatocellular carcinoma and some 1–2 million people will die each year from the long-term complications of this persistent viral infection. A recent serosurvey carried out over three test years, 1995, 2000 and 2005, in Victoria estimated that 1.1% of the population was chronically infected with hepatitis B; the serosurvey also suggested a lower than expected population immunity resulting from current universal vaccination programs.[1]

○ Diagnosis of hepatitis B

The diagnosis of hepatitis B is nearly always based on interpretation of serological assays. During the course of infection the viral surface antigens (HBsAg), core protein (HBcAg) and non-structural secreted 'e' antigen (HBeAg) stimulate the immune system, which responds by producing the corresponding antibodies (anti-HBc, anti-HBs and anti-HBe). The assay for serum HBsAg has proven to be the pre-eminent diagnostic test because the persistence of HBsAg for longer than 6 months defines chronic infection and the presence of its corresponding antibody (anti-HBs) is a marker of immunity and disease resolution. Automated enzyme immunoassays have been adapted for HBsAg and are suitable for the inexpensive screening of large numbers of samples.

Virus structure

For a better understanding of the serological markers of hepatitis B it is necessary to consider the virus structure. Electron microscopy studies by David Dane in 1970 first identified the infectious virus (consequently named the Dane particle) in serum. The virion is approximately 42 nm in diameter. It consists of a 27 nm icosahedral core composed of the HBcAg and is surrounded by a viral envelope composed of protein, lipid and carbohydrate. Exposed on the surface of the envelope is a mosaic of glycoproteins known collectively as HBsAg (Pre-S1, Pre-S2 and S). During infection an excess of HBsAg is secreted into the blood where it circulates as 22 nm diameter spherical and filamentous particles; this excess is one of the reasons why HBsAg has proved to be such a good marker for hepatitis B infection. Within the virion the core encloses the viral genome, which is a circular, incompletely double-stranded piece of DNA bound to a virally-encoded DNA polymerase.

An additional virus antigen, hepatitis B e antigen (HBeAg), also appears in the serum during the course of HBV infection. It is not a structural component. HBeAg is encoded by the core gene from one of two translational start codons. The downstream start codon site allows translation of the core protein while translation from the upstream site produces an HBeAg precursor protein, the precore protein, which is further processed in the endoplasmic reticulum and Golgi of the liver cell to produce the secreted HBeAg.[2]

The immune response subsequently produces antibodies that correspond to the viral antigens, usually in the order anti-HBc, anti-HBe and anti-HBs. Besides HBcAg, which is not usually tested, serological assays of the other respective antigens and antibodies are all of use in the diagnosis of hepatitis B infection (Table 38.1).

Table 38.1 Interpreting diagnostic markers for acute and chronic hepatitis B

Diagnosis	HBs Ag	Anti-HBs	Anti-HBc IgM	Anti-HBc	HBe Ag	Anti-HBe	HBV DNA
Acute	+ (may clear)		+				+ (may be the only marker in the window period)
Chronic	+			+	+ (if negative, check DNA)	+	+ (if HBeAg negative, sequence the precore region)
Response to vaccination		+					

○ Acute hepatitis B infection

Acute infection can result in a clinical course ranging from an asymptomatic or transient subclinical illness to a fulminant infection which can have far more serious consequences including death. In the natural history of the infection the early events in acute and chronic hepatitis B are similar. HBsAg appears early in acute infection and its persistence for a period of 6 months or longer defines chronic infection. HBsAg is usually detected some 6–12 weeks after exposure and is present several days or even weeks before the onset of symptoms or biochemical indications of hepatitis (Fig. 38.1). HBeAg appears soon after and has been shown to be a useful marker of infectivity. Nevertheless it cannot be assumed that patients who are negative for HBeAg do not have acute hepatitis B (see the section on precore mutant HBV). As the titre of the antigens in the blood peaks the level of the serum alanine aminotransferase (ALT) begins to rise and this is the period when symptoms may first become apparent.

The time frame from exposure to the development of symptoms can vary but in most cases ranges from 2 to 4 months. Normally antibodies to the antigens begin to appear during the symptomatic phase. This is consistent with hepatitis B being an immune-mediated disease. The symptoms of hepatitis B are a result of the immune system mounting an attack on infected liver cells, predominantly hepatocytes. The first antibody raised is against the core antigen (anti-HBc). Anti-HBc is found during acute and chronic infection and also with resolved infection. It is the most appropriate marker to test for when trying to determine whether the patient has been previously infected with HBV and is particularly useful in epidemiological studies. In combination with the presence of HBsAg, anti-HBc IgM is the best indicator

Figure 38.1 Course of a typical acute resolving HBV infection showing the clinical, serological and virological response

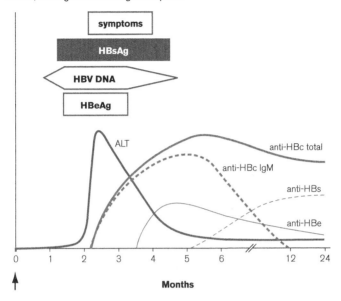

Figure reproduced with permission from Hepatitis B Virus Guide, 2002, p. 148, courtesy of International Medical Press

of acute infection. In the symptomatic phase, anti-HBc IgM is found in high concentrations, peaking in early convalescence and gradually declining over 3–12 months, more or less complementing the increase in titre of anti-HBc IgG. Anti-HBc IgM can sometimes be detected in low titre in chronic infection, usually during exacerbation of disease.

Anti-HBe is the second antibody to be detected after infection and its appearance is associated with the rapid clearance of HBeAg. The seroconversion of HBeAg to anti-HBe coincides with a dramatic increase in ALT, probably because of antibodies causing the immune lysis of infected cells. Often anti-HBe will persist for years but in the absence of any active replication the titre will decline. Finally, anti-HBs (the antibody to HBsAg) appears although it may not be detectable until 3–6 months after infection. Anti-HBs is the neutralising antibody and is recognised as a marker of immunity and thus resolution of disease. In some patients there may be a window period when HBsAg cannot be detected and anti-HBs has not yet appeared; however, anti-HBc IgM can be found at this time. Additionally a

QUICK FLICK 38

proportion of patients do not produce detectable anti-HBs or produce only low levels despite eliminating the virus from the liver. Anti-HBs is also a useful marker for confirming successful vaccination: anti-HBs should be the only hepatitis B antibody to be found (Table 38.1).

With DNA amplification techniques such as the polymerase chain reaction (PCR), HBV DNA is the first viral marker that can be detected, preceding the appearance of antibodies. However, detection of HBV DNA rarely plays a role in the diagnosis of acute infection except perhaps for outbreak investigations or needlestick injury follow-up when transmission is suspected.

◗ Chronic hepatitis B infection

To diagnose chronic infection it is important to establish the presence of HBV markers, just as for acute infection. Any patient who remains HBsAg positive for 6 months or more is considered to have chronic infection and to be a chronic carrier. The age at which infection is acquired is the predominant factor in determining chronicity. If infection occurs early in life (typically from chronically infected mother to baby), chronic infection is the most common outcome. In contrast, with infection as an adult, chronic infection is unlikely to arise. The initial pattern of development of serological markers will correlate with acute infection but as the levels of ALT and anti-HBc IgM decline, HBsAg remains (Fig. 38.2). In the early phase of chronic infection, ongoing replication maintains production of HBsAg and HBeAg as well as HBV DNA. The antibody response consists mostly of anti-HBc IgG, the levels of anti-HBc IgM having declined. Patients with longstanding infection can enter a low replicative phase, characterised by seroconversion of HBeAg to anti-HBe with a corresponding decrease in circulating levels of HBV DNA. This seroconversion occurs at a rate of around 5–20% per year and is sometimes accompanied by a flare in disease activity, known as the seroconversion illness. Often a number of abortive flares of active hepatitis can occur over several years before final anti-HBe seroconversion. In most cases the loss of HBeAg is associated with a significant clinical improvement and normalisation of ALT levels despite the lasting presence of HBsAg. Patients who fail to clear the virus and continue to have active hepatitis are at increased risk of developing cirrhosis and hepatocellular carcinoma.

◗ Precore mutant chronic hepatitis B infection

Despite the loss of HBeAg and development of anti-HBe, sometimes levels of HBV DNA remain high and disease progression continues. This is caused by HBV variants that limit the expression of HBeAg due to mutations in

Figure 38.2 Course of a typical chronic HBV infection showing the clinical, serological and virological response

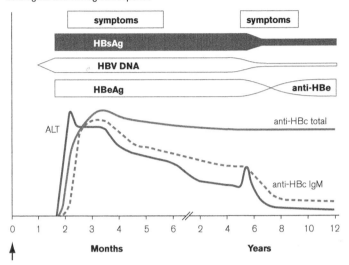

Figure reproduced with permission from Hepatitis B Virus Guide, 2002, p. 148, courtesy of International Medical Press

the precore region of the HBV core gene. The most common mutation is a single base substitution of G>A at nucleotide 1896, which gives rise to a stop codon (TAG) in place of the usual amino acid tryptophan (TGG). Translation of the core protein is unaffected by the mutation because the start codon for the core gene is downstream from this stop codon, allowing virus production.[3]

Further common mutations are seen in the core promoter region (also known as the basal core promoter) at nucleotide positions 1762 and 1764 (A1762T and G1764A) which lead to a reduction in HBeAg synthesis.[4] The G1896A and basal core promoter mutations can occur separately or all mutations can coexist together in the virus genome. The mutant viruses tend to emerge during seroconversion to anti-HBe because the immune response targets infected hepatocytes expressing HBeAg on their surface. Those hepatocytes infected with the precore mutant virus survive, producing more virus which eventually predominates. This strategy of limiting production of the HBeAg is a very efficient mechanism for allowing persistent virus replication. This HBeAg negative chronic hepatitis makes up a large proportion of the hepatitis B disease seen in Australia. While there is no clear information as to whether disease due to infection with precore mutant virus has a more severe course, spontaneous remission of precore mutant chronic disease is uncommon and response to interferon therapy is poor.

Despite the many advantages of HBV serological testing, relying solely on serological markers can have drawbacks. All samples will not necessarily fit into standard serological profiles. For example there are patients with detectable HBV DNA in the absence of HBsAg, which is the so-called occult HBV infection.[5] In such cases there may only be one or two hepatitis B markers present to indicate infection.

○ HBV viral load assays

Deficiencies in HBV DNA testing have been the lack of standardisation between assays and their limited dynamic range. More recently new HBV DNA quantification assays, using real-time PCR or improved signal amplification, have become available (Table 38.2).[6] An international HBV reference standard has been established allowing assay results to be correlated.[7] Mathematical modelling of the kinetics of the decline in viral load has allowed the efficacy of antiviral drugs to be compared.[8] Additionally it may be possible to make predictions about the mechanism of drug action from viral load data.

The results from the large Taiwanese REVEAL-HBV study showed that there was a correlation between HBV DNA levels and the risk of disease progression, including cirrhosis and hepatocellular carcinoma.[9] This study reinforced the importance of viral suppression and the world's three major liver societies now provide guidelines for the management of chronic hepatitis B with levels of HBV DNA playing a pivotal role in defining antiviral treatment eligibility and monitoring. The development of resistance to nucleos(t)ide analogues can also be identified by an increase in the level of HBV DNA, generally considered to be a greater than one $\log_{10}$ increase

Table 38.2 The dynamic range of commonly used HBV DNA load assays

Assay (manufacturer)	Lower limit of quantification (IU/mL)	Upper limit of quantification (IU/mL)
VERSANT HBV bDNA 3.0 (Siemens)	3.5×10^2	1.7×10^7
COBAS TaqMan HBV test v2.0 (Roche)	2×10^1	1.7×10^8
Artus HBV TM PCR Kit (QIAGEN)	1×10^1	5.6×10^9
RealTime HBV Kit (Abbott)	1×10^1	1×10^9

from nadir in a compliant patient.[10] Taken together, this information shows that viral load testing is essential in the clinical management of patients with chronic hepatitis B and this has been recognised by the Government with the Medicare Benefit Schedule providing funding for one HBV DNA quantification assay per year for patients with chronic hepatitis B and not on antiviral therapy and four tests for those patients on therapy.

◗ Quantification of hepatitis B surface antigen

HBsAg seroclearance represents the preferred endpoint of therapy for chronic hepatitis B, as it is believed to signify successful immunological control of active HBV replication. Recent developments in the treatment of chronic hepatitis B have led to interest in alternative biomarkers for predicting treatment response. Quantitative serology for hepatitis B surface antigen (HBsAg) is one promising candidate and preliminary data have supported its clinical utility in treatment protocols for pegylated interferon and nucleos(t)ide analogues.[11,12] In HBeAg negative patients treated with pegylated interferon, the decline in HBsAg titre at week 12 and 24 has been shown to be a useful predictor of achieving an undetectable viral load at 24 weeks post therapy.[13] The results of such studies have implications for future treatment algorithms evaluating the decline on treatment of HBsAg titres in both HBeAg positive and negative patients. It may be that quantification of HBsAg at baseline and/or on treatment will identify those patients most likely to achieve HBsAg seroconversion. Quantitative HBsAg assays are commercially available; they are non invasive, easy to perform and inexpensive.

◗ Vaccination and revaccination for hepatitis B

HBV vaccines consist of recombinant HBsAg, which contains the so-called 'α' determinant, the group-specific determinant. HBV vaccines are highly antigenic and protect against all HBV genotypes. Vaccination against HBV was introduced to control the morbidity and mortality associated with the virus. Until 1997 most Western countries including Australia had policies aimed at limiting the spread of the virus only in at-risk individuals rather than using population-based immunisation strategies (i.e. universal infant immunisation with a catch-up program). As part of the World Health Organization (WHO) program for the control of hepatitis B this selective policy has now been abandoned and a wider program of universal infant immunisation has been adopted (see the National Health and Medical Research Council Immunisation Handbook, available on their website at www1.health.gov.au/immhandbook).[14,15]

HBV immunisation has now been incorporated into multivalent childhood vaccination programs. However, any adolescents who have not previously been vaccinated should receive three doses of standard HBV vaccine. At-risk infants—such as those with a HBsAg positive mother or those from high prevalence (> 2%) communities (e.g. Aboriginal or Torres Strait Islanders and migrants from Africa, Oceania and other endemic areas)—should start a course of three vaccinations within 7 days of birth. In addition to the vaccine the children of HBsAg positive mothers should receive 100 IU hepatitis B immune globulin (HBIG) intramuscularly into the lateral thigh within 12 hours of birth. Occupational risk groups and other at-risk adults must also be considered for HBV vaccination.

Natural HBV variants and mutants selected for following vaccination and passive prophylaxis can have important clinical consequences. HBV vaccines are composed of recombinant HBsAg which carries the predominant antigenic epitope, the α determinant. This determinant covers residues 115 to 145 and is common to all HBV subtypes, and the immune response to the α determinant induces protective immunity. Mutations have appeared in this epitope under pressure generated by vaccine-induced antibodies, the most common encoding a glycine to arginine change at position 145 (G145R), the so-called 'vaccine escape' mutant. Similar mutations have been detected after treatment of liver transplant patients with hepatitis B immune globulin. The vaccine-induced antibodies do not protect against these mutants.

Revaccination

Most people who seroconvert to the vaccine develop antibody titres greater than 100 IU/mL within 8–12 weeks of completing the schedule, the time regarded as most appropriate to check anti-HBs titres. The antibody response in adults is generally detectable for longer than 11 years and can exceed 15 years in children. The NH&MRC advises that booster doses are no longer required for immunocompetent people.[14]

Approximately 5–15% of healthy immunocompetent individuals either fail to mount an antibody response on the primary course of immunisation (they are non-responders) and remain at risk of infection or respond poorly to the vaccine (these people were previously known as hypo-responders).

A non-responder is a person who, despite a correctly administered full course of standard vaccine, does not mount an anti-HBs response when tested 8–12 weeks after the third vaccination. Occasionally failure to respond to HBV vaccine is due to HBV infection itself. For at-risk patients, a check for HBsAg and anti-HBc can avoid a delayed diagnosis. Several published reports have demonstrated that repeated vaccination (up to 10 individual shots) is required in order to promote anti-HBs seroconversion. An anti-HBs titre of less than 10 IU/mL indicates a failure to respond to vaccination. When using this latter schedule the individual should be checked for seroconversion 2 weeks after each additional dose. The next generation of vaccines is likely to incorporate other envelope components (Pre-S1 and Pre-S2) of HBsAg. One partially-controlled trial of a candidate vaccine has shown seroconversion in 70% of non-responders after a single dose of vaccine.[16] These vaccines should be approved for use in Australia in the next few years.

○ Postexposure prophylaxis in non-responders

Any individual who has not responded to HBV vaccination or responded poorly and later has an identifiable or high-risk exposure to HBV (e.g. needlestick injury) should be offered HBIG within 72 hours of exposure. A course of HBV vaccine should also commence within 7 days. While some individuals will have a response to this vaccination others will be at risk of acute or chronic infection until better vaccines become available. There is as yet no evidence-based role for antiviral drug prophylaxis but it may be an option in the future after appropriate trials.

References

1. Cowie B., Karapanagiotidis T., Enriquez A. and Kelly H. Markers of hepatitis B virus infection and immunity in Victoria, Australia, 1995–2005. *Aust NZ J Publ Heal* 2010; 34: 72–8.

2. Hollinger F.B. and Liang T.J. Hepatitis B Virus. In: Knipe D.M., Howley P.M. et al., eds. *Fields Virology.* Philadelphia: Lippincott Williams & Wilkins, 2001. Vol 2, pp. 2971–3036.

3. Lok A.S., Akarca U. and Greene S. Mutations in the pre-core region of hepatitis B virus serve to enhance the stability of the secondary structure of the pre-genome encapsidation signal. *P Natl Acad Sci USA* 1994; 91: 4077–81.

4. Laras A., Koskinas J. and Hadziyannis S.J. In vivo suppression of precore mRNA synthesis is associated with mutations in the hepatitis B virus core promoter. *Virology* 2002; 295: 86–96.

5. Brechot C., Thiers V., Kremsdorf D., Nalpas B., Pol S. and Paterlini-Brechot P. Persistent hepatitis B virus infection in subjects without hepatitis B surface antigen: clinically significant or purely 'occult'? *Hepatology* 2001; 34: 194–203.

6. Pawlotsky J.M. Molecular diagnosis of viral hepatitis. *Gastroenterology* 2002; 122: 1554–68.

7. Saldanha J., Gerlich W., Lelie N., Dawson P., Heermann K. and Heath A. An international collaborative study to establish a World

QUICK FLICK 38

Health Organization international standard for hepatitis B virus DNA nucleic acid amplification techniques. *Vox Sang* 2001; 80: 63–71.

8. Tsiang M., Rooney J. F., Toole J.J. and Gibbs C.S. Biphasic clearance kinetics of hepatitis B virus from patients during adefovir dipivoxil therapy. *Hepatology* 1999; 29: 1863–9.

9. Chen C.J., Yang H.I., Su J., Jen C.L., You S.L., Lu S.N. et al. Risk of hepatocellular carcinoma across a biological gradient of serum hepatitis B virus DNA level. *JAMA* 2006; 295: 65–73.

10. Pawlotsky J.M., Dusheiko G., Hatzakis A., Lau D., Lau G., Liang T.J. et al. Virologic monitoring of hepatitis B virus therapy in clinical trials and practice: recommendations for a standardized approach. *Gastroenterology* 2008;134: 405–415.

11. Wiegand J., Wedemeyer H., Finger A., Heidrich B., Rosenau J., Michel G., Bock C.T. et al. A decline in hepatitis B virus surface antigen (HBsAg) predicts clearance, but does not correlate with quantitative HBeAg or HBV DNA levels. *Antivir Ther* 2008; 13: 547–554.

12. Brunetto M.R., Moriconi F., Bonino F., Lau G.K., Farci P., Yurdaydin C. et al. Hepatitis B virus surface antigen levels: a guide to sustained response to peginterferon alfa-2a in HBeAg-negative chronic hepatitis B. *Hepatology* 2009; 49: 1141–50.

13. Moucari R., Mackiewicz V., Lada O., Ripault M.P., Castelnau C., Martinot-Peignoux M et al. Early serum HBsAg drop: a strong predictor of sustained virological response to pegylated interferon alfa-2a in HBeAg-negative patients. *Hepatology* 2009; 49: 1151–7.

14. Hepatitis B. In: *The Australian Immunisation Handbook.* 8th ed. Canberra: Australian Government Publishing Service, 2003. pp. 120–33.

15. European Consensus Group on Hepatitis B Immunity. Are booster immunisations needed for lifelong hepatitis B immunity? *Lancet* 2000; 355: 561–5.

16. Zuckerman J.N., Sabin C., Craig F.M., Williams A. and Zuckerman A.J. Immune response to a new hepatitis B vaccine in health care workers who had not responded to standard vaccine: randomised double blind dose-response study. *BMJ* 1997; 314: 329–33.

39 Hepatitis C: laboratory diagnosis and monitoring*

D.S. Bowden

Synopsis

Diagnosis of hepatitis C virus (HCV) infection relies on both serological assays for the detection of specific antibodies (anti-HCV) and on molecular assays for the detection of HCV RNA. New generation anti-HCV assays have high sensitivity and specificity and they have made a substantial improvement to public health. However, while anti-HCV assays can indicate exposure to HCV they cannot be used to diagnose chronic infection, which requires detection of HCV RNA by nucleic acid amplification technology. The first marker to appear in acute hepatitis C is HCV RNA, which precedes the elevation of serum transaminase levels and the development of anti-HCV serology. In resolving infection, anti-HCV remains while HCV RNA clears and transaminase levels fall to the normal range. However, most HCV infections progress to chronicity characterised by the persistence of HCV RNA and fluctuating levels of serum transaminases. Additional molecular-based assays including HCV genotyping and HCV RNA quantification have proven useful as predictors of the response to interferon-based therapy. Further advances brought about by the study of HCV replication and human pharmacogenomics are likely to help in the development of other assays and in establishing new antiviral treatment regimes.

○ Introduction

Infection with HCV has become a global health problem with estimates of over 175 million people chronically infected and up to four million new infections per year. In Australia, mathematical modelling carried out in 2006 estimated that 264 000 people had been infected with HCV (i.e. had anti-HCV), and about 200 000 were living with chronic HCV infection.[1] It was

---

*   This chapter updated by D.S. Bowden.

further estimated that there were 9 700 new infections in 2005 with most being newly acquired among injecting drug users. The number of people with chronic hepatitis C and their respective stages of liver disease were also assessed in this study by Razali and colleagues.[1] The authors proposed that there were 154 000 individuals with early disease (77% of the 200 000 people with chronic hepatitis C), 38 000 with progressive disease (19% with moderate to severe fibrosis) and 5 300 (3%) with cirrhosis. Based on such models, the burden of advanced liver disease is expected to double over the next 20 years if there is no substantial increase in the number of people seeking treatment.

HCV is transmitted primarily by percutaneous exposure to infected blood. As expected, injecting drug use accounts for about 80% of all HCV infections in Australia and for 90% of newly acquired HCV cases.[1] Before screening became available (for Australia, February 1990) transfusion of blood and blood products was also a common source of infection. Other less common modes of transmission include from chronically infected mothers to their babies and needlestick injury in the healthcare setting. The latter are not efficient mechanisms of transmission, with rates of around 5%. Sexual transmission of HCV appears to be rare although recent molecular studies have shown an increase in rates of acute hepatitis C among HIV-positive men who have sex with men. This seems to be unrelated to injecting drug use and implies a role for HIV as a cofactor in transmission. Interestingly the incidence of HCV infection with no known risk factors in Australians born overseas is relatively high and likely reflects past unsafe medical and dental procedures in their country of origin.[2]

⊙ Virus structure and genome organisation

HCV is an enveloped single-stranded RNA virus and is the sole member of the Hepacivirus genus of the *Flaviviridae*. The genome is plus-sense RNA, 9.6 kb in length and contains a single open reading frame (ORF) encoding a polyprotein of approximately 3 000 amino acids. The polyprotein is cleaved by both host cell and viral proteases to produce three structural proteins and at least seven non-structural (NS) proteins. The structural proteins are at the N-terminal portion of the polyprotein and include the core protein and two envelope glycoproteins. The NS proteins are involved in processing the polyprotein as well as viral RNA replication and include the RNA-dependent RNA polymerase.[3] While there is little sequence homology between HCV and other viral sequences, the genome organisation and functions of the NS proteins are most similar to the pestiviruses in the *Flaviviridae*.

○ Diagnosis of hepatitis C

The diagnosis of hepatitis C relies on both serological assays for the detection of specific antibodies and on molecular assays for the detection of HCV RNA. Serological assays have been developed for detecting anti-HCV to recombinant antigens and since their introduction they have been frequently modified by the manufacturers to improve sensitivity and specificity. They represent the most cost-effective screening method for determining exposure to HCV but have limitations in that they cannot be used to diagnose chronic HCV infection. This role can be provided by the molecular assays that detect the presence of HCV RNA either qualitatively (detected or not detected) or quantitatively (viral load measurement).

Serological assays

The first anti-HCV screening assay became available in Australia in early 1990 and was based on a single recombinant antigen expressed from the original clone used to identify the virus. The development of this enzyme immunoassay (EIA) was a major breakthrough; however, the assay had substantial specificity problems with a high false positive rate in low-risk populations such as blood donors. Sensitivity was also an issue because it detected only 60–80% of infected individuals in high-risk populations and the window period for seroconversion could be lengthy. Improved second generation assays, which included recombinant core protein, became available in Australia in mid-1991. The addition of further recombinant antigens and reconfiguration of these antigens has led to the current assays which have high sensitivity and specificity. The newer assays have also reduced the window period before seroconversion substantially from around 3 months to an average of 6–7 weeks. Individuals tested with the so-called first generation assay need to have their diagnosis confirmed with the current assays.

The National Hepatitis C Testing Policy offers a number of recommendations to diagnostic laboratories:

- Samples that were non-reactive in an initial screening EIA can be reported as anti-HCV not detected.
- Samples reactive in the initial screening EIA should be re-tested in a different EIA using alternative recombinant antigens and a different assay format. If the second assay also shows reactivity, the sample can be considered to have detectable anti-HCV.
- In the case of a discordant result, if there are no risk factors it is likely the individual is anti-HCV negative. If risk factors are present, a follow-up sample should be tested for anti-HCV and then by a qualitative nucleic acid test (see below).[4]

The serological assays have played an important role in improving public health but they also have their limitations. Other than discordant results between two different EIAs, some samples give equivocal readings (not clearly negative or positive) which are difficult to interpret. Some discrimination may be achieved by supplemental assays for anti-HCV such as immunoblots. The immunoblots have the recombinant antigens separated and bound on a strip, which allows for detection of specific reactivity to an individual antigen. These supplemental assays can play a role in the blood transfusion services where the immunoblot may help determine false reactivity in a low-risk population. However, in most diagnostic laboratories they offer little assistance to resolving problem samples and because the assays are expensive most laboratories find it more cost effective to use the molecular based assays.

HCV RNA–qualitative testing

Does the patient have current infection? The serological assays are highly sensitive at detecting antibodies and thereby indicating exposure to HCV, however, they cannot distinguish resolved infection from active infection or identify individuals in the window period before seroconversion. These deficiencies can be largely overcome by the molecular assays used to detect HCV RNA. The relatively low titre of HCV RNA in the blood of infected individuals makes it difficult to detect by conventional hybridisation techniques and most qualitative and quantitative assays have been developed using the technology of signal or target amplification. These assays vary in their sensitivity and dynamic range (Table 39.1).

Table 39.1 Dynamic range of HCV RNA assays

Comparison of HCV RNA Assays		
Assay (manufacturer)	Lower limit of detection (IU/ml)	Upper limit of detection (IU/ml)
COBAS AMPLICOR HCV test–qualitative (Roche)	5×10^1	Not applicable
VERSANT® HCV RNA TMA test–qualitative (Siemens)	1×10^1	Not applicable
VERSANT HCV bDNA 3.0 (Siemens)	6.1×10^2	7.7×10^6
COBAS HCV MONITOR test (Roche)	6×10^2	7×10^5
COBAS TaqMan HCV test (Roche)	1.5×10^1	6.9×10^7
RealTime HCV test (Abbott)	1.2×10^1	1×10^7

HCV RNA–quantitative testing

There does not appear to be any association between disease activity, progression to chronicity and HCV viral load; however, load has been shown to be a prognostic indicator of therapy outcome. Viral load measurements of serial bleeds from infected patients show that virus levels are maintained at a relatively constant level. This means that there is a dynamic equilibrium between virus production and virus clearance. There can be a large variation in this individual threshold level of viral load between patients. On commencement of interferon-based therapy, monitoring of the viral load shows that the decrease is biphasic.[5] The first phase corresponds to the rate of clearance of the virus from the circulation: this is usually rapid and takes place in the first few days. This is followed by a slower decline in load in the second phase which corresponds to the death of HCV-infected hepatocytes.

The rate of decline in viral load varies among the different HCV genotypes and can be correlated to the sustained viral response (SVR) rate. The likelihood of an SVR is largely determined by the degree of suppression of HCV replication during the early treatment period. Patients who achieve a rapid viral response (RVR; HCV RNA negative at week 4) have a greater prospect of an SVR than those with an early viral response (EVR; HCV RNA negative at week 12) who in turn have a greater chance of an SVR than those who have a partial EVR (pEVR; a minimum 2 $\log_{10}$ decrease in viral load at week 12). It is recommended that patients who do not have a 2 $\log_{10}$ decrease in viral load at week 12 or who remain HCV RNA positive at week 24 discontinue treatment. Monitoring viral load has proven most useful for treatment of the more refractory genotype 1 infection. The importance of viral load monitoring has been recognised in Australia and an allowance in the Medicare Benefits Schedule has now been made for two viral load tests per 12-month period.

Surprisingly, the magnitude of the viral load does not appear to be a major factor in transmission of infection although a high viral load in the mother at the time of delivery has been reported to increase the likelihood of perinatal transmission.[6]

○ Diagnosis–acute hepatitis C infection

Symptomatic acute hepatitis C infection is uncommon and the diagnostic tools are limited, relying on algorithms of anti-HCV detection and qualitative detection of HCV RNA in conjunction with measurement of serum liver transaminases levels, in particular alanine aminotransferase (ALT). Despite concerted efforts by the major companies supplying serological screening tests, no reliable IgM assay is available to assist in the diagnosis of acute hepatitis C. The course of events that follow presentation of symptoms in acute hepatitis C has been well documented but due to the paucity of patients to follow in the presymptomatic stages most data have come from animal studies or from case studies.[7]

The first marker to be detected in acute infection is HCV RNA which can appear as early as 1 week after exposure but is more reliably detected at 2–3 weeks (Fig. 39.1). The level of HCV RNA continues to rise, peaking around 4–5 weeks, and precedes the peak of serum ALT and the onset of symptoms. The rise in ALT and appearance of symptoms are indicative of liver damage and represent an assault on infected hepatocytes by the immune system. If symptoms develop, their onset is on average 6 weeks after exposure, generally ranging from 4 to 10 weeks. Anti-HCV is detectable in the majority of patients at symptom onset although there can be a large variation in the time required before seroconversion. Often the level of antibodies can be seen to rise as early as 4 weeks postexposure even though they may not be clearly positive or above the designated cut-off of the assay. In the immunocompetent patient, equivocal antibody levels, or a lack of antibodies, and the presence of HCV RNA are strong indications of acute hepatitis C. However, equivocal or indeterminate antibody levels alone can occur in other circumstances, and testing of such samples for HCV RNA can help elucidate the clinical significance (Table 39.2).

When testing samples with indeterminate serology for the presence of HCV RNA it is important to obtain a dedicated aliquot rather than using one which has been tested for antibodies in an EIA autoanalyser. This is because these instruments have not been designed to prevent the contamination

Figure 39.1 Course of a typical acute resolving HCV infection showing the clinical, serological and virological response

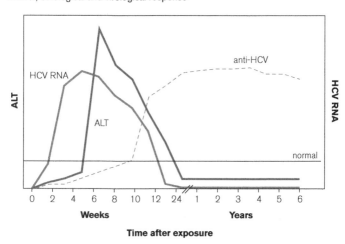

Time after exposure

Table 39.2 Interpretation of equivocal serology results

No.	Reason	HCV RNA	Comment
1	False positive	Not detected	Non-specific reactivity to recombinant antigens. Check risk factors.
2	Waning antibody	Not detected	In acute resolved infection, antibody levels may eventually wane.
3	Maternal antibody	Not detected	Antibody are present up to 12–15 months of age, when seroreversion should be seen.
4	Immunosuppressed or immuncompromised	Detected or not detected	Individuals may not develop an appropriate immune response. Often HCV RNA is detectable.
5	Early seroconversion	Detected	Ensure the sample is a dedicated aliquot for PCR. Request a follow-up sample and test for anti-HCV and HCV RNA.

carryover that can lead to false positive results in the sensitive nucleic acid amplification assays.

In acute resolving hepatitis C, symptoms typically last for several weeks and their disappearance coincides with a drop in HCV RNA and normalisation of ALT levels. Although HCV RNA may become undetectable much earlier a lack of HCV RNA at 6 months postinfection is indicative of resolving hepatitis C. Some patients who go on to develop chronic infection also may have a transient loss of HCV RNA so it is important not to rely on the result of a single HCV RNA measurement to differentiate acute resolving hepatitis from possible chronic infection.

○ Diagnosis–chronic hepatitis C infection

Interestingly patients who develop symptoms are more likely to resolve their infection as this is a reflection of a more potent immune response. The majority of patients who acquire HCV infection go on to develop chronic infection but the chronicity rate has been difficult to determine. In a study conducted at Fairfield Infectious Diseases Hospital (FIDH) in Victoria it was found that 78% (251/323) of anti-HCV positive patients had HCV RNA.[8] However, these figures may have some bias as this was a tertiary referral centre. In contrast, in a natural history study of patients admitted to FIDH between 1971–75 and followed up after a mean of 25 years only 54% of the anti-HCV positive were HCV RNA positive. The route of transmission was presumed to be injecting drug use.[9]

Any patient who remains HCV RNA positive for at least 6 months after infection is considered to have chronic infection and to be a chronic carrier.

The initial pattern of serological markers will correlate with acute infection but in the transition of acute to chronic infection the levels of HCV RNA and ALT can fluctuate (Fig. 39.2). In the early phase of chronic infection a proportion of patients may even have normal levels of serum transaminases and no detectable HCV RNA.[7,8] As chronic infection progresses, the levels of HCV RNA increase and eventually become stable. ALT levels continue to fluctuate but in a narrower range and usually just above the normal range. Nevertheless a proportion of patients with chronic infection and detectable HCV RNA have consistently normal ALT levels. Anti-HCV levels peak after seroconversion and remain high throughout.

Hepatitis C virus genotyping

HCV replication requires the viral RNA-dependent RNA polymerase to copy the RNA genome but this enzyme lacks proofreading ability. As a consequence there is a high error rate which leads to substantial genetic variability in the HCV genome. In an infected individual, HCV circulates as a swarm of genetically-related variants known as quasispecies. Over time this has allowed the virus to adapt to the population it infects, resulting in the evolution of related but distinct groupings also known as genotypes.

Since the discovery of HCV, nucleotide sequence data have accumulated and show that HCV can be divided into six phylogenetically distinct groups. Each phylogenetic group has been assigned a numerical genotype, HCV genotypes 1 to 6, designated in the order of their discovery.[10] Each genotype

Figure 39.2 Course of a typical chronic HCV infection showing the clinical, serological and virological response

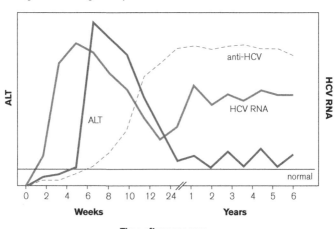

Time after exposure

in turn can be further divided into a number of more closely related subtypes, denoted by a lower case letter (e.g. 1a). Some of the genotypes are widely distributed. For example, HCV genotypes 1, 2 and 3 are found in most industrialised countries while other genotypes are more geographically restricted (e.g. HCV 4 and 5 are found predominantly in the Middle East and South Africa, respectively). In Australia, HCV genotype 1 accounts for over half of the infections and HCV genotype 3a about another third (Fig. 39.3). Evolutionary analysis suggests that the spread of the common HCV subtypes found in high-income countries was relatively recent, with the first wave of spread associated with the introduction of modern medical practices using injection devices such as blood transfusion and vaccinations. The second wave began in the 1960s with the practice of injecting drug use, and HCV genotypes 1a and 3a infections are more likely to be associated with individuals of a younger age with injecting drug use as a risk factor.[10]

Figure 39.3 Distribution of HCV genotypes in Australia (n=6 854)

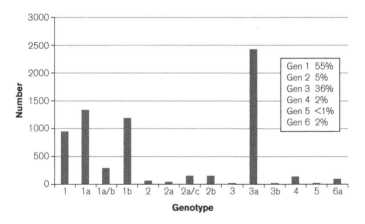

C Clinical significance of genotypes

Largely it appears that virus genotype does not influence clinical presentation, progression to chronicity or severity of disease. However, HCV genotype has been identified as a major predictor of therapy outcome.[11,12] Sustained viral response rates to interferon-α and ribavirin therapy for patients with HCV genotypes 2 or 3 are significantly higher than in those patients with HCV genotype 1. Furthermore optimal outcome for patients infected with HCV genotypes 2 and 3 can be achieved by 6 months of therapy versus 12 months for patients infected with HCV genotype 1.

Little information is available to determine optimal therapy time for other HCV genotypes and in Australia the treatment regime used is the same as that for genotype 1.

◗ **Future trends**

Current EIAs for the detection of anti-HCV show excellent specificity and sensitivity and have provided an important indication of the prevalence of HCV in Australia . The development of real-time PCR techniques has allowed molecular assays for HCV RNA to be introduced which can detect as little as 10 IU/mL and this has allowed thresholds of viral suppression to be used as a guide to therapy dose and duration. Improvement in both the antibody assays and molecular assays will continue as commercial companies seek to gain an edge in this increasing market. Diagnostic testing for hepatitis C does still have some deficiencies. There are limited tools and a simple, inexpensive assay for the diagnosis of acute hepatitis C remains a priority.

The molecular-based assays have also played a role in tailoring therapy to infected individuals. Further examination of antiviral response among the commonly distributed genotypes and investigation of antiviral response to the less characterised genotypes is required. Closer study of viral dynamics on therapy may allow the duration of interferon-based therapy to be determined by the magnitude of the viral suppression rather than genotype. This would have economic consequences as well as consequences for patient welfare, as present therapies can have adverse side effects.

HCV remains a focus of much research. With the recent finding of HCV growth in cell culture, further studies of viral replication will expand our knowledge of the viral lifecycle and may allow the discovery of future targets for antiviral therapy.[13] Already a new catalogue of directly acting agents against the viral polymerase and protease are under evaluation and these show promise for improving SVR rates and reducing duration of therapy. Probably the most exciting breakthrough in HCV therapy is the recent discovery of a polymorphism on the human chromosome near the IL28B gene, which encodes for interferon lambda 3. These polymorphisms are associated with statistically significant differences in how patients infected with HCV genotype 1 respond to interferon-based therapy. In the largest study to date, genotype 1 HCV patients who had the 'good response' polymorphism had an SVR of 69%, compared to only 33% and 27% in patients with the 'poor response' variants.[14] The characterisation of viral and host genetics will hopefully lead to improvements in therapy outcome and a commensurate increase in the number of patients considering therapy.

References

1. Razali K., Thein H.H., Bell J., Cooper-Stanbury M., Dore G., George J. et al. Modelling hepatitis C virus epidemic in Australia. *Drug Alcohol Depen* 2007; 91: 228–35.

2. Caruana S., Bowden S. and Kelly H. Transmission of HCV in the Vietnamese community. *Aust NZ J Public Heal* 2001; 25: 276.

3. Penin F., Dubuisson J., Rey F. A., Moradpour D. and Pawlotsky J. M. Structural biology of hepatitis C virus. *Hepatology* 2004; 39: 5–19.

4. Australian Government Department of Health and Ageing. *National Hepatitis C Testing Policy.* Hepatitis C Subcommittee of the Ministerial Advisory Committee on AIDS, Sexual Health and Hepatitis; the Blood Borne Virus and Sexually Transmissible Infections Subcommittee of the Australian Population Health Development Committee. 2007.

5. Davis G.L. Monitoring of viral levels during therapy of hepatitis C. *Hepatology* 2002; 36: S145–51.

6. MacDonald M., Crofts N. and Kaldor J. Transmission of hepatitis C virus: rates, routes and cofactors. *Epidemiol Rev* 1996; 18: 137–48.

7. Hoofnagle J. H. Course and outcome of hepatitis C. *Hepatology* 2002; 36: S21–9.

8. Kelly H., Maskill W., Sievert W. and Bowden S. Serum alanine aminotransferase levels and the detection of hepatitis C virus (HCV) in chronic HCV infection. *MJA* 2002; 176: 139.

9. Rodger A.J., Roberts S., Lanigan A., Bowden S., Brown T. and Crofts N. Assessment of long term outcomes of community-acquired hepatitis C infection in a cohort with sera stored from 1971–1975. *Hepatology* 2000; 32: 582–87.

10. Simmonds P., Bukh J., Combet C., Deleage G., Enomoto N., Feinstone S. et al. Consensus proposals for a unified system of nomenclature of hepatitis C virus genotypes. *Hepatology* 2005; 42: 962–73.

11. Poynard T., Marcellin P., Lee S. S., Niederau C., Minuk G. S., Ideo G. et al. for the International Hepatitis Interventional Therapy Group (IHIT). Randomised trial of interferon alfa-2b plus ribavirin for 48 weeks or for 24 weeks versus interferon alfa-2b plus ribavirin for 48 weeks for treatment of chronic infection with hepatitis C virus. International Hepatitis Interventional Therapy Group (IHIT). *Lancet* 1998; 352: 1426–32.

12. McHutchison J.G., Gordon S.C., Schiff E.R., Shiffman M.L., Lee W.M., Rustgi V. K. et al. for the International Hepatitis Interventional Therapy Group. Interferon-alfa 2b alone or in combination with ribavirin as initial treatment for chronic hepatitis C. *NEJM* 1998; 339: 1485–92.

13. Wakita T., Pietschmann T., Kato T., Date T., Miyamoto M., Zhao Z. et al. Production of infectious hepatitis C virus in tissue culture from a cloned viral genome. *Nat Med* 2005; 11: 791–6.

14. Thompson A.J., Muir A., Sulkowski M., Ge D., Fellay J., Urban T. et al. IL28B polymorphism improves viral kinetics and is the strongest pre-treatment predictor of SVR in HCV-1 patients. *Gastroenterology* 2010; 139: 120–9.

40 HIV testing in Australia*

A.M. Breschkin, C.J. Birch and M.G. Catton

◯ Introduction

Testing for markers of HIV infection in Australia is delivered by way of
a three-tiered system. Blood banks and approved public and private
laboratories undertake screening tests to detect antibodies to HIV while
blood banks perform nucleic acid testing (NAT) as an additional safeguard
to protect the blood supply. Reactive specimens are referred by these
laboratories to a state reference laboratory (SRL) for confirmatory testing.
SRLs and other approved laboratories also use quantitative NAT to follow
disease progression and monitor HIV antiviral therapy. Some SRLs undertake
testing for HIV antiviral drug resistance. The role of the National Serology
Reference Laboratory (NRL) is to evaluate new diagnostic tests, provide
additional confirmatory tests and facilitate the development of a consensus
on the interpretation of results. In collaboration with the SRLs the NRL also
distributes proficiency panels for HIV antibody testing and nucleic acid testing
to ensure that high-quality testing procedures are maintained in approved
laboratories.

◯ Serological testing

In Australia the most widely used HIV antibody screening assays are enzyme
immunoassays (EIA). A positive test occurs when antibodies in the test serum
bind to purified HIV antigens coating a test well or bead in the presence of
antibodies to human globulin chemically linked to an enzyme or, in some test
formats, to enzyme-labelled HIV antigen. The presence of the bound HIV
antibody/antiglobulin antibody complex is detected by enzymatic cleavage
of an appropriate substrate to yield a colour reaction. The sensitivity and
specificity of the current generation of HIV screening EIA assays is extremely
high. Currently the rate of repeatably reactive test results on sera from healthy
uninfected individuals is between 0.05% and 0.20% depending on the source
of antigen and the format of the test.

---

* This chapter updated by A.M. Breschkin and M.G. Catton.

In 1993, combined screening tests for HIV-1 and HIV-2 antibodies were introduced in Australia and supplemental assays that discriminate HIV-1 and HIV-2 serological reactivity are available and used by the SRLs. At the time of writing there are less than 20 known cases of HIV-2 living permanently in Australia. In 1999, screening assays with enhanced detection of the highly divergent HIV-1 Group O variants were introduced in Australia. Group O strains were isolated from AIDS patients in Cameroon but have not been reported in Australia to date.

In 2001–02 several HIV antigen/antibody combined assays were approved for use in Australia. These assays are designed to detect HIV core antigen in addition to HIV-1 and HIV-2 antibodies in a single screening test thereby improving the diagnosis of early HIV infection. In our laboratory an HIV antibody EIA is still used for routine screening and an HIV antigen/antibody EIA is used as a supplementary test when indeterminate results are obtained. Assays for detecting HIV-1 core (p24) antigen alone remain available. One such assay is used in our laboratory to investigate cases of possible very early stage infection. Samples reactive on p24 antigen assays are confirmed by an additional specific neutralisation step employing an anti-p24 antibody.

Sera found to be repeatedly reactive by HIV screening tests are referred to an SRL for confirmatory testing by Western blot assay. In this assay HIV-specific antibodies from the test serum bind to the major structural proteins of the HIV-1 virus (Fig. 40.1), immobilised as distinct bands on a solid phase, usually a strip of nitrocellulose paper or nylon.

Much of the HIV virion's envelope protein is composed of material derived from the cell membrane. Virus-specific glycosylated proteins in the envelope are gp120 and the transmembrane protein gp41, both of which originate from the same precursor protein. Specific amino acid sequences on gp120 determine cell tropism in vivo. The matrix protein p18 lies directly below the envelope. The core protein p24 is external to the ribonucleoprotein p7, which is itself closely associated with the viral nucleic acid (RNA). The presence of two copies of RNA in each virion is an essential prerequisite for the reverse transcription process, which is carried out by the HIV reverse transcriptase (RT; p66) and involves the conversion of viral RNA to DNA. The HIV DNA is integrated into the cell genome as proviral DNA through the activity of the integrase (p32). Many of these viral components can be detected using assays available to the laboratory. The Western blot assay is capable of detecting antibodies to both structural and non-structural (enzymes) proteins. Nucleic acid assays can detect intracellular HIV-specific DNA following reverse transcription and quantitate the number of copies of RNA present in virions within the blood and other body fluids.

In a Western blot assay HIV antibodies bound to the solid phase are detected using an enzyme-labeled anti-human globulin antibody and an

Figure 40.1 The HIV virion

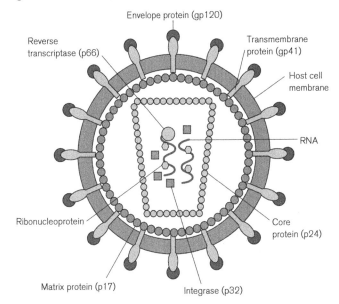

enzyme substrate as described above for EIA. Each protein is located at a different position on the Western blot strip and the appearance of a dark staining band at a specific site indicates the presence of antibody to a particular component of the virus. The commercial Western blot used in Australia also includes an HIV-2 specific peptide that reacts with HIV-2 positive sera. An HIV-2 Western blot is available at the NRL to confirm suspected HIV-2 infections.

According to current Australian guidelines a serum is considered positive for HIV antibodies if it is repeatedly reactive on an HIV screening assay and displays reactivity on a Western blot to at least one envelope glycoprotein and at least three other viral specific proteins. Sera that produce bands not fulfilling the positive criteria are reported as indeterminate. Indeterminate sera may represent partially complete seroconversion during acute HIV infection or spurious reactivity not associated with HIV infection. The indeterminate profiles are grouped as follows:

- group 1—reactivity to viral proteins but not including p18, p24 or any envelope glycoproteins
- group 2—reactivity to viral proteins including p18 but not including p24 or any envelope glycoproteins

- group 3—reactivity to viral proteins including p24 but not to any envelope glycoproteins
- group 4—reactivity to envelope glycoproteins but to less than three other viral proteins.

Figure 40.2 shows a series of three Western blot strips demonstrating seroconversion to HIV over a period of 6 weeks in a recently infected patient. The first specimen, obtained at the time of presentation with a febrile illness suspected to be acute HIV infection, was non-reactive in a screening EIA and gave no bands on a Western blot. HIV RNA was detected by NAT in a specimen of anticoagulated blood obtained at this time and p24 antigen was detected in serum. The second specimen obtained 3 weeks later was reactive by screening EIA for HIV antibody and had a group 4 indeterminate pattern on the Western blot (gp160, gp120 and p24). The patient remained RNA positive but p24 antigen was negative by this time. The final specimen, obtained 6 weeks after the first, was reactive by screening EIA and gave a fully positive Western blot. The patient remained positive by NAT and p24 antigen was again negative.

Experience has shown that indeterminate patterns without antibodies to p24 or an envelope band (groups 1 and 2) are not uncommon in uninfected

Figure 40.2 A series of three Western blot assays demonstrating seroconversion to HIV over a period of 6 weeks in a recently infected patient

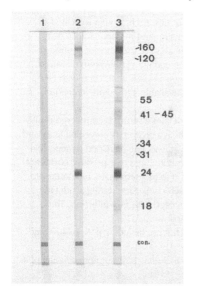

1. At presentation
2. Three weeks
3. Six weeks

individuals and are extremely unlikely to represent HIV seroconversion. At the time of seroconversion antibody to core protein (p24) and/or the glycoproteins are the first markers to be detected, potentially giving rise to group 3 or 4 indeterminate patterns (Fig. 40.2). For this reason individuals whose sera produce these patterns should be monitored over a 12-week period for evidence of seroconversion. In most patients who are seroconverting, samples collected 4 weeks after the first demonstration of a group 3 or 4 indeterminate pattern will show progression to full Western blot positivity. After 12 weeks of follow-up effectively all acutely HIV infected individuals will have developed a positive Western blot. Those showing no progression after 12 weeks are reported as HIV seronegative. On occasion patients treated with antiretroviral drugs at the time of the HIV seroconverting illness may have an altered Western blot response. Their serology should be interpreted on a case-by-case basis in consultation with a SRL.

Sera repeatedly reactive on an HIV screening assay but displaying no bands on a Western blot may be reported as negative by many Australian SRLs. However, it is our practice to re-test such patients after a 4-week interval because the current EIA screening assays are more sensitive at detecting HIV antibodies during early seroconversion than the Western blot. Very rarely a serum with this pattern of reactivity represents the very early stages of HIV seroconversion. If no bands have appeared on a Western blot after 4 weeks, the possibility of early seroconversion is excluded and the patient is reported to be HIV seronegative.

The time between appearance of viraemia and seroconversion, the so-called infectious window period, has been estimated to be 22 days with current generation antibody tests.[1] Although cases of late seroconversion have been reported their occurrence is rare and it is difficult to determine whether these are genuine late seroconversions or represent subsequent exposures to the virus. Circulating p24 antigen and HIV RNA appear early in HIV infection during the antibody negative window. Assays for p24 antigen are usually positive for only a few weeks; p24 antigen then disappears (or declines to very low levels) until the onset of clinical AIDS, at which stage it may become strongly positive.

○ HIV isolation

Virus isolation played an important role in the initial studies of HIV infection. However, the availability of HIV-specific nucleic acid quantitation has to all intents and purposes superseded this method as a means of detecting HIV early in infection and monitoring viral replication late in the disease process. Virus isolation remains an important research tool in the evaluation of new antiviral compounds, the detection of phenotypic antiviral drug resistant strains and the study of the pathogenesis of HIV infection.

◑ Diagnosis of HIV-1 infection using NAT

A strong case exists for the use of HIV nucleic acid testing to provide a diagnosis in situations where the utility of serology is limited but significant risk of HIV infection exists. Examples include: early diagnosis of acute HIV infection when the seroconversion illness is sufficiently severe to warrant treatment with antiretroviral drugs; diagnosis of paediatric HIV infection in children less than 18 months of age; and occasional cases where full seroconversion is delayed by the above-mentioned early intervention with antiretroviral therapy. In addition, early diagnosis of the HIV seroconversion syndrome, with appropriate counselling of the infected individual, may limit further transmission of the virus.

Quantitative RNA assays are now used as the best-available NAT test in the instances above and have the added benefit of providing information on the likely progression of the disease and the subsequent response to antiretroviral therapy. Nevertheless a positive Western blot using the criteria described earlier remains the preferred diagnostic test for HIV infection, and Western blot confirmation of presumptive NAT results should be obtained as soon as practically possible.

◑ Measuring HIV viral load using NAT

The availability of NAT to quantitate HIV-1 in blood has had a significant impact on the management of infected individuals, particularly for prognostication and monitoring the response to antiretroviral drug therapy. Several commercial assays are now available for this purpose in Australia and are widely used. The lower limit of detection of most of these assays can be as low as 50 RNA copies per mL and most practitioners aim to reduce the viral load in their patients to below this level by using antiretroviral therapy. In general the quantitative assays yield similar results when directly compared.[2] They are specific for HIV-1 strains classified as being in the M (major) subtype and appear to be equally efficient in detecting and quantitating each of the HIV clades (A to I) within this subtype. They are also capable of quantifying HIV in sites other than blood, such as cerebrospinal fluid. In Australia the performance of HIV-1 RNA quantitation assays is regulated through participation by laboratories in quality assurance programs overseen by the NRL. An in-house HIV-2 RNA-specific quantitative assay is available at the SRL in Victoria.

○ Antiretroviral drug resistance testing

More than 20 antiretroviral drugs are now available for the treatment of HIV infection in Australia. These drugs fall into the classes of reverse transcriptase (RT; 2 classes), protease (PR), integrase or fusion inhibitors. A fifth class involves inhibition of HIV entry via an essential co-receptor. During HIV replication, errors in the reverse transcription process may generate potentially drug-resistant viruses and these mutant strains may subsequently be selected when suboptimal levels of inhibitor are present. Experience has shown that to achieve maximal suppression of virus replication, and therefore to prevent the development of resistance, antiretroviral therapy should be used in combinations containing at least three drugs, which may include examples from one or more classes.

The presence of drug resistance mutations impacts on virological and clinical responses to therapy. Several prospective studies have demonstrated an improved virological response for periods of up to 12 months in patients who have had resistance testing performed and resistance testing is now recommended in Australian treatment guidelines prior to commencing drug treatment and when there is evidence of drug failure.[3,4]

Currently three methods have been described that fall into the category of antiretroviral drug resistance tests. These are phenotyping, genotyping and virtual phenotyping. Genotyping is the most practical assay available in Australia and is performed by a number of laboratories throughout the country. Its availability is limited by its technical complexity and lack of funding through Medicare.

Genotyping involves the direct sequencing of part of the PR, RT, envelope and integrase genes of the major HIV species present at the time of blood collection. Extraction of RNA from virions in the plasma followed by reverse transcription and amplification of these genes results in a product that can be sequenced. The amino acid sequence is then deduced from this nucleotide sequence and interpreted with respect to the virus's likely drug susceptibility profile. This process of interpretation is not always straightforward although the presence of well characterised mutations can predict resistance to certain inhibitors. A consensus approach to the interpretation of codon changes in HIV proteins targeted by antiretroviral drugs is achieved in Australia by participating laboratories undertaking a quality assurance program coordinated by the NRL.

A now widely recognised issue in the area of antiretroviral drug use and resistance testing is the use of genotyping to detect cases of resistance transmitted at the time of primary infection. Testing over the last few years in Victoria and NSW has shown that up to 12% of newly infected patients have viruses that are resistant to at least one antiretroviral drug. Patients considering commencing antiretroviral drug therapy for the first time should have a genotyping test performed on the first available specimen postinfection.

◗ The future

The combination of screening assays and Western blot for detection of HIV antibody provides sensitivity in excess of 99% and specificity greater than 99.5%. It is unlikely that any significant room for improvement exists in the accuracy or robustness of this diagnostic algorithm. However, change is occurring in the relative emphasis on serological testing and direct viral detection by NAT. Because of their low cost and relative simplicity, antibody screening assays are likely to remain the first-line tests for screening of the general population for HIV infection. However, the great sensitivity of NAT during acute HIV infection and the freedom of these tests from indeterminate results is increasing their role as diagnostic and confirmatory tests for HIV.

References

1. Allain J.P. Genomic screening for blood borne viruses in transfusion settings. *Clin Lab Haem* 2000; 22: 1–10.
2. Schuurman R., Descamps D., Weverling G.J. et al. Multicentre comparison of three commercial methods for quantification of human immunodeficiency virus type 1 RNA in plasma. *J Clin Microbiol* 1996; 34: 3016–22.
3. Durant J., Clevenbergh P., Halfon P. et al. Drug-resistance genotyping in HIV-1 therapy: the VIRADAPT randomised controlled trial. *Lancet* 999; 353: 2195–9.
4. Baxter J.D., Mayers D.L., Wentworth D.N. et al. A randomized study of antiretroviral management based on plasma genotypic antiretroviral resistance testing in patients failing therapy. *AIDS* 2000; 14: F83–93.

41 Testing for sexually transmitted infections

C. Ooi

Synopsis

Rates of sexually transmitted infections (STIs) are increasing worldwide and Australia is part of this trend with increasing notifications. As many STIs are asymptomatic, timely and appropriate testing is needed to avoid the long-term sequelae of infection, halt transmission and improve associated morbidity. Newer testing modalities such as nucleic acid amplification tests (NAATs) offer improved sensitivity and enable non-invasive testing thus augmenting traditional tools such as microscopy and culture.

Introduction

Effective testing for STIs needs to be acceptable to the patient and tailored and targeted appropriately to sexual risk. This risk is determined by factors such as the use of condoms and the number of sexual partners. As many common STIs, such as chlamydia, are largely asymptomatic, doctors need to be aware of local epidemiology and at-risk groups, in order to facilitate opportunistic screening.

To determine which tests to perform, consider the patients' individual needs and concerns, sexual activity, condom use, local epidemiology and any symptoms (Table 41.1). Sexual activity such as vaginal, anal or oral sex will direct sampling and specimen collection site. Pretest counselling and education play important roles in harm minimisation. Serology for HIV should be considered for all patients. Testing for hepatitis B should be considered for those who have not been vaccinated. Men who have sex with men (MSM) should routinely have additional tests for both syphilis and hepatitis A and be vaccinated where appropriate.

With most infections there is a window period (Table 41.2) before laboratory tests become positive. This period must be considered when interpreting results.

Table 41.1 Screening guidelines for different populations*

Who	Routine tests (regardless of condom use)	Other tests to consider	When
Heterosexual men and women	Chlamydia (cervix/urine) Hepatitis B (consider vaccination†)	Depending on sexual practice: – gonorrhoea (cervix/urine/throat/anal) – chlamydia (anal) Depending on local epidemiology: – *Trichomonas* – syphilis – baseline serology for HIV	Consider annual screening for those who have changed partner, or more frequently depending on risk
Men who have sex with men	Gonorrhoea (throat/anal) Chlamydia (urine/anal) Hepatitis A (consider vaccination†) Hepatitis B (consider vaccination†) Syphilis HIV	Anal test indications: – any anal sex with casual partners – any unprotected anal sex – any anal symptoms – HIV positive – past history of gonorrhoea – contact with any STI – requested by patient	Annually if asymptomatic, more frequently depending on sexual risk
Young people (< 25 years)	Chlamydia (cervix/urine) Hepatitis B (consider vaccination†)	Gonorrhoea Baseline serology for HIV	Annually for those who have changed partner, or more frequently depending on risk
Sex workers	Gonorrhoea (cervix/urine) Chlamydia (cervix/urine) Syphilis Hepatitis B (consider vaccination†) HIV Gonorrhoea (throat/anus)	Depending on sexual practice: – chlamydia (anal) – hepatitis A (consider vaccination†)	Every 3–6 months

Who	Routine tests (regardless of condom use)	Other tests to consider	When
People who inject drugs	Chlamydia (cervix/urine) Hepatitis B (consider vaccination†) Hepatitis C Syphilis HIV	Hepatitis A (consider vaccination†)	Annually if asymptomatic, more frequently after particular risk episode

*Adapted from *Clinical Guidelines for the Management of Sexually Transmitted Infections Among Priority Populations*. The Royal Australasian College of Physicians, Australian Chapter of Sexual Health Medicine, 2004
†Once the patient is immunised against hepatitis A/hepatitis B, further serology is unnecessary.

Table 41.2 Tests for sexually transmitted infections

	Test	Specimen	Window period	Indication	Comments
Chlamydia	PCR/LCR	Urine, swab (urethra/cervix/vaginal/rectal)	2–7 days	Screening and diagnosis	PCR at high vaginal and rectal sites not validated Retesting at 1 month post-treatment if indicated Self-collected swabs acceptable
Herpes	PCR	Lesion	Lesion	Diagnosis	Negative PCR or viral culture does not exclude infection
	Viral cultures	Lesion	Lesion	Diagnosis	
	EIA/ELISA	Blood	3–12 weeks	Screening	Type-specific or HSV-2 serology most useful. Beware false results
	Western blot	Blood	3–12 weeks	Screening	

continues

Table 41.2 Tests for sexually transmitted infections *continued*

	Test	Specimen	Window period	Indication	Comments
Gonorrhoea	PCR/LCR	Urine, swab (urethra/ cervix/ rectal)	24 hours	Screening and diagnosis	PCR at high vaginal, throat and rectal sites not validated Self collected swabs acceptable
	Culture	Swab (urethra/ cervix/ throat/ rectum)		Screening/ diagnosis Confirmation of PCR	Culture allows antibiotic sensitivity and specificity testing
Syphilis	Dark ground microscopy	Lesion	3–30 days, if chancre	Diagnosis early syphilis	Only with symptoms
	PCR/LCR	Lesion, tissue, CSF, blood	3–30 days, if chancre	Diagnosis early syphilis	Not widely available
	EIA	Blood	2–12 weeks	Screening	Repeat serology for those with suspected exposure
	RPR/VDRL	Blood, CSF	3–12 weeks	Screening, diagnosis/ staging, treatment response, reinfection	
	FTA-abs, TPPA/ TPHA	Blood	3–12 weeks	Confirmation of diagnosis	
HIV	HIV antibody (EIA, Western blot)	Blood	6–12 weeks	Screening/ diagnosis	Gold standard test
	p24 antigen		Earliest 2 weeks		Transient, may be absent after 2 weeks

	Test	Specimen	Window period	Indication	Comments
	Qualitative PCR HIV DNA (proviral DNA)				Useful for early diagnosis
	Quantitative HIV RNA (viral load)				Beware false positives

CSF cerebrospinal fluid; EIA enzyme immunoassay; ELISA enzyme-linked immunosorbent assay; FTA-abs fluorescent treponemal antibody absorption; LCR ligase chain reaction; PCR polymerase chain reaction; RPR rapid plasma reagin; TPHA *Treponema pallidum* haemagglutination test; TPPA *Treponema pallidum* particle agglutination; VDRL venereal disease research laboratory

○ Chlamydia

Chlamydia trachomatis is the most commonly notified STI in Australia and rates have risen four-fold between 1996 and 2005.[1] In up to 80% of women and 50% of men the infection is asymptomatic.[2] If untreated, chlamydia may have serious sequelae such as pelvic inflammatory disease, ectopic pregnancy and infertility in women, and epididymitis, chronic prostatitis and urethral strictures in men. Screening is recommended for all sexually active individuals younger than 25 years regardless of condom use.

Testing

In Australia, NAATs—polymerase chain reaction (PCR) and ligase chain reaction (LCR)—are accurate and reliable. The chlamydia PCR is highly specific (99–100%) with a sensitivity of 85–90%.[3] These tests allow non-invasive and self-collected sampling. One study evaluating NAATs of self-collected vulval/introital specimens, first void urine samples and clinician-collected cervical samples found the self-collected swabs and urine specimens to be acceptable alternatives to cervical sampling.[4]

A positive result from a chlamydia NAAT is likely to be a true positive. Despite validation for use in urine, cervical and urethral samples only, NAATs have been used extensively to analyse samples from other sites, such as the rectum and vagina.

Chlamydia trachomatis cultures were traditionally the test of choice for use in legal investigations due to high specificity, however, the acceptability of NAATs is increasing. Culture also allows for antibiotic sensitivity testing but has the disadvantage of relatively low sensitivity and high cost. Culture is labour intensive, technically difficult and has a long turnaround time and as such is rarely performed today.

Herpes

Genital herpes is the clinical manifestation of infection with either herpes simplex virus type 1 (HSV-1) or herpes simplex virus type 2 (HSV-2). Infection is common and often asymptomatic. In Australia it is estimated that up to 25–30% of people are seropositive for HSV-2 and 80% are seropositive for HSV-1. Although HSV-1 is traditionally associated with orolabial infection, the majority of which are acquired via non-sexual exposure, the rates of HSV-1 genital infection are on the rise.

Testing

The clinical diagnosis is unreliable and requires confirmation. Testing should be conducted while the patient is symptomatic, indicating viral activity; however, patients who are asymptomatic still shed virus. Type-specific testing should be undertaken to identify HSV type 1 or type 2, as this will provide important prognostic information and may direct education and counselling. Direct detection tests (PCR, viral culture, immunofluorescence) can detect HSV in swabs of lesions or infected secretions. However, viral cultures, immunofluorescence and, to a lesser extent, PCR of swabs may all produce false negative results. A negative test therefore does not rule out genital herpes.

The gold standard test is a NAAT, the HSV polymerase chain reaction test (PCR). If the patient is symptomatic, a direct swab of the lesion will confirm either HSV type 1 or 2 at that site. It is type specific, sensitive and specific. Studies have shown that PCR tests may increase the rate of virus detection by 24–71%.[5,6]

HSV immunofluorescence is rarely performed due to low sensitivity (80%) despite acceptable specificity. The results depend on specimen quality and the experience of the laboratory technician.

With specificity of nearly 100%, viral culture was long regarded as the gold standard but it is slow and labour intensive. Sensitivity varies greatly, dependant on viral shedding, transport conditions, specimen quality and the timing of specimen collection. Indeed, virus isolation may range from 52 to 90% for vesicles to 19 to 27% for crusted lesions.

HSV serology is available and may be useful in epidemiological studies but is of limited benefit for asymptomatic patients. A positive serology test in those with no symptoms is unlikely to change treatment decisions or behaviour and may lead to significant psychological distress. HSV serological tests may be useful in pregnancy, partners of HSV-infected individuals and patients with HIV.

Serological tests that are not type specific have little diagnostic value and are not recommended. HSV type-specific antibody tests are widely available; however, they vary in sensitivity and specificity. Only those based on glycoprotein G have acceptable accuracy with good sensitivity and specificity in high prevalence populations. The positive predictive value (the proportion of positive results that are true positives) is lower in groups with a low prevalence of infection.[7] With some tests for HSV-2 clinicians should be aware of the possibility of cross-reactivity between HSV type 1 and type 2 antibodies. The gold standard for serological tests is the Western blot. This test is highly sensitive and specific for both HSV types 1 and 2 but it is expensive and not widely available. The window period for serological tests ranges from 2 to 12 weeks.

Gonorrhoea

Notification rates for gonococcal infections are increasing. In Australia, MSM, those who have had sexual contact abroad, and rural and remote indigenous communities have the highest rates of gonorrhoea. Most urethral infections are symptomatic; however, the majority of rectal, pharyngeal and cervical infections will be silent, becoming symptomatic when complications such as pelvic inflammatory disease occur.

Testing

Similarly to the chlamydia scenario, NAATs have a high sensitivity (90–95%) and specificity (98–100%) for swab samples.[3] Non-invasive testing with first void urine samples and self-collected anal swabs provide options for patients declining examination. Studies with older generation NAATs reported that endocervical swabs are more sensitive than urine samples (94.2% vs 55.6%). Like NAATs for chlamydia, those for gonorrhoea have only been validated for use with urine, cervical and urethral samples. The positive predictive value of NAATs for gonorrhoea decreases in a low prevalence population resulting in higher proportions of false positive results. With high rates of resistant organisms, positive NAATs should be confirmed with culture allowing for antibiotic sensitivity testing. Traditionally the main stay of diagnosis, culture is highly specific but sensitivity may fall with lengthy delays between collection site and the laboratory. NAATs are more robust.

Syphilis

The rates of syphilis in Australia are about 10/100000 overall, nearly double that in New South Wales and up to 140/100000 in the Northern Territory, with a national indigenous rate of 300/100000.[8] Despite remaining fairly stable in the heterosexual community, syphilis rates continue to rise in MSM.[8] Other groups in Australia at risk of syphilis include rural and remote indigenous communities and those from overseas. Most infections are detected in the late latent phase, when the patient is asymptomatic, having passed the early infectious stages unrecognised.

Testing

National antenatal screening includes syphilis testing. Diagnostic serological tests are widely available, cheap and accurate. For most patients, diagnosis and staging of infection depend upon interpretation of a combination of treponemal and nontreponemal tests.

Serology

The nontreponemal tests are the venereal disease research laboratory test (VDRL) and the rapid plasma reagin test (RPR); both detect non-specific antibodies and are reported as a titre. They are a marker of infectivity; increases may indicate reinfection and decreases may be used to monitor response to treatment. These tests are simple and cheap with sensitivity of 78–86% in primary syphilis, virtually 100% in secondary syphilis and 95–98% in late latent infection. They may cross-react with other treponemal infections and false positive results may occur in 1–2% of the population in association with pregnancy, HIV and other medical conditions. False negative results may occur in patients with very high titres—the prozone phenomenon.

Treponemal tests detect specific treponemal antibodies. The *Treponema pallidum* particle agglutination tests (TPPA), *Treponema pallidum* haemagglutination test (TPHA) and fluorescent treponemal antibody absorption test (FTA-abs) are performed manually and used to confirm the diagnosis. False negatives may occur in early primary infection prior to antibody response, hence the sensitivity is 80% in primary syphilis and nearly 100% thereafter. The automated syphilis enzyme immunoassay (EIA) is both sensitive and specific and is commonly used for screening.[9]

Following treatment nontreponemal tests may become non reactive, however, they may remain at a low titre for life. Similarly, most of those with reactive treponemal specific tests will remain positive for life regardless of treatment or disease activity, with 15–25% of those treated in primary syphilis reverting to negative serology after several years.[10]

Other tests

For symptomatic patients with lesions suggestive of primary or secondary syphilis, direct detection methods such as dark ground microscopy may be used. Despite limited availability, if performed correctly, dark ground microscopy has a sensitivity of up to 74–86% and is 97% specific. Sensitivity will depend on the age and condition of the lesion. Microscopy requires trained laboratory staff, specialised equipment and rigorous conditions for the storage and transport of the sample.

NAATs such as syphilis PCR have sensitivity of 91% and specificity approaching 100%. They have the ability to detect as few as 10 treponemes per lesion. The tests are useful for the diagnosis of congenital syphilis; however, they require serological confirmation once the child reaches a certain age.[9] A reactive treponemal test at 18 months is diagnostic of congenital syphilis. These tests are not widely available in Australia and are not routinely used for screening.

○ HIV

In Australia, the highest risk of HIV exposure occurs in MSM and those from, or those who have had sexual contact in, high prevalence countries. Given the serious sequelae of untreated infection, testing should be offered to everyone presenting for STI screening, those specifically asking for HIV testing and pregnant women. Pre- and post-test counselling is important and should cover associated legal aspects and test limitations including window periods.

Testing

The HIV antibody test or HIV combined antibody/antigen test is used for screening (see Chapter 40). For antibody screening, sera are first tested with an enzyme immunoassay or enzyme-linked immunosorbent assay. If either test is positive, a confirmatory Western blot, the gold standard, is performed. The window period for HIV antibody tests to become positive is 3 months but symptomatic patients may have positive antibody tests 3 weeks after the onset of clinical signs and symptoms. In acute infection, combined antibody/antigen test comprising p24 antigen test with HIV antibody test will become positive before antibody test alone. Viral protein tests such as the p24 antigen may become positive within a few days of symptoms, however, this will be absent after 2 weeks.

Usually requiring a reference laboratory, direct viral detection tests are costly and specialised and should be undertaken only if clinically indicated. PCR detection of viral nucleic acid can be qualitative (proviral DNA testing), or quantitative (viral load). These tests may become positive within days and will remain positive as the antibody develops. For immediate diagnosis, qualitative proviral DNA is recommended. Quantitative HIV RNA testing is not generally recommended as it has a 3% false positive rate in the acute setting.[11]

○ Human papillomavirus

Anogenital human papillomaviruses (HPV) are sexually transmitted and extremely common, with up to 75% of sexually active individuals having evidence of current or past infection.[12] Patients presenting with genital warts may have concurrent STIs and appropriate screening is recommended.

While most infections are subclinical and transient, others may cause a spectrum of disease from genital warts (infection with low risk HPV types e.g. 6 and 11) to cervical cancer (infection with high risk HPV types e.g. types 16 and 18). Although cervical cancer is a rare outcome of HPV infection, over 99.7% of cervical cancers are positive for HPV DNA. Cervical screening programs and guidelines capture many cases of cervical change related to high-risk HPV types; however, the diagnosis of genital warts remains largely clinical.[13]

The National Immunisation Program recommends HPV vaccination for females 10–13 years with either bivalent (HPV types 16 and 18) or quadrivalent (6, 11, 16, 18) vaccine. RACGP guidelines recommend vaccination for females 10–26 years and acknowledge that women 27–45 years may benefit depending on sexual history.

◑ *Trichomonas vaginalis*

There are over 170 million annual cases of *Trichomonas* vaginitis worldwide and, although rates are declining in developed countries and infection remains uncommon in urban Australia, hyperendemic rates have been reported in indigenous women living in remote communities.[14,15] Infection with this protozoan parasite is often asymptomatic but may manifest clinically with vaginal discharge, vaginitis and irritation. It has been associated with pelvic inflammatory disease and infertility, complications in pregnancy including premature rupture of membranes and low birth weight, and increased risk of HIV transmission.[14]

Testing

Conventional testing has relied largely on wet mount microscopy of vaginal fluid. Although cheap and highly specific, the sensitivity of microscopy is poor (50–60%). Culture of high vaginal swabs is rarely conducted due to expense, slow turnaround time and poor sensitivity dependant on transport and fragility of viable organisms. Similarly, while Pap smears may detect *Trichomonas vaginalis*, sensitivity is low (60–70%) with a significant false positive rate.

PCR testing is available at reference laboratories and several have developed multiplex PCR tests to include other STIs. The *Trichomonas vaginalis* PCR is highly specific and sensitive. Like other NAATs it is robust and accommodates non-invasive and self-collected sampling. PCR testing is more expensive than microscopy and turnaround time may be slow.[14]

Point of care tests are now available in the UK and USA and are the recommended testing modality by the US Centers for Disease Control.

This 10 minute dipstick test, which does not require viable organisms, is an immunochromatographic capillary flow enzyme immunoassay. Compared to a combination of wet preparation and PCR, the positive predictive value was 100% and negative predictive value 99.9% in a low prevalence population.[16] Issues in Australia may be availability and cost.

⬭ Lymphogranuloma venereum (LGV)

Chlamydia trachomatis serovars L1 to 3 cause LGV (serovars D to K are responsible for common urogenital infection). Largely an STI of the developing world, in recent years LGV has emerged among groups of MSM in industrialised nations. Infection is usually associated with high risk sexual practices such as unprotected anal sex, fisting and group sex and up to 80% of cases were HIV positive.

LGV chlamydial serovars tend to be invasive and destructive. Patients may present with acute proctitis ('anorectal syndrome') or inguinal lymphadenopathy ('inguinal syndrome') which is less likely to be seen in MSM.[17] Infection may mimic Crohn's disease and cause complications including strictures, chronic fistulas, abscesses and genital elephantiasis.

Testing
PCR is the gold standard for testing; however, it does not distinguish between serovars. If LGV is suspected, genotype testing must be requested. Identification is essential as treatment requirements are different from the non-LGV serovars.

⬭ Summary

Accurate and appropriate screening for STIs is essential to prevent significant individual morbidity and mortality and is highly important for public health. As well as the diagnosis and management of each individual, opportunistic testing for other infections, safe sex advice, education and contact tracing of partners is often required.

References

1. *HIV/AIDS, Viral Hepatitis And Sexually Transmissible Infections In Australia. 2006 Annual Surveillance Report.* Sydney: National Centre in HIV Epidemiology and Clinical Research, 2006.
2. Gaydos C.A., Howell M.R., Pare B., Clark K.L., Ellis D.A., Hendrix R.M. et al. Chlamydia trachomatis infections in female military recruits. *NEJM* 1998; 339: 739–44.

3. Cook R.L., Hutchison S.L., Ostergaard L., Braithwaite R.S. and Ness R.B. Systematic review: noninvasive testing for Chlamydia trachomatis and Neisseria gonorrhoeae. *Ann Intern Med* 2005; 142: 914–25.

4. Carder C., Robinson A.J., Broughton C., Stephenson J.M. and Ridgway G.L. Evaluation of self-taken samples for the presence of genital Chlamydia trachomatis infection in women using the ligase chain reaction assay. *Int J STD AIDS* 1999; 10: 776–9.

5. Scoular A., Gillespie G. and Carman W.F. Polymerase chain reaction for diagnosis of genital herpes in a genitourinary medicine clinic. *Sex Transm Infect* 2002; 78: 21–5.

6. Ramaswamy M., McDonald C., Smith M., Thomas D., Maxwell S., Tenant-Flowers M. et al. Diagnosis of genital herpes by real time PCR in routine clinical practice. *Sex Transm Infect* 2004; 80: 406–10.

7. Strick L. and Wald A. Type specific testing for herpes simplex virus. *Expert Rev Mol Diagn* 2004; 4: 443–53.

8. *HIV/AIDS, Viral Hepatitis And Sexually Transmissible Infections In Australia. 2005 Annual Surveillance Report.* Sydney: National Centre in HIV Epidemiology and Clinical Research, 2005.

9. Peeling R.W. and Ye H. Diagnostic tools for preventing and managing maternal and congenital syphilis: an overview. *B World Health Organ* 2004; 82: 439–46.

10. Centers for Disease Control and Prevention. Sexually transmitted diseases treatment guidelines. *MMWR* 2002; 51: RR-6.

11. *HIV/Viral Hepatitis: A Guide For Primary Care.* Sydney: Australasian Society for HIV Medicine, 2002. pp. 30–6.

12. Koutsky L. Epidemiology of genital human papillomavirus infection. *Am J Med* 1997; 102(S5): 3–8.

13. *Screening To Prevent Cervical Cancer: Guidelines For The Management Of Asymptomatic Women With Screen Detected Abnormalities.* Canberra: National Health and Medical Research Council, 2005.

14. Smith K.S., Tabrizi S.N., Fethers K.A., Knox J.B., Pearce C. and Garland S.M. Comparison of conventional testing to polymerase chain reaction in detection of Trichomonas vaginalis in indigenous women living in remote areas. *Int J STD/AIDS* 2005; 16: 811–5.

15. Marrone J., Fairley C.K., Saville M., Bradshaw C., Bowden F.J., Horvath L.B. et al. Temporal associations with declining Trichomonas vaginalis diagnosis among women in the state of Victoria, Australia, 1947 to 2005. *Sex Trans Dis* 2008; 35: 572–6.

16. Campbell L., Woods V., Lloyd T., Elsayed S. and Church D.L. Evaluation of the OSOM Trichomonas rapid test versus wet preparation examination for detection of Trichomonas vaginalis vaginitis in

specimens from women with a low prevalence of infection. *J Clin Microbiol* 2008; 46: 3467–9.

17. Lee D.M., Fairley C.K., Owen L., Horvath L. and Chen M.Y. Lymphogranuloma venereum becomes an established infection among men who have sex with men in Melbourne. *Aust NZ J Publ Health* 2009; 33: 94.

42 Testing for *Helicobacter pylori*

D. Badov

Synopsis

Helicobacter pylori commonly infects Australians and can cause gastritis, peptic ulcer disease and gastric cancer. Several non-invasive and invasive (requiring endoscopy) diagnostic tests are available. Non-invasive tests (breath tests or serology) are indicated when endoscopy is not required.

◗ Introduction

Helicobacter pylori is a spiral gram negative bacterium found in association with human gastric epithelial cells.[1] Infection of the gastric mucosa by *H. pylori* results in chronic antral gastritis and subsequently atrophic gastritis. Furthermore *H. pylori* is a major pathogenic agent in duodenal and gastric ulcer disease and has recently been implicated in gastric cancer and lymphoma. Seroepidemiological studies show that 30–40% of the Australian-born adult population are infected with *H. pylori*. The prevalence of infection is even higher in older age groups. The indications for *H. pylori* eradication and the optimal therapeutic regimen are still evolving.[1,2] *H. pylori* can be detected using a range of non-invasive and invasive tests (Table 42.1).

Table 42.1 Properties of current clinical tests for *H. pylori*

Test	Sensitivity	Specificity	Availability	Cost (at press)
Invasive				
Histology	95%	98%	A	$97.80
Culture	90%	100%	D	$48.45
Urease test	90%	95%	A	$2.18*

* Test done on fresh specimen at time of biopsy.

Test	Sensitivity	Specificity	Availability	Cost (at press)
Non-invasive				
IgG serology	80–95%	80–95%	A	$17.45
^{14}C or ^{13}C urea breath test	95%	95%	A	$78.15
Stool antigen	95%	95%	D	$28.85

A = excellent, B = good, C = satisfactory, D = poor
Antibiotics, bismuth and proton pump inhibitors should be avoided during the 4 weeks before testing

○ Technical aspects

Non-invasive tests
Breath tests
Several tests are based on the ability of *H. pylori* to produce urease. This enzyme catalyses the degradation of urea to ammonia and bicarbonate. In a breath test, urea that has been labelled with a carbon isotope (^{13}C or ^{14}C) is swallowed. Infected patients rapidly release labelled CO_2 into their breath. Carbon 14 can be easily quantified using a scintillation counter. Carbon 13 has the advantage of being non-radioactive but requires more sophisticated equipment for detection. Although the radioactivity of ^{14}C appears to be minimal, particularly with new protocols using 37 kBq (1 microcurie) dosage, ^{13}C breath tests should be used in pregnant women and children. Breath tests have a sensitivity of about 95% and a specificity of nearly 100%. The breath test usually becomes negative within 1 month after eradication of *H. pylori* and is particularly useful for assessing the efficacy of treatment.

Serology
H. pylori infection causes a local and a systemic immune response. The presence of *H. pylori* can be shown by detecting specific IgG and IgA antibodies in the serum. A number of different serological tests are now commercially available and used routinely in diagnostic laboratories. The sensitivity of these tests is quoted as 80–95% and their specificity as 80–95%.[3]

Rapid office-based serological tests of serum/whole blood have recently become available. These tests have similar sensitivity and specificity to other serological tests and may be useful in diagnosing *H. pylori* in a primary care setting. The precise role of these tests in patients with dyspepsia presenting to general practitioners is currently being evaluated. Serology is not clinically useful for monitoring patients' post *H. pylori* eradication therapy, as antibody titres may persist for many months.

42

Invasive tests

Invasive tests require upper gastrointestinal endoscopy and biopsy.

Histology

H. pylori causes chronic active inflammation within the gastric mucosa. Organisms can be seen on haematoxylin and eosin stained biopsies as well as with special stains including modified Giemsa, Warthin Starry silver and acridine orange. In addition to the stain used, a second factor that influences the histologic detection of *H. pylori* is the uneven distribution of the organism through the gastric mucosa. Two antral biopsies are generally recommended. Sensitivity and specificity are approximately 95% and 98%.[4]

Culture

Culture from gastric mucosal biopsies is considered the gold standard of detection. Cultures are grown on selective and non-selective media at 35°C in a moist environment with CO_2 and hydrogen enrichment and maintained for at least 7 days. Culture of the organisms is particularly useful in identifying the more pathogenic strains of *H. pylori* including cytotoxin production. In addition, antimicrobial sensitivity testing can be undertaken. The sensitivity and specificity of the test are approximately 90% and 100%. The sensitivity of this test is diminished if the number of organisms is small, culture techniques are inadequate or the patient has recently taken antimicrobial, bismuth or proton pump inhibitor therapy.

Because of the cost and the expertise required for culture of *H. pylori*, routine assessment is not currently recommended. The need for culture and sensitivity testing occurs in patients in whom initial eradication regimens fail.

Rapid urease test

Gastric mucosal biopsies can be inoculated onto a urea-containing medium and if *H. pylori* is present, its urease splits the urea into ammonia and CO_2. The ammonia elevates the pH of the medium. This changes the colour of a pH-sensitive indicator. Commercially available agar-based tests such as CLO and HUT require up to 24 hours to become positive with about 70% positive within 2 hours. The sensitivity and specificity of urease tests are comparable to those of histology.

◐ Diagnostic strategies

The test(s) employed depend on the patient's age, suspected diagnosis, previous diagnoses and treatment, the need for gastroscopy, local test availability and resources. Table 42.2 summarises potential approaches to the use of diagnostic testing.

Table 42.2 Clinical disease and *H. pylori* testing

Indications	Test
Dyspepsia	
Children/pregnant women	Serology ¹³C urea breath test
Young adults < 45 years old	Serology Urea breath test
Young adults with suspected malignancy or Barrett's oesophagus	Gastroscopy and biopsy
Older adults > 45 years old	Gastroscopy and biopsy
Duodenal ulcer	
Current	Gastroscopy and biopsy
Previously documented	Urea breath test
Gastric ulcer	
Post-treatment	Gastroscopy and biopsy
Post-*Helicobacter* treatment	
Indication for gastroscopy (e.g. complicated ulcer, gastric ulcer)	Gastroscopy and biopsy
No indication for gastroscopy	Urea breath test
Failed eradication	Gastroscopy and biopsy culture and antibiotic sensitivity

○ Summary

H. pylori infection can be detected by several methods. The choice of a particular test depends on clinical factors including the need for upper gastrointestinal endoscopy and monitoring of eradication therapy and the availability, relative specificity, sensitivity and cost of the test. In most cases, testing should be done only if there is intention to treat if infection is found.

References

1. *Helicobacter pylori: Guidelines for Healthcare Providers.* 3rd ed. Australian Gastroenterology Institute, 1999.
2. Lambert J.R. and Badov D. Gastric acid-related disorders: GORD and peptic ulcer disease. *Aust Fam Physician* 1995; 24: 1889–96.

3. Schembri M.A., Lin S.K. and Lambert J R. Comparison of commercial diagnostic tests for *Helicobacter pylori* antibodies. *J Clin Microbiol* 1993; 31: 2621–4.
4. Lin S.K. et al. A comparison of diagnostic tests to determine *Helicobacter pylori* infection. *J Gastroenterol Hepatol* 1992; 7: 203–9.

Part 5

Immunology Tests

43 Screening for multiple myeloma

F. Firkin

Synopsis

Patients with suspected multiple myeloma should be investigated with tests that have high diagnostic specificity for the disorder. An initial step is to check for the presence of a paraprotein in the serum, Bence-Jones protein in the urine, or both. If these proteins are detected by protein electrophoresis, the patient requires further investigations to distinguish multiple myeloma from monoclonal gammopathy of uncertain significance. Identifying the paraprotein isotype further assists in the diagnosis of multiple myeloma. Assessment of the extent of tumour burden requires a bone marrow biopsy to ascertain the percentage of plasma cells in the marrow.

○ Introduction

Multiple myeloma has a wide range of clinical presentations. It should be considered as the underlying disorder, for example, in patients with vertebral crush fractures, unusually severe osteoporosis, susceptibility to recurrent bacterial infections, renal failure or anaemia that is associated with bone pain.

In multiple myeloma there is a proliferation of malignant plasma cells which typically produce a monoclonal protein. This protein is an immunoglobulin that consists of two light and two heavy polypeptide chains. In almost every instance the malignant plasma cells also produce a monoclonal kappa or lambda light chain that readily passes through the glomerulus, in contrast to the larger monoclonal immunoglobulin molecule, and thus appears in the urine where it is referred to as Bence-Jones protein. Filtered monoclonal light chains can be deposited in the kidney tubules, reducing renal function. Accumulation of plasma cells in the bone marrow eventually leads to anaemia. The diagnosis of multiple myeloma requires investigation of immunoglobulins in the blood and urine and the content and morphology of plasma cells in bone marrow.

○ Initial investigations

Patients suspected of having multiple myeloma should have screening tests and, if these are positive, more specialised tests to confirm the diagnosis. This sequence of investigations identifies the presence of a clonal plasma cell disorder, then differentiates whether it is behaving benignly (monoclonal gammopathy of uncertain significance) or malignantly (multiple myeloma) (Fig. 43.1). All patients are screened with electrophoresis of serum and urine protein. Other basic tests include a full blood count, urea, creatinine and electrolytes including calcium.

Figure 43.1 Screening and diagnosis of multiple myeloma

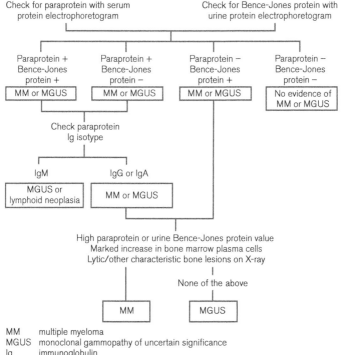

MM   multiple myeloma
MGUS monoclonal gammopathy of uncertain significance
Ig   immunoglobulin

◗ Serum and urine protein electrophoresis

Protein electrophoresis of serum and urine is a sensitive means of detecting the abnormal monoclonal proteins found in myeloma. The test can identify intact monoclonal immunoglobulin and/or free light chains in about 98% of cases. During electrophoresis of serum proteins, intact monoclonal immunoglobulin molecules migrate as sharply defined bands. These bands are called paraproteins and are detected in about 80% of patients with myeloma. They are almost always found in association with Bence-Jones protein in the urine protein electrophoretogram. In most of the remaining 20% of cases of myeloma, where a paraprotein is not detected in the serum electrophoretogram, monoclonal light chains are readily detected by protein electrophoresis of concentrated urine. This form of myeloma is usually referred to as Bence-Jones myeloma.

◗ Paraprotein heavy chain type isotype

Identification of the immunoglobulin isotype of a paraprotein by immunofixation of the paraprotein band should be performed and this procedure enables it to be classified as an immunoglobulin G (IgG), immunoglobulin A (IgA) or immunoglobulin M (IgM) molecule. Other paraprotein isotypes, such as IgD and IgE, are extremely rare. The identity of the isotype is important in differentiating whether production of the paraprotein is by a clonal plasma cell disorder or by a clonal lymphoproliferative condition.

IgG and IgA paraproteins suggest a clonal plasma cell disorder. In myelomas that produce paraproteins, IgG paraproteins occur in approximately 75% and IgA paraproteins in the remaining 25% of cases. An IgM paraprotein is extremely uncommon in myeloma. It is more indicative of a clonal lymphoproliferative disorder, such as low-grade non-Hodgkin's lymphoma. Waldenstrom's macroglobulinaemia is an example of one form of low-grade non-Hodgkin's lymphoma that is characteristically associated with a serum IgM paraprotein.

◗ Serum immunoglobulin quantitation

Measuring total concentrations of IgG, IgA and IgM in serum can reveal elevation of a specific immunoglobulin isotype that is suggestive of the presence of a paraprotein. However, the test does not distinguish between the normal polyclonal and abnormal monoclonal forms of a particular immunoglobulin. This test is therefore not a substitute for the serum electrophoretogram for identifying the presence of a paraprotein in screening for myeloma.

◐ Erythrocyte sedimentation rate

The erythrocyte sedimentation rate (ESR) was used in screening for myeloma before the ready availability of serum and urine protein electrophoresis. Very high values are often observed in association with a serum paraprotein but there are many other causes of a very high ESR and it therefore lacks specificity. Another limitation is that typically the ESR is not markedly elevated in Bence-Jones myeloma.

◐ Differentiating monoclonal gammopathy of uncertain significance from multiple myeloma

Sometimes a patient has a paraprotein but no other features of multiple myeloma. Investigations typically fail to show a substantial tumour burden. This situation is referred to as monoclonal gammopathy of uncertain significance. It is relatively common with a prevalence in the community that increases with age to about 3% in people aged 50–60 years and about 5% in persons over 70 years old.[1] This clonal plasma cell or lymphoproliferative condition is designated as one of uncertain significance, as it can run a non-progressive, clinically benign course, but it can also evolve in an apparently unpredictable manner to multiple myeloma or a lymphoproliferative disorder. The rate of transformation is on average about 1% per year but evolution to clinically aggressive disease appears to be more common in the context of a rising rather than a stable level of paraprotein, or relatively high actual levels of paraprotein.[1] The risk of transformation is however a persistent feature in monoclonal gammopathy of uncertain significance, as one monitoring study showed that the cumulative risk of transformation amounted to 10% after 10 years and 21% after 20 years.[2] Transformation to aggressive disease in a patient with an IgM paraprotein is usually to lymphoproliferative malignancy, while in patients with an IgA or IgG paraprotein the transformation is usually to myeloma.[1]

Consequently, detection of a paraprotein as a lone finding is insufficient to confirm a diagnosis of myeloma. Further information is required to establish whether the paraprotein disorder is monoclonal gammopathy of uncertain significance or clinically aggressive disease, such as myeloma, or a lymphoproliferative disorder.

Serum paraprotein concentration

The serum paraprotein concentration has commonly been considered to differentiate between these conditions. Concentrations below certain threshold values are stated to be more likely to be monoclonal gammopathy of uncertain significance and those above are more likely to be myeloma.[1] These values are:

- IgG paraprotein disorders 30 g/L
- IgA paraprotein disorders 20 g/L.

Patients with Bence-Jones myeloma have very low serum concentrations of the protein. However, they usually excrete more than 1 g of Bence-Jones protein in a 24-h collection of urine.

Experience suggests that these values are only a very approximate guide, especially in the case of the upper half of the stated range, when it is recommended that additional investigations be performed to search for manifestations of clinically active disease.

Skeletal radiology

A major distinction between myeloma and monoclonal gammopathy of uncertain significance is increased lysis of bone resulting from the activation of osteoclasts by myeloma cells. In myeloma a skeletal X-ray survey commonly reveals abnormalities such as multiple discrete lytic lesions, vertebral crush fractures, or even areas of diffusely reduced bone density. These findings are some of the most important means for detecting the malignant characteristics of myeloma.

▷ Bone scan

Conventional bone scanning with technetium-99 labelled methylene diphosphonate measures localisation of the tracer in many tissues, including newly formed bone due to increased osteoblastic activity. The tracer is however not selectively accumulated by myeloma tissue. There can be sites of tracer-positive increased osteoblastic activity with myeloma, but this is likely to reflect increased osteoblastic activity occurring at sites of repair after fracture or sites affected by infection or inflammation. Bone scanning therefore lacks specificity for myeloma and is not a suitable alternative to radiological examination.

▷ Bone marrow examination

A bone marrow aspirate and trephine biopsy is a key procedure in establishing a definitive diagnosis of myeloma. The procedure is usually performed when there is any suggestion from other screening tests of the possibility of underlying myeloma. It provides a direct measure of the degree of plasma cell infiltration in the bone marrow. In myeloma there is an abnormally high percentage of plasma cells (greater than 10%), compared to an approximately normal percentage in monoclonal gammopathy of uncertain significance.

Bone marrow biopsy may be unnecessary as part of initial screening if the patient has the typical features of monoclonal gammopathy of uncertain significance. An example would be the incidental detection of a very low paraprotein concentration in someone with an entirely normal blood count, normal renal function, absence of skeletal X-ray abnormalities and no Bence-Jones protein in the urine.

Approximately 10–15% of patients in whom the degree of plasma cell bone marrow infiltration and concentration of serum paraprotein fulfil the criteria for myeloma have little or none of the skeletal, haematological or renal complications typical of clinically aggressive myeloma. They have a relatively protracted, indolent clinical course in the absence of therapy. This form of myeloma is designated as smouldering or indolent myeloma on the basis of its activity compared to that of the clinically aggressive form of the disorder.[3]

QUICK FLICK 43

◯ **Newer tests**

Assays for free light chains in the serum have become available relatively recently. This type of assay is more sensitive than protein electrophoresis for detection of light chains and can detect the low levels present in normal individuals. Specificity for detection of an abnormal increase in one or other type of free light chain (due to a monoclonal process increasing that type) is established by demonstrating that the ratio of kappa to lambda light chains is outside the normal range. While this assay does not supersede protein electrophoresis in screening for myeloma, it is very sensitive and can detect the small but significantly abnormal elevations in one or other type of free light chain in the rare condition designated non-secretory myeloma. This condition is characterised by showing the classical clinical and morphological features of myeloma, without showing a paraprotein or urinary Bence-Jones protein on electrophoresis. The assay is also of considerable diagnostic value in detecting the very low but significantly increased levels of monoclonal free light chains implicated in light chain amyloidosis.

◯ **Summary**

Multiple myeloma causes widely varied clinical manifestations. Screening tests to detect paraproteins followed by biopsy to confirm an increased presence of plasma cells in the bone marrow can rapidly establish the diagnosis. Failure to recognise progressive myeloma can result in serious complications, which in the case of those affecting bone and kidney can be debilitating and irreversible. Early diagnosis followed by current management will in the majority of patients be followed by major treatment responses which delay development of complications and prolong survival for up to many years.

References

1. Kyle R.A., Therneau T.M., Rajkumar S.V., Larson D.R., Plevak M.F., Offord J.R. et al. Prevalence of monoclonal gammopathy of undetermined significance. *NEJM* 2006; 354: 1362–9.
2. Kyle R.A. and Kumar S. The significance of monoclonal gammopathy of uncertain significance. *Haematologica* 2009; 94:1 641–4.
3. Kyle R.A., Remstein E.D., Therneau T.M., Dispenzieri A., Kurtin P.J., Hodnefield J.M. et al. Clinical course and prognosis of smoldering (asymptomatic) multiple myeloma. *NEJM* 2007; 356: 2582–90.

44 Testing cell-mediated immunity

S. Limaye

Synopsis

Patients with cell-mediated immunodeficiency experience recurrent infections with a broad range of pathogens, and an accompanying humoral immunodeficiency is not uncommon. A persistently low lymphocyte differential on a full blood count may provide a clue and should prompt further testing with quantification of lymphocyte subsets. Measuring total immunoglobulins is a first-line screening investigation in suspected humoral immunodeficiency. Further investigations, which provide an in vitro or in vivo functional assessment, are highly specialised assays which are difficult to perform and interpret. Consultation with a specialist immunologist and the diagnostic laboratory is recommended.

○ Introduction

Defence against potentially harmful pathogens is achieved by physical barriers, such as skin and mucous membranes, and the coordinated efforts of the innate and adaptive immune systems. Innate immune responses are carried out by macrophages, neutrophils and natural killer cells, together with cytokines, complement and acute phase reactants such as C-reactive protein. Adaptive immunity relies upon B and T lymphocytes which express antigen-specific surface receptors. It can be divided into humoral (antibody mediated and dependent upon B lymphocytes) and cellular (coordinated by T lymphocytes) immunity. While this distinction is oversimplified and somewhat inaccurate in that both types of responses are dependent upon helper T lymphocytes, it provides a useful model for classifying and evaluating suspected immunodeficiency.

○ Immunodeficiency

This occurs when failure of any part of the immune system leads to an increased predisposition to infection and associated sequelae such as autoimmunity and malignancy. Primary immunodeficiency results from genetic mutations of components intrinsic to the immune system. Clinical diagnosis should be accompanied by molecular identification of a genetic mutation wherever possible to confirm the diagnosis, identify genotype-phenotype correlation, assist with genetic counselling and identify suitable candidates for gene-specific therapy. Secondary immunodeficiency results from defective immune function as a consequence of another condition such as HIV infection. Drugs such as corticosteroids, azathioprine, methotrexate or cyclosporine can also cause secondary immunodeficiency. Subtle impairment of immune function can also accompany certain chronic medical conditions including diabetes and chronic renal failure.

Immunodeficiency can be classified functionally into humoral or cell-mediated arms, as dysfunction of either pathway is characterised by specific clinical presentations (Table 44.1). Possible investigations for suspected immunodeficiency are presented in Table 44.2. These tests should be performed when the patient is clinically well, and not during an acute infective illness.

Table 44.1 Characteristic clinical presentations of immunodeficiency

Type of immunodeficiency	Clinical presentation
Humoral immunodeficiency	

Hypogammaglobulinaemia	Recurrent sinopulmonary infection:
	     Streptococcus pneumoniae
	     Haemophilus influenzae
	     Neisseria species
	 Other bacterial infections such as gastrointestinal, central nervous system, joint
	 Evidence of end-organ damage such as bronchiectasis, conductive hearing loss

Cellular immunodeficiency	
T cell dysfunction	Infections with: – intracellular bacteria (mycobacteria, salmonella) – viruses (Epstein Barr, cytomegalovirus, varicella zoster, herpes simplex) – fungi (Candida, Aspergillus, Cryptococcus, Histoplasma, Pneumocystis) – protozoa (Toxoplasma, Microsporidia, Cryptosporidium)

Type of immunodeficiency	Clinical presentation
Interleukin-12–interferon gamma axis deficiency	Atypical mycobacterial and salmonella infections
Impaired response to *Candida* species	Persistent mucocutaneous candidiasis Autoimmune endocrinopathy
Combined immunodeficiency	
Combined T and B cell dysfunction	Combined features of T cell deficiency and hypogammaglobulinaemia
Severe combined immunodeficiency syndromes	Failure to thrive in children Opportunistic infection Overwhelming sepsis
Wiskott-Aldrich syndrome	Thrombocytopenia Eczema Infection with encapsulated bacteria
Ataxia telangiectasia	Sinopulmonary disease Cerebellar ataxia Oculocutaneous telangiectasia
DiGeorge syndrome	Hypocalcaemia Recurrent infection Cardiac disease Abnormal facial features
Hyper IgM syndromes	Recurrent pyogenic infection Opportunistic infection
Natural killer cell dysfunction	Recurrent herpes virus infection Recurrent papillomavirus infection (warts)
Phagocyte defects	Recurrent pyogenic infections Recurrent abscesses

QUICK FLICK 44

◌ Humoral immunodeficiency

Antibody deficiency, or hypogammaglobulinaemia, can occur as a result of a primary intrinsic defects of humoral immunity or be secondary to another pathological condition. It is the most common manifestation of primary immunodeficiency and encompasses a broad range of clinical diagnoses. Clinical presentation can range from asymptomatic to recurrent, atypical or life-threatening infections. Encapsulated bacteria, such as *Streptococcus pneumoniae*, *Neisseria* species and *Haemophilus influenzae* pose a particular threat, as do other bacterial species including *Staphylococcus aureus*, *Pseudomonas aeruginosa*, *Campylobacter fetus* and *Mycoplasma*

Table 44.2 Investigations for suspected immunodeficiency

Suspected immunodeficiency	Screening tests	Advanced investigations
Humoral immunodeficiency	IgG, IgA, IgM Full blood count and differential* Lymphocyte subsets*	IgG subclasses Specific antibody titres and response to vaccination
Cellular immunodeficiency	Full blood count and differential* Lymphocyte subsets* HIV testing if indicated IgG, IgA, IgM	Delayed-type hypersensitivity skin tests Lymphocyte proliferation assays Natural killer cell cytotoxicity

Ig immunoglobulin
*Defer testing until resolution of acute infective illness

species. Recurrent or unusually severe sinopulmonary infection, other infections (gastrointestinal, skin, joint or central nervous system) or evidence of end-organ damage such as bronchiectasis should alert the doctor to the possibility of an underlying humoral immunodeficiency.

Measuring humoral immunity
The simplest initial investigation for this condition is to quantify immunoglobulin (Ig) concentrations (IgG, IgA and IgM). Normal levels, however, do not exclude a humoral defect and if clinical suspicion is high, more advanced investigations can be undertaken. This includes measuring antibodies to specific antigens following vaccination to assess whether the patient produces a functional antibody response. This is usually performed in conjunction with assessment by a clinical immunologist. Immunoglobulin G subclasses can also be quantified—however, the clinical utility of this investigation is somewhat controversial.

○ Cell-mediated immunodeficiency

Defective T cell-mediated immunity predisposes patients to a broader range of infections than humoral immunodeficiency, including intracellular pathogens, persistent superficial candidiasis or recurrent viral, fungal or protozoal infections (Table 44.1). Defects can again be classified as either primary or secondary to extrinsic factors. HIV infection resulting in progressive depletion of CD4 T cells is a particular consideration. As helper T cells are required for B cell-mediated antibody production, T cell immunodeficiency can result in functional B cell defects; thus patients with cell-mediated immunodeficiency often have an accompanying hypogammaglobulinaemia. This is termed combined immunodeficiency.

Measuring cellular immunity

Measurement of cell-mediated immunity can be undertaken by both in vitro and in vivo methods. It is, however, more problematic than humoral assessment as assays are plagued by difficulties in standardisation, biological variability, imprecision and technical complexity. Most tests are highly specialised and referral to a clinical immunologist is recommended.

Flow cytometry

The first step in the evaluation of cell-mediated immunity is to quantify circulating immune cells and their subsets by flow cytometric analysis. Patients' blood cells are incubated with fluorochrome-labelled monoclonal antibodies directed against cell surface molecules and analysed by a flow cytometer, which measures light scatter and fluorescence emission from individual cells. Different cell populations (B cells, CD4/CD8 T cells and natural killer cells) can be distinguished based on their scatter profile and surface molecule expression. Absolute cell numbers are calculated as a percentage of the total white cell count and results are compared to age-matched reference ranges. It is important to note, however, that analogous to immunoglobulin measurement, quantification of lymphocyte numbers does not give an indication of their functional capacity. Lymphocyte subset analysis aids in the diagnosis and classification of paediatric severe combined immunodeficiency syndromes and is also recommended in the evaluation of hypogammaglobulinaemia in common variable immunodeficiency. Quantifying CD4 T lymphocytes provides prognostic information and gives an indication of susceptibility to opportunistic infections in patients with HIV infection.

Delayed-type hypersensitivity skin testing

Delayed-type hypersensitivity skin testing provides a functional in vivo assessment of cellular immunity. The skin response following intradermal inoculation of antigen is dependent on antigen-specific memory T cells and results in local inflammation after 48–72 hours due to the recruitment of mononuclear cells (lymphocytes, monocytes) and neutrophils. By convention, a diameter of 5 mm induration is accepted as a positive result. The most widespread use of this type of test is the Mantoux test, which assesses previous exposure to *Mycobacterium tuberculosis* or Bacillus Calmette-Guérin (BCG) vaccination by evaluating the skin response to intradermal tuberculin. Other ubiquitous antigens that can be tested include tetanus, Candida and certain bacterial antigens. Skin responses are dependent upon previous exposure to the antigen and thus this test is of little use in infants less than 6 months of age.

Skin testing identifies functional memory T cells to a particular antigen or the presence of cutaneous anergy. The latter is defined as an impaired cutaneous hypersensitivity response to a panel of common antigens and is consistent with cellular immune dysfunction. Causes of cutaneous anergy are listed in Table 44.3.

Table 44.3 Causes of cutaneous anergy*

Cause	Examples
Drugs	Corticosteroids (usually high dose) Immunosuppressants Chemotherapy
Immunodeficiency	Ataxia telangiectasia DiGeorge syndrome Severe combined immunodeficiency syndrome Wiskott-Aldrich syndrome
Infection	HIV Influenza Measles Mumps Active tuberculosis
Other conditions	Malignancy Chronic lymphocytic leukaemia Sarcoidosis Chronic renal failure Chronic liver disease
Testing errors	Poor technique Inadequate antigen dose

*Impaired skin response to antigen

Lymphocyte proliferation assays

Lymphocyte proliferation assays are indicated if there is a suspicion of a defective cellular immune response either globally or to a specific antigen such as Candida. The patient's peripheral blood mononuclear cells are incubated in vitro for 3–5 days with either a mitogen (substance that induces cellular division) or a recall antigen (to which the patient has been previously exposed). Radioactive thymidine is added to the culture and subsequently incorporated into the DNA of dividing cells. Radioactivity of the cell culture is measured after 24 hours and is directly proportional to the degree of induced cellular proliferation. Peripheral blood mononuclear cells from a healthy control are evaluated in parallel for comparison.

These assays are technically complex and are only performed by specialist laboratories. As the investigation can be time consuming, it is advisable to first discuss the appropriateness of testing and choice of assay with the laboratory. Results are affected by immunosuppressive drugs, severe nutritional deficiencies and intercurrent illness and these factors must be considered when interpreting results.[1] As with skin testing, the patient must have been previously exposed to the antigen, thus antigen proliferation assays are not feasible in babies less than 6 months of age. Response to mitogens, however, can be performed at any age from birth onwards.[2]

Other assays measuring lymphocyte activation

Other functional in vitro measures of lymphocyte activation include determining changes in surface marker expression (CD25, CD69, CD71) following activation or measurement of intracellular cytokines of T lymphocytes.[3]

T cell proliferation following stimulation can be measured by succinimidyl ester of carboxyfluorescein diacetate (CFSE) dilution techniques or T cell cytokine production quantified by ELISPOT assays.[4] These assays, however, are not in routine use and are confined to research or specialised reference immunology laboratories.

The recently introduced interferon gamma (IFNγ) release assays measure T lymphocyte production of IFNγ in response to antigen exposure, thereby providing an assessment of cell-mediated immunity. As with delayed-type hypersensitivity skin testing, clinical application is currently confined to the domain of tuberculosis latency and exposure.

Natural killer cell cytotoxicity assays

Assessing natural killer cells is indicated in patients suffering recurrent infection with herpes virus or papillomavirus (associated with cutaneous warts). Natural killer cell cytotoxicity is assessed by a ⁵¹Cr-release assay in which the patient's natural killer cells are incubated with ⁵¹Cr-labelled target cells. Lysis of the target cells by natural killer cells leads to the release of radioactivity which can be measured. Natural killer cell dysfunction may occur in patients with CD16 genetic mutations, chronic mucocutaneous candidiasis, severe combined immunodeficiency and other cellular immunodeficiency syndromes.[5] These conditions need to be considered and excluded if natural killer cell dysfunction is confirmed. As with T and B lymphocytes, functional natural killer cell deficits can occur even when natural killer cell counts are normal. Natural killer cell assays are technically complex and are rarely performed in diagnostic immunology laboratories.

○ Summary

The evaluation of suspected immunodeficiency is guided by clinical presentation. Screening tests of humoral and cellular immune function are initially performed, followed by referral to a specialist for more advanced investigations if clinically indicated (Table 44.2). Secondary causes of immunodeficiency, including HIV infection, need to be considered and excluded. When interpreting results, confounding factors such as immunosuppressive drug therapy and patient comorbidities, as well as analytical variables such as assay precision and reproducibility, need to be considered.

References

1. Bonilla F.A. Interpretation of lymphocyte proliferation tests. *Ann Allerg Asthma Im* 2008; 101: 101–4.

2. Hicks M..J, Jones J.F., Thies A.C., Weigle K.A. and Minnich L.L. Age-related changes in mitogen-induced lymphocyte function from birth to old age. *Am J Clin Pathol* 1983; 80: 15–63.

3. Caruso A., Licenziati S., Corulli M., Canaris A.D., De Francesco M.A., Fiorentini S. et al. Flow cytometric analysis of activation markers on stimulated T cells and their correlation with cell proliferation. *Cytometry* 1997; 27: 71–6.

4. Fulcher D.A. and Wong S.W.J. Carboxyfluorescein succinimidyl ester-based proliferative assays for assessment of T cell function in the diagnostic laboratory. *Immunol Cell Biol* 1999; 77: 559–64.

5. Bonilla F.A., Bernstein I.L., Khan D.A., Ballas Z.K., Chinen J., Frank M.M. et al. Practice parameter for the diagnosis and management of primary immunodeficiency. *Ann Allerg Asthma Im* 2005; 94: S1–63.

K. Cartwright

Synopsis

Cell markers serve as a monogram to help identify and classify cells. The majority are molecules or antigens within the plasma membrane of cells. Specific combinations of markers are unique to different cell types. These molecules are not merely markers but also have important functional roles. Knowing which molecules are present can help in the diagnosis of disease or in directing treatment.

○ Introduction

Most cell markers are molecules in the cell membrane which can be used to identify cell types. They are classified by their clusters of differentiation (CD) which are recognised by specific antibodies.

Table 45.1

Immunophenotyping of cells allows us to:
Identify cell lineages
• Classify abnormal cell populations identified by microscopy to help diagnose leukaemia and lymphoma
• Assess the level of immunosuppression in HIV and other immunodeficiency states
Identify the presence of disease specific targets for therapy (e.g. CD20 for rituximab or Her2 for trastuzumab)
Detect paroxysmal haemoglobinuria
Identify foreign cell populations
• Feto-maternal haemorrhage
• Detection of 'blood doping' by identifying homologous blood cell antigens
Monitor for minimal residual disease
Assess cell proliferation
Provide prognostic information in some disease states

◯ How does the laboratory analyse cell surface markers?

The common methods of analysis include immunophenotyping by flow cytometry performed on fresh, unfixed cell suspensions and immunohistochemistry performed on fixed specimens. These tests can be performed on blood as well as bone marrow, lymph node and other tissue samples.

An understanding of these tests and the necessary specimen preparation is important for practitioners collecting fine needle aspirates and surgical biopsies, to ensure optimal processing and interpretation.

◯ Flow cytometry

Flow cytometry uses a laser light source to analyse the size, complexity and physical properties of fresh viable cells in suspension after labelling with multiple fluorescent monoclonal antibodies. One to two thousand cells can be analysed per second.

The advantages of flow cytometry include the ability to rapidly and simultaneously analyse multiple cell parameters. The disadvantage is the inability to directly assess the cellular morphology of the cell population under analysis. A smear of the specimen must be stained and reviewed in correlation with flow cytometry to ensure analysis of the correct cell population, to guide the selection of antibodies to be tested and to assess cell viability.

The population of interest on light microscopy is isolated or 'gated' based on cell size and granularity. These inherent properties determine the degree of forward and side scatter. The gated population is then subjected to a panel of different antibodies which interact with specific antigens to determine whether there is an aberrant population present.

Although the acquisition of data can be automated, haematologists' input and critical judgment are required to interpret the results and determine their clinical significance. Results should be analysed in conjunction with the clinical presentation, morphological features, cytogenetics and molecular studies when appropriate. Results may be severely compromised if the samples contain insufficient material or too many dead cells.

◯ Immunohistochemistry

Immunohistochemistry is the phenotyping method of choice for tissue biopsies and is an integral component of routine diagnostic histopathology. The staining process involves a series of enzymatic reactions leading to brown pigmentation if the cell expresses the characteristic antigen. The selection of antibodies available for use on paraffin section is more limited and the turn around time is slower than for flow cytometry. However, immunohistochemistry allows direct visualisation of the antigen label and cellular morphology, permitting the pathologist to use light microscopy to determine whether the cell in question expresses the characteristic antigen.

Results may be severely compromised if the samples are too small or inadequately fixed. This is particularly true for patients with suspected lymphoma. An excisional or incisional biopsy is highly preferable to a core biopsy or fine needle aspirate for diagnosing lymphomas because the architecture of the lymph node is critical to the diagnosis. Core biopsies are frequently crushed and small, hampering the pathologist's interpretation.

�‣ When are these tests useful?

1. To assess abnormal cell populations

Generally this analysis is requested by haematologists or pathologists to further investigate aberrant cell populations in blood, marrow, lymph nodes or other tissues found upon microscopic review of the specimen. Flow cytometry is now an essential tool in the diagnosis of haematological malignancies such as leukaemia and lymphoma.

For example, immunophenotyping may be recommended to investigate persistent peripheral blood lymphocytosis. Lymphocytosis may be due to a reactive state such as resolved viral infection, prior splenectomy or an underlying lymphoproliferative disorder such as chronic lymphocytic leukaemia (CLL). CD8 T-lymphocytes predominate in reactive lymphocytosis whereas B-CLL has a distinctive immunophenotype characterised by the expression of mature B cell markers (CD19, CD20 and CD23), weak expression of monoclonal surface immunoglobulin and co-expression of the cell marker CD5. Expression of other markers such as CD38, ZAP70 and p53 correlates with a poor prognosis.[1]

Flow cytometry is not useful in the diagnosis of Hodgkin's lymphoma and other fibrotic tumours. This is due to the low number of malignant cells compared to the numerous surrounding reactive cells, whereas immunohistochemistry easily identifies the malignant cells among the reactive background.

2. To monitor for minimal residual disease

Flow cytometry is one of several methods used to detect minimal residual disease in patients with no clinical or morphological evidence of disease. In patients with a known haematological malignancy such as acute lymphoblastic leukaemia, flow cytometry may be useful to detect low levels of persistent disease following therapy although molecular techniques are generally preferred due to greater sensitivity.

3. To quantify cell populations

Clinicians may also request the analysis of specific markers to help guide therapy, for example using flow cytometry to measure CD4 counts in immunosuppressed or HIV positive patients. Patients with low CD4 counts are at greater risk of opportunistic infections. This is particularly true when the CD4 count in peripheral blood falls below 200 cells/microL or 0.2×10^9/L.

4. To assess cell proliferation

Ki-67 (MIB1) is an important marker of cell proliferation which can be assessed by immunohistochemistry or flow cytometry to assist diagnosis and guide therapy.[1] For example, Burkitt lymphoma is characterised by a very high growth fraction with nearly 100% of cells positive for Ki-67. This is much higher than seen in other lymphomas. Because of this high proliferative index, Burkitt lymphoma can frequently be cured with intensive chemotherapy.

5. To identify disease-specific targets for therapy

Targeted therapies are an important but expensive advance in cancer therapy. Positivity for the target antigen is required for efficacy and pharmaceutical reimbursement. Over the past 10 years rituximab, an anti-CD20 antibody, has become an integral component in the treatment of B-cell non-Hodgkin's lymphoma. Similarly, trastuzumab, which targets the human epidermal growth factor receptor 2 protein (HER2), is an exciting new therapy for breast cancer. Testing patient specimens for these antigens helps to determine whether patients may benefit from the using these targeted therapies. CD20 may be found on B lymphocytes by either immunophenotyping or immunohistochemistry while HER2 is found by immunohistochemistry or fluorescent in situ hybridisation.

6. To identify foreign cell populations

In some laboratories the Kleihauer assay, used to detect feto-maternal haemorrhage, is now performed by flow cytometry, which is more sensitive than the standard Kleihauer assay, leading to a more accurate quantification of the volume of haemorrhage and the required anti-D dose if the mother is at risk for developing Rh antibodies. Similar methodologies have been developed to detect blood doping in athletes.[2]

7. To detect paroxysmal nocturnal haemoglobinuria

Paroxysmal nocturnal haemoglobinuria is a rare haematological disorder characterised by marrow aplasia, intravascular haemolysis and an increased risk of venous thrombosis. It is due to an acquired inability to produce the molecule that anchors certain cell membrane proteins. This leads to a deficiency in specific membrane proteins. Flow cytometric analysis can detect clonal populations of blood cells deficient in these proteins, greatly simplifying the diagnosis.

Summary

Analysis of blood and tissue for cell surface markers is a widely accepted and useful tool to assist clinicians to diagnose and manage a variety of conditions, particularly haematological malignancies. These tests are generally requested by specialists and general practitioners involved in the diagnostic process. An understanding of these tests and the necessary specimen preparation is important for practitioners performing fine needle aspirates and surgical biopsies to ensure optimal processing and interpretation.

References

1. Gudgin E.J. and Erber W.N. Immunophenotyping of lymphoproliferative disorders: state of the art. *Pathology* 2005; 37: 457–78.
2. Nelson M., Popp H., Sharpe K. and Ashenden M. Proof of homologous blood transfusion through quantification of blood group antigens. *Haematologica* 2003; 88:1 284–95.

QUICK FLICK 45

Further reading

Leisner R.J. and Goldstone A.H. ABC of clinical haematology: the acute leukaemias. *BMJ* 1997; 314: 733.

Herdson P.B., Scolyer R.A. and McGregor A.R. Defining moments in medicine: pathology. *MJA* 2001; 174: 11–12.

Fleisher T.A. and Tomar R.H. Introduction to diagnostic laboratory immunology. *JAMA* 1997; 278: 1823–34.

46 Skin prick testing and in vitro assays for allergic sensitivity

R.M. O'Brien

Synopsis

Specific IgE-mediated allergic reactivity can be tested for by an in vivo skin prick test or by an in vitro enzyme or fluorescence-based immunoassay, commonly called a radioallergosorbent test. Many people have circulating specific IgE but do not have clinical allergic disease. The relevance of a positive or abnormal test result therefore depends on the clinical scenario. Skin prick testing is more sensitive than radioallergosorbent tests for detection of IgE reactivity, as the majority of specific IgE in the body is bound to mast cells or other cells bearing high-affinity IgE receptors with little in the circulation. In the majority of clinical situations a negative skin prick test excludes an IgE-mediated allergic basis for a potentially allergic condition, such as asthma or rhinitis.

○ Introduction

Since the early years of the last century, before the aetiology of allergic reactivity had been established, in vivo techniques—including conjunctival instillation and skin testing—had been used to identify triggers of allergic reactions. The key mediator of allergic disease, IgE, was the last class of immunoglobulin to be discovered, partly because it is highly bound to mast cells, basophils and other cells and only small amounts are present in the serum. It was therefore easy to detect IgE by skin testing but difficult to isolate or measure it in the serum. IgE was only conclusively identified and confirmed to be the elusive 'reagin' of allergy in 1967.[1,2] At about the same time, laboratory testing was expanding in all medical disciplines and it was not long before immunoassays for allergen-specific IgE were designed and commercialised. The first radioallergosorbent tests (RAST) appeared in 1974 and tests not unlike the current ones were in use by the late 1970s. Since then the relative merits of in vivo skin testing and in vitro RAST measurements have been argued by their respective proponents.

○ Tests for allergen-specific IgE

Skin prick testing

Skin prick testing is the conventional way to test for the presence of allergen-specific IgE. It detects IgE bound to the surface of mast cells in the skin. Allergen in solution is applied to the skin, generally the volar surface of the forearm. When the skin is pricked with a lancet the allergen comes into contact with specific IgE bound to the surface of cutaneous mast cells. The binding of the allergen leads to cell activation and the immediate release of mediators including histamine (other mediators are released but histamine appears to be the critical one as skin prick tests become negative after taking antihistamines). The release of mediators results in a wheal and flare type reaction and the test is generally reported as the maximal wheal diameter after 15 to 20 minutes. A wheal with a diameter three or more millimetres greater than the control is generally regarded as positive. The amount of specific IgE present can be estimated by the size of the wheal. These tests are simple, quick and the most sensitive method of detecting specific IgE. Skin prick tests are particularly helpful in excluding potential allergens as a cause of symptoms because false negatives are uncommon.

Although these tests are extremely safe, with only rare reports of generalised reactions, the risk of systemic absorption remains and anaphylaxis is a remote possibility in highly sensitised individuals. Testing should therefore always be performed under the supervision of a trained and experienced clinician who has resuscitation equipment immediately available.

Patch testing

As distinct from skin prick testing, which measures specific IgE, patch testing is used to detect the presence of antigen-specific T cells. The main clinical application for patch testing is in detecting antigens responsible for contact dermatitis rather than atopic disorders such as asthma, rhinitis or eczema.

In vitro immunoassays for specific IgE

Although serum tests for specific IgE are still frequently referred to as radioallergosorbent tests, they are generally not performed by traditional radio-immunoassay. They more frequently use a commercial, solid phase, enzyme-linked immunoassay or ELISA with the antigen bound to some form of solid support, such as a paper disc. Following incubation of the test serum with the bound antigen, specific IgE is detected by adding labelled antibodies specific for human IgE. Results are usually presented in a semi-quantitative fashion: 0 = no specific IgE detected, 1 = low level, 2 = significant level, and 3, 4, 5 (and sometimes 6) indicating increasingly high concentrations. As numerous allergens can potentially be tested for, most laboratories also test for reactivity to batches of somewhat related allergens, for example food mix or inhalant mix.

Only nanograms of specific IgE are present in the serum; therefore even in highly allergic individuals RAST testing is not as sensitive as skin prick testing and low-level reactivity may not be detected. Tests using the mixes are even less sensitive and more difficult to quantitate than tests for individual allergens so false negative results are common. In addition to this low sensitivity there is variability between the allergen preparations used for RAST testing. Different laboratories may therefore report different results for the same serum sample. Variability is even greater between allergen mixes as standardisation is difficult. This variability between laboratories has been documented by the Quality Assurance Program of the Royal College of Pathologists of Australia.[3] A recent review of testing in US laboratories also showed considerable variation in results between laboratories testing the same serum sample.[4]

⊙ When and how to test for allergen-specific reactivity

An underlying atopic state, defined as the capacity to produce specific IgE to ubiquitous allergens, is more common than the presence of symptomatic allergic disease. Consequently if individuals were randomly tested for allergic reactivity many irrelevant positive results would be found. Furthermore if a patient is sensitive to one allergen it is more likely that reactivity will be present to other allergens even if there is no clinical sensitivity. The detection of specific IgE in the absence of a reasonable clinical suspicion of an allergy is hard to interpret. This may create problems; for example, if tests are used to investigate fairly vague symptoms, such as abdominal bloating or fatigue, and a specific food sensitivity is detected, drastic and unhelpful dietary modification may be advised. It is therefore essential that testing should only be done when there is a reasonable clinical suspicion (high pretest probability) that sensitivity to a particular allergen is present.

An underlying atopic state is more common than the presence of symptomatic allergic disease.

Most of the allergens in Table 46.1 can be tested for by either RAST or skin prick testing.

For perennial respiratory symptoms, the most likely allergens are house dust mite, pet hair and dander, and mould spores. For seasonal symptoms grass pollens, particularly rye grass, are most frequently implicated although tree and weed pollens and even mould spores can cause seasonal symptoms. Food allergens are rarely implicated in respiratory disease but can cause systemic reactions, including anaphylaxis and angioedema, and on occasions

Table 46.1 Common allergens

Inhalants	House dust mite, grass pollens, pet (especially cat) hair and dander, and mould spores (especially *Alternaria* and *Cladosporium*) are the most commonly recognised allergens
Foods	Important particularly in children with eczema and in adults where there is a strong clinical suspicion. The most important foods are peanuts and tree nuts, egg, milk, seafood, wheat, soy and fruits. Avoidance is the mainstay of treatment. If doubt exists about the relevance of a particular finding, a double-blind oral food challenge is the most definitive test.
Insects	Honey bee (*Apis mellifera*), European wasp (*Vespula germanica*) and paper wasp (*Vespula polistes*) are the main insect stings tested for in Australia. Allergy to jumper ants (*Myrmecia pilosula*) is also very important in rural south-eastern Australia but no test is currently available.
Medications	Antibiotics (mainly beta-lactams) and a number of anaesthetic agents
Others	Latex and a variety of occupational allergens. While tests for latex are now available there are few routine tests for most occupational allergens.

can also be relevant in eczema. In the case of serious generalised reactions the causative food is usually obvious from the patient's history, and testing is only undertaken to confirm the clinical suspicion. For severe eczema or for eczema where there is a strong suspicion that particular foods aggravate the condition, skin testing is appropriate and is generally undertaken in specialised multidisciplinary centres. Oral challenge tests are sometimes still used for confirmation of a positive skin prick test.

Skin prick testing remains more sensitive and more specific than in vitro tests for allergen-specific IgE and in general remains the method of first choice for detection of reactivity. It is quicker and simpler than undertaking a RAST but on the negative side it requires a trained clinician with access to resuscitation equipment. These requirements may result in delays before the test is carried out. If a RAST is requested it is important to specify which allergens are to be tested, as a positive result to an allergen mix does not identify the specific sensitivity and further tests are required to find the relevant (or most relevant) allergen. There are some situations where a RAST may be preferable to a skin prick test (Table 46.2).

○ Summary

Either skin prick tests or RAST can accurately determine the presence of allergen-specific IgE. Skin prick testing is the preferred method as it is more sensitive, faster and simpler. False negatives are very unusual and a negative skin prick test makes the presence of IgE mediated allergic

Table 46.2 Indications for in vitro RAST measurement rather than skin prick testing

Patients with extensive skin disease with no suitable site for testing
Dermatographism where wheals are produced by any minor trauma
Current administration of antihistamines
Risk of anaphylaxis, especially certain foods and latex
Confirmation of an unexpectedly negative skin prick test

reactivity most unlikely. Conversely, specific IgE may well be present in the absence of clinical sensitivity, and positive tests must always be interpreted in conjunction with the clinical findings.

References

1. Wide L., Bennich H. and Johansson S. G. Diagnosis of allergy by an in vitro test for allergen antibodies. *Lancet* 1967; 2: 1105–7.
2. Ishizaka K. and Ishizaka T. Identification of gamma-E-antibodies as a carrier of reaginic activity. *J Immunol* 1967; 99: 1187–98.
3. Roberts-Thomson P J., McEvoy R., Gale R., Jovanovich S. and Bradley J. Quality assurance of immunodiagnostic tests in Australia: II. Five year review. *Asian Pac J Allergy Immunol* 1993; 11: 29–37.
4. Yunginger J.W., Ahlstedt S., Eggleston P.A., Homburger H.A., Nelson H.S., Ownby D.R. et al. Quantitative IgE antibody assays in allergic diseases. *J Allergy Clin Immun* 2000; 105: 1077–84.

47 Antinuclear antibodies (ANA)*

S.M. Chatfield

Synopsis

The main use of the antinuclear antibody (ANA) test is in screening for multisystem autoimmune diseases, the prototype of which is systemic lupus erythematosus (SLE). When interpreting ANA results, it is important to consider the limitations of the test in particular its modest specificity. ANAs are sometimes found in a number of other conditions and in low titre in approximately 5% of healthy people. A positive ANA result in the right clinical scenario may prompt more specific extractable nuclear antigen (ENA) and double-stranded DNA (dsDNA) testing.

○ Introduction

Antinuclear antibodies (ANAs) are strongly associated with connective tissue disorders and are important in their diagnosis. The first recognition of ANA was through the lupus erythematosus (LE) cell, a characteristic cell type found in SLE which was discovered in the 1940s. Modern methods of detection have replaced the LE cell test.

○ Technical aspects

Antinuclear antibodies are directed against various antigenic components of nuclei in cells, including proteins and DNA itself. The usual method for detection employs a cultured human cell line (originally Hep-2 cells and more recently the Hep-2000 cell engineered to be more sensitive for certain ENAs). These are fixed on glass slides and incubated with the patient's serum. The cells are then washed and if ANA is present in the serum it will remain adherent to the cell nuclei. The second stage is a further incubation of the slide with a fluorescein-labeled antiserum to human gammaglobulin. If ANA is present this serum will adhere to the patient's antibody at the

---

*   This chapter represents an update by S.M. Chatfield of Chapter 38 of the second edition by L. Roberts and D. Barraclough. (Editor)

sites where it is attached to nuclei and can subsequently be detected by fluorescent light microscopy. The antibody titre can be determined by serial dilution (1:40, 1:80 etc). In addition to the titre, the pattern of staining can be assessed (Table 47.1). Apart from the centromere pattern, ANA staining patterns are usually not clinically helpful and have been superseded by testing for antibodies to extractable nuclear antigens (ENA) and double-stranded DNA (see below).

Table 47.1 Patterns of immunofluorescence in antinuclear antibodies

Homogeneous

Homogeneous means the whole of the nucleus is evenly stained; this may be shiny or matt. This pattern may occur in many of the connective tissue diseases and in drug-induced SLE. A shiny homogeneous pattern suggests the specificity is anti-double-stranded DNA.

Speckled

There are many patterns of speckling ranging from 'diffuse grainy', which may be seen in scleroderma, to coarse speckles representative of the anti-Sm of SLE and the anti-UI ribonucleoprotein of mixed connective tissue disease, to sparse discrete dots seen in primary biliary cirrhosis and many discrete dots seen in the anticentromere antibodies of limited cutaneous scleroderma. Often the specificities of speckled pattern ANAs are unknown and the disease associations not yet recognised.

Nucleolar

The patterns within the nucleolus may be homogeneous, speckled or clumpy, each representing different specificities. About 50% of those patients with antinucleolar antibodies have scleroderma.

Centromere

The dots seen in this pattern represent centromeres. The pattern occurs in about 90% of patients with the limited cutaneous (CREST) type of scleroderma and less commonly in other scleroderma patients.

Miscellaneous

Several other patterns have been described which do not fit into the above classification. Anti-spindle, anti-mid-body, anti-lamin and anti-centriole patterns are some examples. Anti-proliferating nuclear cell antigen (PCNA) reacts only with the nucleus of dividing cells.

○ What does a positive ANA screening test mean?

The main use of the test is in screening for multisystem autoimmune diseases, particularly SLE. As with any test, it is vital to interpret the results in conjunction with other clinical and laboratory information. Screening tests are often employed to 'rule out' conditions. Highly sensitive tests are useful for ruling conditions out. ANA is a very sensitive test for SLE (i.e. it has very few false negatives). ANA-negative SLE does occur but this is very uncommon. In SLE the ANA test will usually be positive in high titre (≥ 1:640) and in general the higher the titre, the more likely that it represents a connective tissue disease.

A positive ANA test, however, may occur in a number of other conditions (Table 47.2) and is only modestly specific. Tests with higher specificity are needed to help confirm the diagnosis (i.e. a specific test is useful for ruling a diagnosis in).

ANA titres do not reflect disease activity and do not need to be followed in patients with established connective tissue diseases.

ANA in juvenile idiopathic arthritis

One other disease in which ANA testing may be useful is juvenile idiopathic arthritis (JIA). ANA positive patients, often with an oligoarticular pattern of joint involvement, are at higher risk of uveitis that can be asymptomatic but vision threatening. More frequent screening may be warranted by an ophthalmologist in this patient group.

Table 47.2 Some conditions which may have a positive ANA test

Systemic lupus erythematosus (SLE)
Rheumatoid arthritis (RA)
Juvenile chronic arthritis
Primary Sjögren's syndrome
Scleroderma
Mixed connective tissue disease
Autoimmune chronic active hepatitis
Apparently healthy people (especially in the elderly)
Some drugs e.g. hydralazine, procainamide

○ Drug-induced antinuclear antibodies

Antinuclear antibodies may be induced in significant numbers of patients on certain drugs. These include hydralazine, procainamide, tumour necrosis factor inhibitors and uncommonly some other drugs. Only a small proportion of patients with ANAs induced by these drugs will go on to develop SLE. These ANAs are directed against histones and are usually associated with rheumatoid factor. Antihistone antibodies also occur in a minority of patients with idiopathic SLE (20–30%) when these drugs are not implicated. Antibodies to double-stranded DNA are rarely detected in drug-induced SLE.

◗ Further identification of ANA

A positive ANA result reflects the presence of circulating autoantibodies against a number of different nuclear antigens. These antibodies may be more specific than ANA alone and can also have associations with particular connective tissue diseases. They can be detected using a number of techniques. These antibodies should not be routinely tested (poor sensitivity) but may be helpful when a preliminary ANA screening test is positive with a significant titre (e.g. ≥ 1:320) in a patient who has clinical features consistent with a multisystem autoimmune disease. The results must always be interpreted in the context of other clinical and laboratory data.

Some examples are:

1 Antibodies to double-stranded (ds) DNA

A number of assays test for antibodies to dsDNA. Enzyme-linked immunosorbent assay (ELISA) is the simplest. Radioimmunoassay (Farr assay) and indirect immunofluorescence using Crithidia are more difficult to perform and done less commonly although they may be more specific. Anti-dsDNA is requested when the clinical features suggest SLE and a positive ANA screening test has been obtained. Although positive tests have been reported in several conditions other than SLE, it is a highly specific test (≥ 95%), particularly if strongly positive. Positive results are present in approximately 60–70% of patients with active SLE. The levels do fluctuate with disease activity in some patients and are occasionally used when following patients with SLE.

2 Antibodies to extractable nuclear antigens (ENA antibodies). These may be tested using an ELISA platform, counter immunoelectrophoresis (CIEP) line assays and more recently fluorescent bead-based platforms.

- *Antibodies to Ro (SS-A)*. These are found in Sjögren's syndrome, SLE and some other connective tissue diseases. Neonatal SLE and congenital heart block are associated with maternal antibodies to Ro, although only a small proportion of women with these antibodies will have children who develop these problems.

- *Antibodies to La (SS-B)*. As with antibodies to Ro these may occur in primary Sjögren's syndrome and Sjögren's syndrome associated with SLE. The ANA is positive in speckled pattern.

- *Antibodies to Scl-70 (topoisomerase 1)*. These antibodies are seen in approximately 20–30% of patients with scleroderma and are highly specific for this illness. The ANA is positive in speckled pattern.

- *Antibodies to Sm.* This antibody is highly specific for SLE but is present in only 4% of Caucasians with SLE. It is found in 30% of patients of Asian descent with SLE. The ANA pattern is speckled.
- *Antibodies to U1 ribonucleoprotein (U1RNP).* These are found in mixed connective tissue disease (MCTD; an illness often consisting of overlapping features of SLE, scleroderma and polymyositis) but may also occur in SLE, especially in patients of Asian descent. The ANA screening test is positive with a speckled pattern in high titre.
- *Antibodies to Jo1.* These antibodies are seen in approximately 30% of patients with polymyositis. In this case, the ANA is negative as this antigen is not of nuclear origin. An ENA should be ordered if there is a high clinical suspicion of polymyositis.

Summary

The ANA test is a very sensitive test for the diagnosis of SLE but has low specificity, being positive in a number of other conditions and in some apparently healthy individuals. A negative ANA is useful in ruling out SLE. A positive ANA must always be interpreted in conjunction with other clinical information and sometimes by more specific testing with ENA and dsDNA.

Acknowledgment

The author gratefully acknowledges the authors (Drs Barraclough and Roberts) of the previous version of this article, which forms the basis of the current one.

48 Rheumatoid factor and anti-citrullinated peptide antibody*

S.M. Chatfield

◌ Introduction

It was noted by Waaler in 1937 that a high proportion of sera from patients with rheumatoid arthritis (RA) agglutinated sheep erythrocytes sensitised with rabbit immunoglobulin G (IgG) antibodies to sheep erythrocytes. The term 'rheumatoid factor' (RF) was coined and it has formed part of the diagnostic work up for patients with suspected RA ever since. In fact, the presence of RF is one component of the widely used American College of Rheumatology classification criteria. Rheumatoid factors are antibodies specific to antigenic determinants on the Fc fragments of human or animal IgG. The rheumatoid factor commonly tested for is an immunoglobulin M (IgM) although immunoglobulins of several other classes have been demonstrated by special techniques.

Despite its widespread use, RF has significant limitations, the most prominent being its relatively poor specificity (i.e. high false positive rate) which coupled with a modest sensitivity limits its usefulness as a diagnostic test. Recently antibodies to various citrullinated proteins (so-called anti-citrullinated peptide antibodies or ACPA) have been described that are highly specific for the diagnosis of RA. They were initially identified as anti-perinuclear factor antibodies back in 1964 and it has only been over the last 10 years that the importance of these antibodies has been fully appreciated and reliable easy-to-perform tests have been designed and validated.

◌ Technical aspects

A number of different methods for testing RF have been used. Nephelometry is the most common method although the latex test is still sometimes used. Sheep erythrocyte agglutination (the Rose Waaler test) is rarely used today. Whatever method is employed it is important that a titre or some quantitative measure of the degree of positivity is obtained. Positive test results are

---

* This chapter represents an update and consolidation by S.M. Chatfield of Chapter 39 of the second edition by L. Roberts and D. Barraclough and the *Australian Prescriber* article by D. Langguth and R.C.W. Wong. (Editor)

defined by choosing a cut-off value that best discriminates between people with RA and those without.

Nephelometric method for RF

Heat-aggregated human IgG is used. Interaction of RF with the human IgG causes an increase in the scatter of light. This alteration in light scatter may be quantitatively measured and forms the basis of this test.

Latex test for rheumatoid factor

Particles of polystyrene are coated with human IgG. Patients' sera containing RF will bind to the IgG and consequently precipitate the polystyrene particles. Serial dilutions are subsequently done.

ELISA for cyclic citrullinated peptide

Some proteins are modified after their formation in the cell. Citrullination is one such modification process in which arginine residues are converted into citrulline residues (a non-essential amino acid). This process, which may be necessary for proper protein function, also causes a number of proteins (e.g. fillagrin, vimentin and keratin) to become targets for autoantibody formation. These antibodies are highly specific for RA and may be easily measured in serum using an enzyme-linked immunosorbent assay (ELISA). The ELISA uses artificially derived cyclic citrullinated proteins as the antigen. This is then incubated with patients' sera and if antibodies are present they will bind. The presence of binding is indicated by an enzymatically induced colour change in the well with the degree of colour change providing quantitation. The most commonly used version is the anti-CCP2 which demonstrates the best test performance characteristics.

◗ What does a positive test mean?

For a more detailed description of the statistical usefulness of RF and ACPA in various clinical scenarios, please see reference 1.

◗ Rheumatoid factor

Apart from RA, RF can be detected in otherwise normal people and also in a number of other diseases (Table 48.1). These include other connective tissue diseases (which may share some of the clinical features of RA), some hepatic and pulmonary diseases and also some infections. RF is more prevalent with age and low titre RF is present in up to 10% of the elderly population. High titre RF is less common in normal individuals. Approximately 70% of individuals with RA have a positive RF test. Hence, the presence of RF must be interpreted in the clinical context and not used as a diagnostic test in isolation.

QUICK FLICK 48

Table 48.1 Disease which may be associated with a positive rheumatoid factor

Connective tissue diseases	Rheumatoid arthritis Sjögren's syndrome Scleroderma Systemic lupus erythematosus Mixed connective tissue disease
Viral infections	Infectious mononucleosis Hepatitis B or C Others
Bacterial infections	Tuberculosis Subacute bacterial endocarditis Leprosy Brucellosis Syphilis Bronchiectasis
Parasitic infections	Malaria
Miscellaneous	Some neoplasms Cryoglobulinaemia Chronic liver disease Sarcoidosis Chronic pulmonary fibrosis

If a patient has a symmetrical inflammatory polyarthritis involving appropriate joints, that has been present for more than 6 weeks, if RF is present, and if there is nothing on clinical or laboratory grounds to suggest an alternative diagnosis, then seropositive RA is highly likely. *The absence of RF in this setting does not exclude rheumatoid arthritis* (in this case 'seronegative') but should stimulate a thorough check for alternative diagnoses. RF is less likely to be positive early in the disease.

Although of use in confirming a clinical diagnosis of RA, RF is of no use in following the course of the disease. If a significantly positive result has been obtained, there is no indication for serial measurements. RF has prognostic implications, with patients with RF exhibiting more severe disease, erosions and extra-articular manifestations.

○ Anti-citrullinated peptide antibodies (ACPA)

Unlike RF, ACPA are rarely seen in conditions other than RA (specificity 95–98%), making this a very useful test when positive.[2] The sensitivity of the assay is lower in earlier disease and is approximately 70% overall (similar to RF). The presence of ACPA also correlates with a poorer prognosis. It is still unclear whether it is best to test for one or the other or both. Some CCP positive patients are RF negative and vice versa.

ACPA is of no use in following disease activity and does not need to be re-tested. Like RF, ACPA-positive RA tends to be more severe.

◑ Summary

RF and ACPA testing provide valuable diagnostic and prognostic information in patients presenting with an inflammatory arthritis. The results of these tests must be interpreted in the light of clinical findings. A positive RF provides supporting evidence for the diagnosis of RA and a positive ACPA test provides very strong evidence for this diagnosis. RA may still occur in patients with a negative RF and ACPA test. As there is now strong evidence to support the early use of disease-modifying therapy in rheumatoid arthritis, testing for ACPA and RF has assumed a more important role in diagnosing RA accurately and early.

Acknowledgment

I would like to thank the authors of previous reviews of this topic, Drs Barraclough, Roberts, Langguth and Wong, whose work provided the basis for this update.

References

1. Chatfield S.M., Wicks I.P., Sturgess A.D. and Roberts L.J. Anti-citrullinated peptide antibody: death of the rheumatoid factor? *MJA* 2009; 190: 693–5.
2. Whiting P.F., Smidt N., Sterne J.A., Harbord R., Burton A., Burke M. et al. Systematic review: accuracy of anti-citrullinated peptide antibodies for diagnosing rheumatoid arthritis. *Ann Intern Med* 2010; 152: 456–64, W155–66.

Part 6

Genetic Tests

49 BRCA testing for familial breast cancer

C. Lau and G. Suthers

Synopsis

Mutations in the BRCA1 and BRCA2 genes are associated with hereditary breast and ovarian cancer. Genetic testing is available in specialised laboratories but is expensive and presents a significant technical and interpretative challenge. Identification of a causative mutation carries lifelong health and psychosocial implications for the woman and her relatives. It also influences surveillance and treatment options. Testing should therefore only be considered with professional genetic counselling by specialists in familial cancer clinics.

◗ Introduction

Breast cancer is the most common form of cancer among women in Australia. A woman has approximately a 1 in 10 chance of developing breast cancer at some point in her life. Most of these breast cancers are sporadic, reflecting the inevitable accumulation of errors in a person's DNA with age. However, 5–10% of affected women have a strong underlying and heritable predisposition to develop breast cancer.

Mutations in many different genes can cause a predisposition to develop breast cancer. For most women with familial breast cancer, the causative mutation is unknown and cannot be identified. However, the mutations most commonly identified in women with familial breast cancer are breast cancer susceptibility gene 1 (BRCA1) and breast cancer susceptibility gene 2 (BRCA2). Together these mutations are found in approximately 20% of familial cases (that is, 1–2% of all breast cancers). Mutations in other genes, for example TP53, CDH1, PTEN and STK11, are associated with rare genetic syndromes which can also predispose to breast cancer.

○ BRCA1 and BRCA2 genes

The BRCA1 gene is found on chromosome 17 and the BRCA2 gene is found on chromosome 13. They are tumour suppressor genes. The proteins encoded by these genes are part of a multi-protein complex that repairs damaged DNA. The complex normally repairs double-strand breaks in the DNA by homologous recombination. A cell which has lost BRCA1 or BRCA2 activity is unable to repair this damage and can rapidly accumulate mutations that eventually lead to cancer.[1]

A heritable mutation in either gene greatly increases the chance that a cell will become malignant. These mutations are inherited as autosomal dominants and there is a 50% chance that a child will inherit the abnormal gene from a carrier parent. The child will also inherit a normal copy of the gene from the other parent which will function, but the cell lacks a backup should this normal copy fail. With the inevitable accumulation of genetic errors with age, the normal copy may eventually become mutated (sometimes called the 'second hit') and the cell is left with no functioning BRCA gene. The resulting rapid accumulation of uncorrected errors in the cell's DNA usually leads to cancer.

For reasons that are not clear, the loss of BRCA1 or BRCA2 function increases the risk of some but not all cancers. Female carriers of a mutation in BRCA1 or BRCA2 are at high risk of developing breast cancer and ovarian cancer, while male carriers are at increased risk of breast and prostate cancer. In addition there is also a slightly increased risk of a wide range of other cancers, but the predominant cancer risk by far is that of breast and ovarian cancer.[1]

It is possible for someone to carry both a BRCA1 and BRCA2 mutation (double heterozygote) but this is very rare, accounting for less than 1% of all BRCA mutation carriers. For reasons that are not clear, double heterozygotes do not have a higher risk of cancer or more severe disease compared to single mutation carriers.

○ Indications for BRCA testing

A family history of breast or ovarian cancer is the basis for making a clinical diagnosis of familial breast or ovarian cancer in a specific patient. The family history can also provide an indication of the risk of breast or ovarian cancer in an unaffected woman. Simple guidelines for assessing and interpreting a family history of breast and ovarian cancer are available from the National Breast and Ovarian Cancer Centre (www.nbocc.org.au).[2]

The clinical diagnosis of familial breast or ovarian cancer is not necessarily an appropriate indication for genetic testing for mutations in the BRCA1 and BRCA2 genes, as the majority of women with familial breast cancer do

QUICK FLICK 49

not have an identifiable mutation in a known gene. Mutation analysis of the BRCA1 and BRCA2 genes is complex and expensive and is not justified in many women with familial breast or ovarian cancer. The current cost to the Australian healthcare system is $2–3000 per patient screened. There are a number of algorithms to estimate the likelihood of finding a BRCA1/BRCA2 mutation in a patient, but the positive predictive value of these algorithms is generally poor. The general consensus among familial cancer specialists in Australia is that a woman should be offered genetic testing for the BRCA1 and BRCA2 mutations if the estimated probability of finding a mutation is greater than 10%. The mutation search usually starts with testing the blood from an affected individual. Once a mutation has been identified, genetic testing of unaffected relatives (often called presymptomatic testing) may provide useful information regarding the risk of cancer and allow carriers to undertake specific cancer prevention and detection strategies before the development of disease.

Genetic testing of an unaffected person for a BRCA1 or BRCA2 mutation is generally not recommended unless a mutation has already been identified in a family member. If a mutation has not already been identified in a relative, it is impossible to interpret a normal result in an unaffected person. The normal result could mean that the person tested has not inherited the family's (unidentified) BRCA mutation or that the person tested has inherited the family's non-BRCA mutation.

Genetic testing for a BRCA1 or BRCA2 mutation raises challenges in identifying which women should be tested, interpreting a complex test result and managing the medical and psychological consequences of the result for both the patient and her relatives. For these reasons, the guidelines of the National Health and Medical Research Council recommend, and Australian laboratory standards require, that the testing is limited to specialists in familial cancer clinics. There are clinics across Australia and their services can be accessed by referral from medical practitioners.[3]

◯ Mutation detection methodology

Analysis of the BRCA1 and BRCA2 genes is not simply 'two tests'. The BRCA1 and BRCA2 genes together consist of approximately 20 000 nucleotides. Analysis of each nucleotide in this length of DNA sequence presents a significant technical and interpretative challenge. There are approximately 10 laboratories in Australia that provide this service. DNA is extracted from a patient's blood sample and each exon of each gene is amplified by the polymerase chain reaction. Bidirectional sequencing is then performed on the products of the polymerase chain reaction. Any variation from the normal reference sequence must be assessed to determine if it is a benign variant, pathogenic mutation or a variant of unknown clinical significance.

Direct sequencing does not detect large deletions or duplications that might involve many consecutive exons. Some laboratories can quantify the copy number of each exon relative to normal controls.

○ Interpreting results

A normal person can have thousands of variations in their genetic code. In analysing the 20 000 nucleotides of the BRCA1 and BRCA2 genes, the laboratory will find many genetic variants. Some of these will be common variants that are well documented as being benign. The laboratory may also identify a variant that inactivates the gene and is documented as being pathogenic, that is, places a woman at high genetic risk of developing breast or ovarian cancer. There are international databases that catalogue variants and assist the laboratory in determining the significance of a particular variant. The laboratory may also identify one or more rare variants that are of unknown clinical significance.

The identification of a pathogenic variant carries significant implications for both the woman tested and members of her family. For this reason, the interpretation of a variant requires a high degree of scientific skill and accountability.

Failure to identify a pathogenic variant does not exclude the diagnosis of familial cancer. This is because the majority of women with familial breast or ovarian cancer do not have an identifiable mutation in the BRCA1 or BRCA2 genes.

The identification of a variant of unknown clinical significance is troubling for both the clinician and patient. However, such variants should not be the basis for clinical decision making because, as more information is accumulated worldwide, many of them will turn out to be rare benign variants.

Once a pathogenic variant has been identified, other at-risk adult family members (male or female) can have a presymptomatic/predictive genetic test to determine their cancer risk. In this situation, the interpretation is much simpler. The relative has either inherited the pathogenic variant or not. This type of testing carries significant medical, psychological, ethical and social consequences. National clinical and laboratory standards require that such testing be accompanied by expert genetic counselling. For men, the principal reason for knowing their carrier status is to clarify the risk of their daughters' inheriting the mutation.

○ Management

The main benefit of finding the familial BRCA mutation is the prevention or early detection of cancer in at-risk relatives. The care of someone carrying a BRCA1 or BRCA2 mutation must be individualised because the issues and options vary with the gene involved and the gender and age of the person.[4] Options include breast cancer surveillance, risk-reducing surgery and chemoprevention with drugs such as tamoxifen. Management involves the general practitioner and potentially multiple specialists and genetic counsellors. At this time, BRCA mutation status usually makes little difference to the treatment of the cancer for the affected individual but this may change with the availability of new drugs.

◯ Genetic counselling

Genetic testing differs from most routine laboratory tests in that the detection of a mutation carries lifelong implications for the patient as well as relatives. The testing for BRCA1/BRCA2 mutations must always be accompanied by appropriate genetic counselling. This counselling should commence before any genetic testing and should be provided by a practitioner with professional genetic counselling training and experience.

◯ Summary

BRCA1 and BRCA2 mutations are an important cause of familial breast and ovarian cancer. Genetic testing should take place in the context of appropriate pretest and post-test genetic counselling, as provided by familial cancer clinics. Identification of pathogenic mutations has important implications for the clinical management of the patient and family members. However, a normal test result must be interpreted with caution. On the one hand, the absence of an identified mutation in an affected woman does not exclude the clinical diagnosis of familial breast cancer. It is likely that the woman has a mutation in a different yet-to-be-identified gene. On the other hand, once a mutation has been identified in the family, a normal test result means that the person has not inherited the family's predisposition to develop cancer and does not require special cancer surveillance.

References

1. Petrucelli N., Daly M.B., Culver J.O.B. and Feldman G.L. BRCA1 and BRCA2 hereditary breast/ovarian cancer. *Gene Reviews*. 1998, updated 2007. www.ncbi.nlm.nih.gov/bookshelf/br.fcgi?book=gene&part=brca1 [cited Oct 13, 2010].
2. National Breast and Ovarian Cancer Centre. *Advice About Familial Aspects Of Breast Cancer And Ovarian Cancer*. 2006. http://nbocc.org.au/view-document-details/bog-advice-about-familial-aspects-of-breast-cancer-and-ovarian-cancer [cited Oct 13, 2010].

3. Centre for Genetics Education, NSW Health. *Family Cancer Services.* www.genetics.com.au/services/canclin.asp [cited Oct 13, 2010].
4. Suthers G.K. Cancer risks for Australian women with a BRCA1 or a BRCA2 mutation. *Aust NZ J Surg* 2007; 77: 314–9.

Index